Lecture Notes in Computer Science 6135

Nassir Navab   Pierre Jannin (Eds.)

Information Processing in Computer-Assisted Interventions

First International Conference, IPCAI 2010
Geneva, Switzerland, June 23, 2010
Proceedings

Springer

Volume Editors

Nassir Navab
Technische Universität München
Institut für Informatik 16, CAMPAR
Boltzmannstr. 3, 85748 Garching, Germany
E-mail: navab@cs.tum.edu

Pierre Jannin
Montreal Neurological Institute and Hospital
McGill University, Montreal, Canada
and
INSERM-INRIA-Université de Rennes 1
Faculté de Médecine
2 Avenue du Pr. Léon Bernard, CS 34317, 35043 Rennes Cedex, France
E-mail: Pierre.Jannin@univ-rennes1.fr

Library of Congress Control Number: 2010928334

CR Subject Classification (1998): I.6, I.4, J.3, I.5, I.2.10, I.2.9

LNCS Sublibrary: SL 6 – Image Processing, Computer Vision, Pattern Recognition, and Graphics

ISSN	0302-9743
ISBN-10	3-642-13710-5 Springer Berlin Heidelberg New York
ISBN-13	978-3-642-13710-5 Springer Berlin Heidelberg New York

springer.com

Printed in Germany

Typesetting: Camera-ready by author, data conversion by Scientific Publishing Services, Chennai, India
Printed on acid-free paper 06/3180

Preface

Thanks to scientific and technological advances in many parallel fields, medical procedures are rapidly evolving towards solutions which are less invasive and more effective. In the previous decades, information processing in diagnostic imaging provided many solutions to physicians in particular within radiology, neurology, cardiology, nuclear medicine and radiation therapy departments. In the last decade, progress in computer technology, imaging and mechatronics has allowed computer-assisted intervention (CAI) systems and solutions to penetrate the intervention and operating rooms.

CAI's major challenge in the beginning of the twenty-first century is real-time processing, analysis and visualization of large amount of heterogeneous, static and dynamic patient data, and understanding of surgery for designing intelligent operating rooms and developing advanced training tools. Excellent scientists, engineers and physicians have created many advanced research groups around the world and are starting to provide innovative, breakthrough solutions. *Information Processing in Computer-Assisted Interventions* (IPCAI) aims at gathering the best work in this field and allowing authors to present and discuss it in detail. IPCAI wishes to select and present the highlights of research in CAI and aims at distinguishing itself for the quality of the presented papers and the excitement and depth of the discussions they generate.

How Is IPCAI Positioned Related to Other Conferences in This Area ?

Medical Image Computing and Computer-Assisted Intervention (MICCAI) has established itself as both a society and an annual event where a set of selected paper in both fields of medical image computing (MIC) and are presented. MICCAI often gathers around 1,000 participants presenting mostly MIC, but also CAI papers. The Computer Assisted Radiology and Surgery (CARS) series of conferences, on the other hand, focus mostly on the CAI community. It gathers a large number of interested scientists and engineers in this field. It bases itself mostly on long abstract submissions and aims at gathering a large number of players and at creating a place of encounter for academic and industrial researchers in this field. IPCAI considers itself as a complementary event to both MICCAI and CARS, filling an existing gap.

IPCAI 2010: The Review Process

This year, there were 40 full paper submissions (40% from North America, 39% from Europe and 21% from Asia). Four editors managed the assignment of the anonymous submissions to the reviewers. There were 61 reviewers: 85% of the papers had 3 reviewers, 10% had 2 reviewers, and 5% had 4 reviewers. Additionally, each editor reviewed the papers he had in charge. Reviewers were asked to provide detailed, journal-quality reviews. After the review phase, 16 papers were initially selected according to a weighted score only. A threshold of 3 on 4 was used. Papers out of the scope of the conference were rejected automatically. The editors asked the authors of 'conditionally accepted' papers to revise their manuscript according to reviewers' and editor's suggestions. A final version was then submitted. These final versions were reviewed by the editors only. They checked whether the reviewers' suggestions were taken into account. All the authors integrated the reviewers' suggestions and improved the manuscript accordingly. The final distinction between oral presentation and short oral plus poster was made according to the average scores given by the anonymous reviewers.

IPCAI: It Is Your Conference

We want to thank all authors who submitted to IPCAI for their effort in submitting high-quality long papers. We also want to thank the reviewers for providing detailed high-quality reviews, very helpful for the authors, whether their papers were accepted or not. Both authors and reviewers contributed to the quality of the conference.

IPCAI 2010: The Idea

IPCAI aims at being extremely selective in order to present only the highlights in CAI. Co-located with the CARS conference, IPCAI 2010 presented the first in a series of events to be organized in the upcoming years. We hope that IPCAI keeps its promises and offers its participants and the CAI community a series of strong and innovative contributions. We also aim at creating a friendly and constructive atmosphere to share ideas and concepts for enhancing research and innovations in this area.

June 2010

Nassir Navab
Pierre Jannin

Organization

IPCAI Executive Committee

Nassir Navab	Computer Aided Medical Procedures (CAMP), Technische Universität München, Germany (General Chair)
Pierre Jannin	INSERM/INRIA, Rennes, France and MNI-McGill, Montréal, Canada (Co Chair)
Dave Hawkes	University College London, UK
Leo Joskowicz	Hebrew University, Israel
Kensaku Mori	Nagoya University, Japan
Russell Taylor	Johns Hopkins University, USA

Area Chairs

1) Clinical Applications, Systems, Software, and Validation

Kevin Cleary	Georgetown University, USA
Yoshinobu Sato	Osaka University, Japan
Thomas Langø	SINTEF, Norway
Jocelyne Troccaz	TIMC/CNRS, France
Gabor Fichtinger	Queen's University, Canada
Peter Kazanzides	Johns Hopkins University, USA
Luc Soler	IRCAD, France
Noby Hata	Brigham and Women's Hospital, USA
Kirby Vosburgh	Massachusetts General Hospital, USA
Wolfgang Birkfellner	University of Vienna, Austria
Lutz Nolte	University of Bern, Switzerland

2) Interventional Robotics and Navigation

Ichiro Sakuma	Tokyo University, Japan
Brian Davies	Imperial College London, UK
Koji Ikuta	Nagoya University, Japan
Kiyoyuki Chinzei	National Institute of Advanced Industrial Science and Technology, Japan

3) Surgical Planning, Simulation, and Advanced Intra-Op Visualization

Benoit Dawant	Vanderbilt University, USA
Terry Peters	Imaging Research Laboratories, Robarts Research Institute, Canada

Gábor Székely	ETH Zürich, Switzerland
Hervé Delingette	INRIA Sophia-Antipolis, France
Tim Salcudean	University of British Columbia, Canada
Sebastien Ourselin	University College London, UK

4) Interventional Imaging

Alison Noble	Oxford University, UK
Purang Abolmaesumi	University of British Columbia, Canada
Ali Kamen	Siemens Corporate Research, USA
Joachim Hornegger	Friedrich-Alexander University Erlangen-Nuremberg, Germany
Pierre Hellier	INRIA Rennes, France
Louis Collins	McGill University, Canada

5) Cognition, Modeling and Context Awareness

Guang-Zhong Yang	Imperial College London, UK
Greg Hager	Johns Hopkins University, USA
Ken Masamune	Tokyo University, Japan

Industrial Liaisons

Wolfgang Wein	Siemens Corporate Research, USA
Ameet Jain	Philips Healthcare, USA
Tom Vercauteren	Mauna Kea, France
Simon DiMaio	Intuitive Surgical, USA
Joerg Traub	SurgicEye, Germany

IPCAI 2010 Local Organization

Martin Groher	Computer Aided Medical Procedures (CAMP), Technische Universität München, Germany
Martin Horn	Computer Aided Medical Procedures (CAMP), Technische Universität München, Germany
Marco Feuerstein	Nagoya University, Japan

Steering Committee

Dave Hawkes, Nassir Navab, Pierre Jannin, Leo Joskowicz, Kensaku Mori, Kevin Cleary, Terry Peters, Tim Salcudean, Gábor Székely, Russell Taylor, Guang-Zhong Yang, Ichiro Sakuma, Ron Kikinis

Reviewers

Purang Abolmaesumi
Wolfgang Birkfellner
Emad Boctor
Kevin Cleary
Louis Collins
Benoit Dawant
Herve Delingette
Eddie Edwards
Marco Feuerstein
Gabor Fichtinger
Moti Freiman
Guido Gerig
Penney Graeme
Hayit Greenspan
Gregory Hager
Noby Hata
Dave Hawkes
Leo Joskowicz
Ali Kamen
Peter Kazanzides
Takayuki Kitasaka
Thomas Lango
Ken Masamune
Jamie McClelland
Todd McNutt
Kensaku Mori
Yukitaka Nimura
Alison Noble
Masahito Oda
Sebastien Ourselin
Terry Peters
Tobias Reichl
Ingerid Reinertsen
Joseph Reinhardt
Kawal Rhode
Daniel Rueckert
Tim Salcudean
Yoshinobu Sato
Ruby Shamir
Luc Soler
Gabor Szekely
Russ Taylor
Jocelyne Troccaz
Bram Van Ginneken
Theo van Walsum
Tom Vercauteren
Kirby Vosburgh
Guang-Zhong Yang
Ziv Yaniv

Table of Contents

CAI: Imaging, Modeling and Visualization

Clinical Applications and Validation

Medical Robotics, Instrumentation, and Modeling

Cardiovascular Modeling and Navigation

Planning, Simulation, and Guidance

Visualization and Planning of Neurosurgical Interventions with Straight Access

Nikhil V. Navkar[1], Nikolaos V. Tsekos[1], Jason R. Stafford[2], Jeffrey S. Weinberg[2], and Zhigang Deng[1]

[1] University of Houston, Department of Computer Science, Houston, TX
[2] University of Texas, MD Anderson Cancer Center, Houston, TX
{ntsekos,zdeng}@cs.uh.edu

Abstract. Image-guided neurosurgical interventional procedures utilize medical imaging techniques to identify the most appropriate path for accessing a targeted structure. Often, preoperative planning entails the use of multi-contrast or multi-modal imaging for assessing different aspects of patient's pathophysiology related to the procedure. Comprehensive visualization and manipulation of such large volume of three-dimensional anatomical information is a major challenge. In this work we propose a technique for simple and efficient visualization of the region of intervention for neurosurgical procedures. It is done through the generation of access maps on the surface of the patient's skin, which assists a neurosurgeon in selecting the most appropriate path of access by avoiding vital structures and minimizing potential trauma to healthy tissue. Our preliminary evaluation showed that this technique is effective as well as easy to use for planning neurosurgical interventions such as biopsies, deep brain stimulation, ablation of brain lesions.

1 Introduction

Currently, we witness the rapid evolution of minimally invasive surgeries and image guided interventions that can lead to improved and cost effective patient treatments. It is becoming apparent that sustaining and expanding this paradigm shift would require new computational methodology that could assist surgeons in planning these procedures. A major challenge at either the preoperative or the intraoperative stage of an image guided procedure is visualization, comprehension and manipulation of a large volume of three-dimensional (3D) anatomical data.

Most often, 3D models of the brain tissue are generated after segmentation and rendering of the different anatomies. The operator may use those models for manual or computer-assisted selection of appropriate paths to access the targeted anatomy/structure. When a straight tool such as a biopsy needle or an applicator is used, the interventional task maybe approached as a two-point access practice, i.e. the point representing the entrance and the target. Since the target location is well known from the original inspection of images, it would be

N. Navab and P. Jannin (Eds.): IPCAI 2010, LNCS 6135, pp. 1–11, 2010.

helpful to visualize the outer surface of the patient by incorporating information about the underlying tissue. In this work we present a preliminary technique to such a visualization allowing for quantitative or semi-quantitative comparison among various points of entrance for neurosurgical procedures that require straight access. The main contribution of our work is the generation of access maps on the surface of patient's head which provide a neurosurgeon with plethora of meaningful information about the anatomy of the region of intervention and safety of selected insertion paths. In addition, our preliminary evaluation results showed that our method was intuitive and easy to use for neurosurgeons, which makes our technique clinically applicable. Meanwhile, the approach can be used in conjunction with existing visualization techniques to further improve the preoperative planning process.

A large volume of work in the field of neurosurgical planning is primarily focused on the development of computational methods to process and visualize multi-modality 3D data sets and generate 3D models of the brain (e.g. [10,13,11, 12]). The models are generated by using either multi volumetric or iso-surface rendering methods. Although, these approaches have been proved efficient in generating realistic and highly accurate 3D representations of the anatomy of the brain, they do not provide the extra quantitative information (apart from visualization) which would help neurosurgeons in making decisions during preoperative planning.

For neurosurgical interventions, many studies have introduced approaches for path planning [7,9,5,8,6]. Lee et al. [7] and Nowinsky et al. [5] have incorporated the use of brain atlases for improving stereotactic neurosurgery. Although such an approach may allow for high fidelity tissue classification, it requires manual selection of the entry points. Bourbakis et al. [8] proposed another approach for 3D visualization pertinent to image guided brain surgery based on replicating surgeon behavior and decision-making. This approach requires user input to set appropriate parameters for calculating insertion points. Fujii et al. [9] proposed an automatic neurosurgical path-searching algorithm that requires assigning importance values to the cutting and touching of different tissues based on anatomical knowledge and the experience of neurosurgeons, which might not be very intuitive. This approach also incorporates blood vessels into the path searching algorithm by assigning them a cost value. For this part, it extracts a centerline for the vessels and then assumes a cylindrical shape that may not be close to the real anatomy. The algorithm finds a curvilinear path, which is not suited for straight-access interventions by current interventional tools. Most closely related to our work is that of Brunenberg et al. [6] which automatically calculates the possible trajectories for implantation of electrodes to selected targets for deep brain simulation. This algorithm calculates safe paths automatically without significant user input. However, it requires segmenting the insertion path at regular intervals. The distance from each point at given regular intervals to every point on the vessels needs to be calculated. This is time consuming. In our work, we use a mesh-based representation of the anatomical structures that does not require segmenting the path; the minimum distance of the path to any point on the vessel is then directly computed and visualized.

2 Materials and Methods

2.1 Generation of Access Maps

In a generalized approach, the performance of a minimally invasive intervention with a straight tubular tool can be viewed as defining two points in a 3D space: the point of insertion of the tool and the targeted structure. Those two points define a path of insertion. Tomographic modalities, such as MRI or CT, offer 3D imaging thereby providing the means of such stereotactic approach. Since the target is a well-defined point in space (selected by inspecting the images), the problem of path planning is to select an entry point on the skin of the patient's head. We hypothesize that, by projecting the underlying brain tissue on the skin, it is possible to have a simple and intuitive selection of access paths. Since the preparatory stage of our approach (as discussed in section 2.2) renders anatomical structures with a mesh, without the loss of generality, the task of path planning is to find a vertex which is most suitable for incision. We assume that $\mathbf{M_s} = (\mathbf{V_s}, \mathbf{F_s})$ is a mesh that corresponds to the reconstructed skin on patient's head with vertices $\mathbf{V_s}$ and faces $\mathbf{F_s}$. The insertion vertex $\mathbf{v}$, where $\mathbf{v} \in \mathbf{V_s}$, is selected such that a line drawn from this vertex to a target point $\mathbf{t}$, where $\mathbf{t} \in \mathbf{R^3}$, defines a safe insertion path. In our approach, to achieve a high efficiency in the manual portion of planning, i.e. when the point of entrance is selected by the neurosurgeon, all the computationally intensive parts will be performed during the preparatory phase. Every vertex in the mesh $\mathbf{M_s}$ corresponds to a possible incision point on the surface of the patient's head.

In order to find a set of vertices $\mathbf{V_{safe}} \subset \mathbf{V_s}$ that corresponds to safe incision points, our approach entails the generation of three access maps on the surface of the patient's head that can be used by the neurosurgeon to select an optimal path of insertion. These access maps, individually or in accord, provide an intuitive visualization of the region of intervention. The generation of these maps is described in more details in the follow-up paragraphs.

Direct Impact Map: The first map in our path-planning approach generates the projection of vital brain structures. The vertices on the skin surface whose path trajectory passes directly through the vital tissue should be considered unsafe and discarded. We start by considering all the vertices as safe incision points, thus initializing $\mathbf{V_{safe}} = \mathbf{V}$. Vital tissues are represented in form of a triangular mesh $\mathbf{M_v} = (\mathbf{V_v}, \mathbf{F_v})$, with $\mathbf{V_v}$ vertices and $\mathbf{F_v}$ faces. A line segment is drawn from the target point $\mathbf{t}$ to each vertex $\mathbf{v}$, where $\mathbf{v} \in \mathbf{V_s}$. If the line segment intersects any triangular face $\mathbf{f}$, where $\mathbf{f} \in \mathbf{F_v}$, the corresponding vertex is treated unsafe and removed from $\mathbf{V_{safe}}$. Thus, at the end of this step $\mathbf{V_{safe}}$ consists of only those vertices, which guarantees that the path drawn from them never hits the vital tissue.

Proximity Map: The above direct impact map ensures that the trajectory of the pre-planned path will not intersect the vital tissue. There are situations when the direct impact map may not be sufficient and additional information or processing may be needed. One such situation is when for a particular path the interventional tool passes very close to a region of the vital tissue without directly impacting it. In such a case, even a minute deviation from the pre-planned path could result in a serious damage to the vital tissue. Another challenge is that the different interventional tools have different diameters or thickness. The direct impact map does not take into account the thickness of the tool; thereby only using the direct impact map may bring the tool to very close proximity and even puncture the vital tissue. To address this issue, we incorporate a safe 3D buffer region that encloses the vital structures.

For every vertex $\mathbf{v} \in \mathbf{V_{safe}}$ on the skin surface, we try to compute the proximity for the vertex as:

$$PR(\mathbf{v}) = \arg \min_{e_{ij} \in E_v} (f_{v,t}(v_i, v_j)) \tag{1}$$

where $\mathbf{E_v}$ correspond to set of edges of the mesh $\mathbf{M_v}$. $\mathbf{e_{ij}}$ is the edge between vertices $\mathbf{v_i} \in \mathbf{V_v}$ and $\mathbf{v_j} \in \mathbf{V_v}$. If there exist a line which intersects and is orthogonal to the line segments with end points $< \mathbf{v_i}, \mathbf{v_j} >$ and $< \mathbf{v}, \mathbf{t} >$, function $f_{v,t}()$ returns the minimum distance between these two line segments. Otherwise we check, if there exists any orthogonal projection from vertex $\mathbf{v_i}$ or $\mathbf{v_j}$ on the trajectory of the path defined by the line segment with end points $\mathbf{v}$ and $\mathbf{t}$, function $f_{v,t}()$ returns $min(d_i, d_j)$ where d_i or d_j is the shortest distance of the vertex $\mathbf{v_i}$ or $\mathbf{v_j}$ from the line segment.

For a path with the starting point at vertex $\mathbf{v}$, $PR(\mathbf{v})$ is the minimum distance between the vital tissue and the line segment representing the trajectory of the insertion path. It ensures that if any insertion is made through vertex v there will not be any vital structure at least at a distance $PR(\mathbf{v})$ from the insertion path. Thus, a safe buffer region can be created around the vital structures by removing those vertices from the set $\mathbf{V_{safe}}$ whose $PR(\mathbf{v})$ falls below a given threshold PR_T.

The same concept is used for considering the thickness of surgical instruments. If we consider a cylinder with radius equal to $PR(\mathbf{v})$ and central axis aligned along the path trajectory starting from vertex $\mathbf{v}$ to target $\mathbf{t}$, there won't be any vital structure in the vicinity of the cylinder. Thus, it is safe to insert a surgical instrument at $\mathbf{v}$ whose thickness is less than $PR(\mathbf{v})$.

Path Length Map: The above two maps ensure that the interventional tool maintains a minimum distance $PR(\mathbf{v})$ from the vital structures. An additional concern in an intervention might be the depth of traversed tissue; in general, the shorter the distance, the less the risk of trauma even to non-vital structures. Therefore, we introduce a third map that shows the traversed length from the target to the skin. This map is generated by calculating the path length $PL(\mathbf{v})$, of the target from each vertex $\mathbf{v} \in \mathbf{V_{safe}}$. Those vertices are excluded from $\mathbf{V_{safe}}$ for whom the value of $PL(\mathbf{v})$ is greater than a given threshold PL_T.

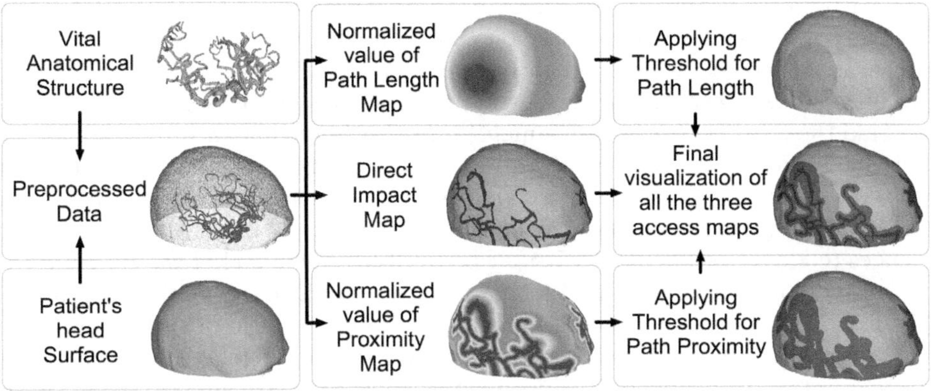

Fig. 1. Illustrates the generation of the access maps. In case of 'Normalized value of Proximity Map' the red color corresponds to insertion points whose access path is closer to the vital structure. In 'Normalized value of Path Length Map' red color corresponds to shorter distances of the target from the surface.

The process of generating the above access maps is schematically illustrated in Fig. 1. For the sake of a clear explanation, we assign blood vessels as one of the vital anatomical structures. The preprocessed data consist of the patient's head surface, blood vessels and the target point registered together. The steps involved in data preprocessing are explained in details in section 2.2. A suitable set of insertion points $\mathbf{V_{safe}}$ can be found on the patient's head for a given neurosurgical interventional procedure by setting the values of the two thresholds PR_T and PL_T for the normalized value of the proximity map and the path length map, respectively. The final set of insertion points is given as:

$$\begin{aligned}\mathbf{V_{safe}} &= \{\mathbf{v}|\mathbf{v} \in \mathbf{V_s}\} \\ &- \{\mathbf{v} \in \mathbf{V_s} \text{ which directly intersect vessels}\} \\ &- \{\mathbf{v}|\mathbf{v} \in \mathbf{V_s}\ ,\ PR(\mathbf{v}) < PR_T\} \\ &- \{\mathbf{v}|\mathbf{v} \in \mathbf{V_s}\ ,\ PL(\mathbf{v}) > PL_T\}\end{aligned}$$

2.2 Data Preprocessing

We tested this approach using MRI data. A high resolution T2 weighted 3D spin-echo multislice set and a time-of-ight (TOF) MRA of the same subject was used for extracting the surface of the head and the brain vasculature, respectively. The extracted brain vasculature is assigned as the vital tissue in this work.

The multi-contrast MR data were subjected to a three-step pre-processing to be used in the planning and visualization algorithms. The first step entails segmentation of the MRA and T2-weighted images. Specifically, to segment the blood vessels from the MRA, we used a region-oriented segmentation techniques of thresholding and region growing [1]. In the original TOF images, the vessels appear brighter relative to the surrounding tissue. First, we applied thresholding and then a connectivity filter based on region growing by selecting the base of the vessel as the seed point. Subsequently, the outer surface of the head was extracted from the T2-weighed MR images by applying a threshold to segment the region outside the head (like a negative mold) and then applying an inversion filter to get the inside region. Segmentation of the head surface stopped just above the nose and ears. In the second step, we used the marching cube algorithm [3] to construct 3D iso-surfaces that surround the high intensity pixels of the segmented images (e.g. vessels from the MRA). The resulting 3D model of the skin and the vessels is represented in form of a triangular mesh. Since the mesh generated by the marching cube algorithm also includes noise in the form of surface artifacts, we first applied the Laplace+HC mesh smoothing algorithm [4] followed by a low pass filter [2]. To avoid possible excess smoothing that may cause shrinkage of the mesh, the number of iteration steps for both algorithms was carefully chosen to ensure no or minimal volume shrinkage. The final step involves the co-registration of the two 3D models. This was straightforward in our studies, since we used the inherent coordinate system of the MR scanner that is shared among all the image sets and there was no patient's head motion during MR scans. At the end of the pre-processing step, we had two 3D models of the angiograms from the MRA and the skin surface from the T2-weighted images. The data-preprocessing step may led to formation of mesh with non uniform sample density of triangles. In such a case, isotropic remeshing algorithms could be used. Secondly, to ensure fine-scale discretization of the head surface, the resultant mesh could be further subdivided as per the requirement of the interventional procedure. Those data along with the target point were then used as input to the path planning approach detailed in section 2.1.

3 Results

This proposed method was applied to test cases representing a wide range of target morphologies, i.e. the positions of the target points were selected as per the requirements of given surgical procedures. Below we describe and discuss two specific cases to illustrate its performance for different proximities of the target relative to a vital anatomy (e.g., blood vessel).

Test Case 1: In the first case, the target was positioned in the cerebrum region of the brain. A maximum threshold of 40.26 mm for path length and minimum threshold of 4.00 mm for the distance from blood vessels were specified. The minimum value of the path length from the head surface to the target point is 37.21mm. Three insertion points namely IP1, IP2, IP3 were selected (as shown in Figure 2) on the outer surface of the head. Among all the insertion points, point IP1 is the closest to the target from the surface at a distance 37.99 mm. Although an insertion made through that point would have shorter path length, the path of insertion of the interventional tool passes directly through the blood vessel. Therefore a path might be shorter but not safe. The insertion path from

Point IP2 (positioned at the boundary of the proximity map) to the target although being at the safe distance of 4.00 mm, the interventional tool need to travel a long distance of 59.64 mm. For the given threshold value, IP3 is the optimal point with a minimum distance of 4.74 mm from the insertion path and a path length of 39.67 mm.

Test Case 2: In the second test case, the target was positioned very close to the vessel. Path length threshold is set to a value of 34.93mm. Threshold for a minimum distance of the insertion path from the vessel is set to 1.48 mm. The minimum value of the path length from the head surface to the target point is 34.37 mm. In the right of figure 2, the blood vessel that is very close to the target, has a broader proximity map, compared to other blood vessels. In spite of the vessel being very close to the target, the buffer region ensures that the interventional tool maintains a minimum distance from the vessel and is still able to hit the target. In this test case, IP1 is the optimal insertion point.

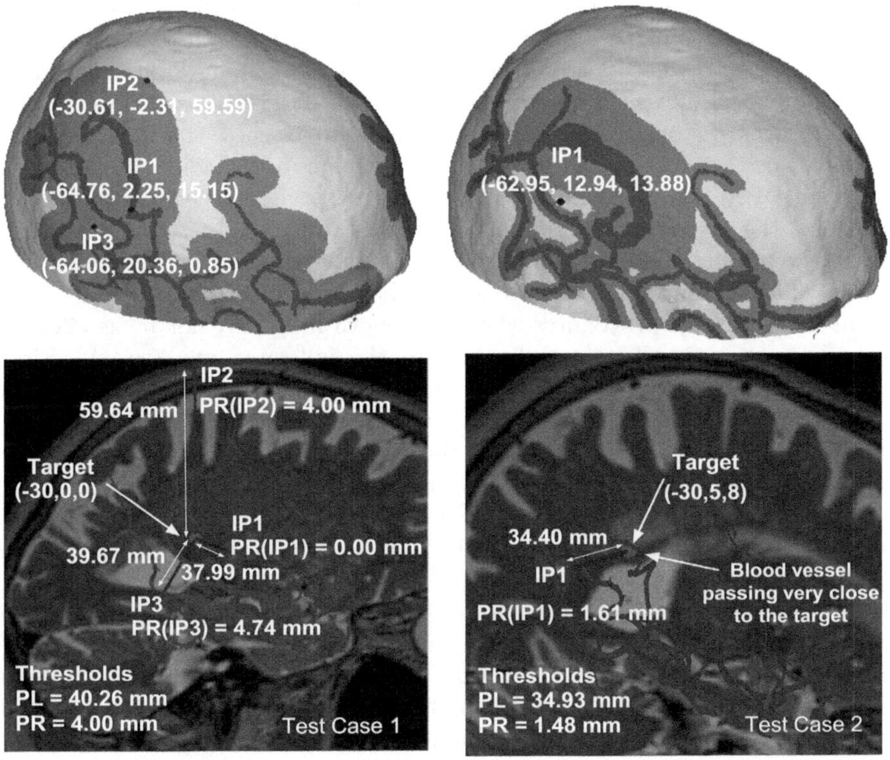

Fig. 2. Test Cases: test case 1 (left) and test case 2 (right). Top figures shows 3D model of patient's head illuminated with access maps and selected insertion points. The bottom figure shows the morphology of the area relative to MR images.

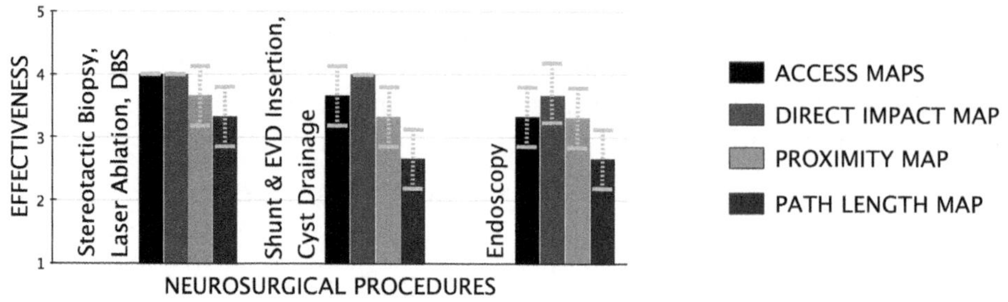

Fig. 3. Shows the effectiveness of the access maps (in conjunction as well as individual) for different neurosurgical interventional procedure.

Preliminary Evaluation: To evaluate the effectiveness of our approach, we performed a preliminary evaluation by collecting feedback from neurosurgeons. As suggested by Brunenberg et al. [6], we also invited three neurosurgeons for our preliminary evaluation. The three neurosurgeons were asked to rate the effectiveness of the access maps for different neurosurgical interventional procedures on a scale of 1 to 5 where 1 stands for 'not very effective' and 5 for 'extremely effective'. Figure 3 shows the means and the standard deviations of the effectiveness in the form of a bar graph. The results (in figure 3) show that neurosurgical procedures such as stereotactic biopsy, laser ablation of tumors, and deep brain stimulation(DBS) could be planned more effectively with the help of our access maps. Also, the given approach is relatively easy to be used by a neurosurgeon in an interventional suite as it only requires tuning the two parameters (PR_T and PL_T) for a given vital structure as per the neurosurgical procedure.

In all neurosurgical procedures, the path length map may not be as effective as other access maps. This mainly dues to the following two reasons. First, the path length can be adequately determined manually during preoperative planning. Second, it is not necessary that the path traversed by an intervention tool should be the shortest. In case of the endoscopic procedure, the target is usually large (comparing to the single point used in the approach) and the entry points are standardized. Therefore, image guidance is not as helpful as that in other stereotactic procedures. As a result, the access maps tend to be ineffective in planning these kinds of procedures.

Most of the neurosurgical interventions are planned by analyzing the 3D data of brain images in sagittal, coronal and transverse planes. The neurosurgeon finalizes the path by inspecting the image slices perpendicular to the bird's-eye view along the insertion path and looking for any abnormalities. Image guidance systems (such as from BrainLab and Radionics) are used for the purpose of preoperative planning. The survey also included questions regarding the integration of the proposed approach with existing systems. If the proposed visualization technique is used in conjunction with the existing systems, it would provide improvement in terms of time required for trajectory planning as it has the potential to make the process less fiddly. However, the access maps do not provide any improvements in terms of accuracy or precision of how the interventional tool would follow the pre-planned path. The accuracy solely depends upon the kind of stereotactic frame system used during the time of intervention.

4 Discussion

In the current test cases, we limited the vital tissue to blood vessels only. Although blood vessels are vital structures, other important anatomical structures need to be considered, depending on specific neurosurgical procedures and the targeted areas. Considering other soft tissues and neuronal pathways would further improve the work. The work of [14, 16] shows the use of brain atlases for path calculation. Incorporating information derived from different atlases and surgeon experience level [15] would help in better risk assessment. We plan to expand this work by incorporating data from other modalities including functional Magnetic Resonance Imaging (fMRI) and Diffusion Tensor Imaging (DTI) and thus extend our classification component depicting the neural and metabolic activities of the brain. However, as this is a feasibility study, this limitation does not affect the generality of our method. Another limitation of the current work is the inclusion of only healthy volunteers, and as a consequence, we used virtual targeted tissues and artificial thresholds. In the future we will expand the work to include cases of patients.

The current work assumes that the brain tissue is rigid; we did not consider any possible tissue shifting when the patient is transferred from the imaging to the surgical suite, or to the procedure (i.e. intra-operative changes). As it may be appreciated, even a slight shift of a deeply seated brain structure during the incision or the advancement of the interventional tool may result in the damage of the vital tissue or missing the target. Apart from brain shift, registration errors could occur. The possible reasons of the registration errors could be either slipping of the fiducial markers or the displacement caused by patients' baggy skin. Some of the neurosurgical needles tend to bent as they penetrate into the tissue layer. In the future, we plan to expand and investigate appropriate safety margins to account for such deformations.

5 Conclusion

In this work, we present a method for visualizing and planning a neurosurgical intervention with straight access. The basic concept of our approach is the generation of various access maps on the surface of the skin of the patient's head. These access maps can guide a neurosurgeon in selecting an entrance point for accessing a specific targeted anatomical structure inside brain. The basis for generating these maps is the classification of tissue from images of different contrast suitable for tissue identification, segmentation and eventual classification. With the help of the direct impact map, impingement of the interventional tool on a vital anatomical structure can be avoided. Subsequently, with the help of the proximity map, the trajectory of a straight line of access from the incision point to the target can maintain a minimum distance from the vital structures, thereby creates a safe buffer region.

While this method was implemented using brain MRI and neurosurgical interventional paradigms, it might be applicable to other anatomical areas and other imaging modalities. Our preliminary user study results showed that our approach is effective and visually intuitive for neurosurgeons. Moreover, the concept of projecting vital information on the surface of the skin was proved efficient for alleviating the challenge associated with the visualization, understanding and manipulation of 3D medical data sets. Such kind of visualization is a critical factor in the interventional suite to reduce the workload and increase accuracy.

Acknowledgments. This work was supported in part by NSF CNS-0932272, NSF IIS-0914965, and Texas NHARP 003652-0058-2007. Any opinions, findings, and conclusions or recommendations expressed in this material are those of the authors and do not necessarily reflect the views of the funding agencies.

References

1. Luo, S., Zhong, Y.: Extraction of Brain Vessels from Magnetic Resonance Angiographic Images: Concise Literature Review, Challenges, and Proposals. In: Proc. of IEEE EMBS, pp. 1422–1425 (2005)
2. Taubin, G.: A signal processing approach to fair surface design. In: Proc. of SIGGRAPH'95, 351-358 (1995)
3. Lorensen, W.E., Cline, H.E.: Marching Cubes: A High Resolution 3D Surface Construction Algorithm. In: Proc. of SIGGRAPH'87, 163-169 (1987)
4. Vollmer, J., Mencl, R., Muller, H.: Improved Laplacian Smoothing of Noisy Surface Meshes. In: Proc. of Eurographics 1999, pp. 131–138 (1999)
5. Nowinski, W.L.: Virtual Reality in Brain Intervention. In: IEEE Symp. on Bioinformatics and Bioengineering, 245-248 (2004)
6. Brunenberg, E.J.L., Bartroli, A.V., Vandewalle, V.V., Temel, Y., Ackermans, L., Platel, B., Romenij, B.M.H.: Automatic Trajectory Planning for Deep Brain Stimulation: A Feasibility Study. In: Ayache, N., Ourselin, S., Maeder, A. (eds.) MICCAI 2007, Part I. LNCS, vol. 4791, pp. 584–592. Springer, Heidelberg (2007)
7. Lee, J.D., Huang, C.H., Lee, S.T.: Improving stereotactic surgery using 3-D reconstruction. IEEE Eng. in Med. and Bio. Mag., vol. 21, 109-116 (2002)
8. Bourbakis, N.G., Awad, M.: A 3-D visualization method for image-guided brain surgery. IEEE Trans. on Systems, Man, Cybernetics, vol. 33, 766-781 (2003)
9. Fujii, T., Emoto, H., Sugou, N., Mito, T. Shibata, I.: Neuropath planner-automatic path searching for neurosurgery. In: Proc. of Computer Assisted Radiology and Surgery (CARS), vol. 1256, 587-583 (2003)
10. Beyer, J., Hadwiger, M., Wolsberger, S., Buhler, K.: High-Quality Multimodal Volume Rendering for Preoperative Planning of Neurosurgical Interventions. IEEE Trans. on Vis. and Comp. Graph., vol. 13, 1696-1703 (2007)
11. Joshi, A., Scheinost, D., Vives, K.P., Spencer, D.D., Staib, L.H., Papademetris, X. Novel interaction techniques for neurosurgical planning and stereotactic navigation, IEEE Trans. on Vis. and Comp. Graph., vol. 14, 1587-1594 (2008)
12. Seigneuret, J.F., Jannin, P., Fleig, O.J., Seigneuret, E., Mor, X., Raimbault, M., Cedex, R.: Multimodal and Multi-Informational Neuronavigation. In: CARS - Computer Assisted Radiology and Surgery, 167-172 (2000)

13. Serra, L., Kockro, R.A., Guan, C.G., Hern, N., Lee, E.C.K., Lee, Y.H., Chan, C., Nowinski, W.L.: Multimodal Volume-based Tumor Neurosurgery Planning in the Virtual Workbench. In: MICCAI'98, 1007-1015 (1998)
14. Vaillant, M., Davatzikos, C., Taylor, R. H., Bryan, R. N.: A path-planning algorithm for image-guided neurosurgery. In Proc. of Computer Vision, Virtual Reality and Robotics in Medicine and Medical Robotics and Computer-Assisted Surgery, 467-476 (1997)
15. Tirelli, P., De Momi, E., Borghese, N.A., Ferrigno, G.: An intelligent atlas-based planning system for keyhole neurosurgery. Int'l. J. of Computer Assisted Radiology and Surgery (IJCARS) 4, 85–91 (2009)
16. Popovic, A., and Trovato, K.: Path planning for reducing tissue damage in minimally invasive brain access. In Computer Assisted Radiology and Surgery (CARS 2009), supplemental S132-S133, (2009)

Active Multispectral Illumination and Image Fusion for Retinal Microsurgery

Raphael Sznitman, Seth Billings, Diego Rother, Daniel Mirota, Yi Yang, Jim Handa, Peter Gehlbach, Jin U. Kang, Gregory D. Hager, and Russell Taylor

Johns Hopkins University
3400 North Charles Street, Baltimore, MD, 21218, USA
{sznitman,sbillin3,yyang30,jthanda,pgelbach,jkang,hager,rht}@jhu.edu

Abstract. It has been shown that white light exposure during retinal microsurgeries is detrimental to patients. To address this problem, we present a novel device and image processing tool, which can be used to significantly reduce the amount of phototoxicity induced in the eye. Our device alternates between illuminating the retina using white and limited spectrum light, while a fully automated image processing algorithm produces a synthetic white light video by colorizing non-white light images. We show qualitatively and quantitatively that our system can provide reliable images using far less toxic light when compared to traditional systems. In addition, the method proposed in this paper may be adapted to other clinical applications in order to give surgeons more flexibility when visualizing areas of interest.

1 Introduction

Retinal microsurgery is one of the most demanding types of surgery. The difficulty stems from the microscopic dimensions of tissue planes and blood vessels in the eye, the delicate nature of the neurosensory retina and the poor recovery of retinal function after injury. Many micron-scale maneuvers are physically not possible for many retinal surgeons due to inability to visualize the tissue planes, tremor, or insufficient dexterity. To safely perform these maneuvers, microscopes are required to view the retina. A central issue for the surgeon is the compromise between adequate illumination of retinal structures, and the risk of iatrogenic phototoxicity either from the operating microscope or endoilluminators, which are fiber-optic light sources that are placed into the vitreous cavity to provide adequate illumination of the retina during delicate maneuvers.

Retinal phototoxicity from an operating microscope was first reported in 1983 in patients who had undergone cataract surgery with intraocular lens implantation [1]. Retinal phototoxicity is now a well recognized potential complication of any intraocular surgical procedure, and the frequency is reported to occur from 7% to 28% of patients undergoing cataract surgery [2, 3]. As a result, the International Commission on Non-Ionizing Radiation Protection (ICNIRP) now

N. Navab and P. Jannin (Eds.): IPCAI 2010, LNCS 6135, pp. 12–22, 2010.

provides safety guidelines for illumination of the fundus in both phakic and aphakic subjects [4]. Blue wavelength and ultraviolet light induce the greatest degree of retinal injury. In fact, in [5] it was found that commercially available light sources for endoillumination exceeded the ICNIRP guidelines for retinal damage by visible light within 3 minutes, and in 9 of 10 sources, the safe exposure time was exceeded in less than 1 minute. In vitrectomy for macular hole repair, up to 7% of the patients have been reported to have experienced visually significant phototoxicity [6–8].

Phototoxicity can be either thermal or photochemical in nature from excessive ultraviolet (UV) or blue light toxicity. Ham et al. showed the action spectrum or relative risk of UV or blue light toxicity when the retina was exposed to various wavelengths of light [9]. The action spectrum was then used to create a relative risk of phototoxicity associated with a given wavelength of light. The current state of the art endoillumination systems have taken advantage of these data. The new systems are significantly brighter and when compared to earlier systems, they appear to be safer. Previously, halogen light sources containing significant blue wavelength light have been replaced by xenon and mercury illumination systems, with reduced blue wavelengths. The risk, while reduced, is still significant for intraocular surgery. Given the advancing age of the population and increasing prevalence of retinal diseases, further improvements aimed at reducing iatrogenic retinal phototoxicity would be a welcome addition.

To address this issue, we present a novel visualization system that can be used to significantly reduce the emission of highly toxic wavelengths over existing systems. While changing the spectral composition of the illumination toward longer wavelengths could help reduce phototoxicity, we have created a new device which cyclicly illuminates the retina using white and less damaging non-white light, allowing for maximal phototoxicity reduction. Consequently, images provided by this device are either fully colored or monochromatic.

To avoid visually straining any potential user (*i.e.* surgeon) this device is used together with an image recoloring scheme. Computer colorization schemes have existed since the 70's [10] and have since been further developed [11, 12]. In general, however, such systems rely on a user to pre-select regions of the image that correspond to specific colors, making them ill-suited for this application. More recently, a time series analysis was proposed to model the retinal image scene [13]. This methods however relies on having all visual cues (*e.g.* color and texture) available at all times to maintain an accurate retina model. To our knowledge, no previous work has focused on fusing images taken under varying spectrum illumination to form continuous and coherent image sequences.

Therefore, in order to facilitate the use of this device for surgical procedures, we have developed a fully automated algorithm for colorizing non-white light images, so that they appear fully colored. Our method is simple and requires little parameter tuning making it easy to use. We have experimentally shown that our method provides a quantitative and qualitative improvement in coloring accuracy over naive recoloring schemes.

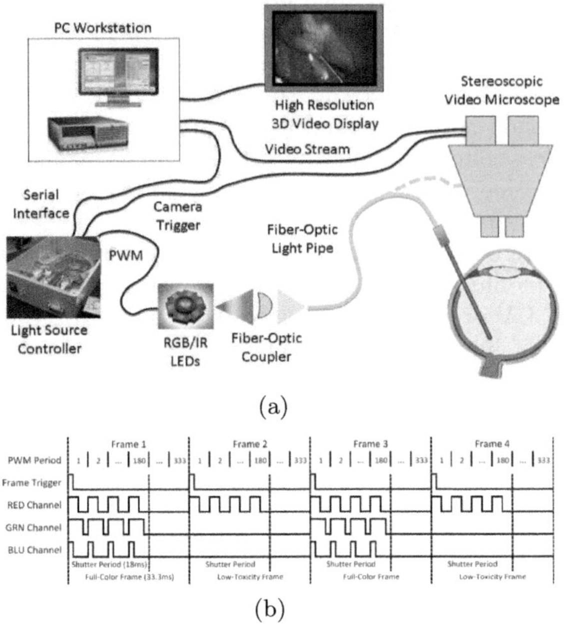

Fig. 1. (a) System overview and (b) example light source control signals

The remainder of this article is as follows: in section 2 we present the system overview and our device. In section 3 our colorization algorithm is presented. Section 4 details in depth experiments on our system, while we discuss some of the pit-falls of our system and future works in section 5.

2 Light Source

Figure 1(a) shows an overview of the system. Visualization of the retina occurs via a 3D LCD display, which accepts a video feed from high-resolution cameras mounted on a surgical microscope. Illumination is provided using high power LEDs in RGB configuration, and may be delivered either through a fiber-optic probe or through a surgical microscope. A control box, housing an embedded microcontroller and LED driver electronics, controls illumination activity via independent pulse-width modulation (PWM) of each LED channel. A serial command interface between the control box and a PC provides user-level control of the light source from a GUI application. The control box also sources a trigger signal to the cameras for synchronizing illumination activity with the shutter periods of the cameras.

The system reduces white light exposure by two means. Firstly, illumination is deactivated during the shutter closed period of each camera frame. For a typical shutter period of 18 milliseconds and a frame rate of 30 frames per second, the light exposure time is reduced by 50%. Secondly, rather than illuminating every frame with white light, some frames are rendered under limited spectrum light having low toxic potential, such as red or infrared light. The result is a video feed interleaving full-color frames, when white light is active, with limited-spectrum (red) frames, when low toxicity light is active. Thus, the exposure period of highly toxic wavelengths is reduced by a further fraction equal to the repeat rate of white light images in the frame sequence. Figure 1(b) shows control signals from the light source controller for generating a sequence of alternating full color and monochrome images.

3 Image Recoloring

From the device described above, white and red light images are cyclicly produced at a fixed rate. Naturally, emitting fewer white light images allows for lower levels of phototoxicity for the patient. However, reducing the number of white light images increases the difficulty of the procedure for the surgeon. Hence, a method which restricts the number of white light images used, and still provides a *typical* view for the surgeon, is required. Ultimately, it is necessary to produce an accurate colored image of the retina at any given time, irrespective of which illumination was used.

To provide a coherent colored image sequence, we present two methods: a *naive* (section 3.1) and an *active scene rendering* (section 3.2) approach. Due to the lack of previous work on this particular topic, we treat the naive approach as a baseline algorithm. This algorithm is simple and only useful in cases with high fractions of white light. In section 4.1 we compare both methods on image sequences where ground truth is available, thus demonstrating improvements produced by non-naive methods.

At each discrete time step, t, we denote the type of illumination the device is triggering as L_t, where $L_t = 1$ when white light is used, and $L_t = 0$ for non-white light. Associated with each illumination, $I_t = \{R_t, G_t, B_t\}$ is the corresponding RGB image acquired. The rate at which white light illuminates the retina is then defined as $\phi = \frac{\sum_{i=1}^{t} L_i}{t}$.

In order to perform recoloring, it is necessary to correctly account for the color of the non-white illuminant. We define the color space of the acquired images as the usual RGB color space denoted by $S \subset R(3)$. Following [14], we define a separate color space $S' \subset R(3)$ such that the color of the non-white illuminant is (1,0,0). We relate S and S' by a linear transformation F of the form $F = sR$, where s is a scale factor and R is a rotation. Then for any RGB value $p \in S$, we can compute $p' \in S'$ as $p' = Fp$. The optimal F can be computed by first acquiring a non-white illuminated image, finding the largest principal component, x, and subsequently constructing two orthogonal components y and z as in [14]. R is constructed from these components. The scale s can then be computed by comparing a while light and non-white light image under the (color) rotation R.

Since our non-white illuminant is largely red, in the remainder of the paper we will continue to refer to the non-white image as the "red" image and the two orthogonal components as green and blue with the understanding that these are, in general, not the raw color values from the camera.

We denote $\mathcal{I}_t$ as the final fully colored image rendered by our system. As the device sequentially provides us with images, we will maintain a color model for the retina, $\mathcal{M} = \{m_G, m_B\}$, where m_B and m_G are the green and blue color models (represented in the form of images), respectively. Such a color model will be maintained over time, and we thus denote $\mathcal{M}_t$ as the color model at time t. In order to have a color model at any given time, t, let I_1 be a white light image.

3.1 Naive Approach

Perhaps the simplest method to create and maintain a colored image model, $\mathcal{M}$, is to assume that images do not significantly change over time. In other words, a strong continuity in the appearance in color from I_t to $I_{t+\delta t}$ is assumed.

The corresponding algorithm is simple: if $L_t = 1$, then the model $\mathcal{M}_t$ is updated, $\mathcal{M}_t = \{G_t, B_t\}$ and $\mathcal{I}_t = I_t$. Otherwise, $L_t = 0$ and we let $\mathcal{I}_t = (R_t, m_G, m_B)$. Following such a procedures ensures that all $\mathcal{I}_t$ are fully colored images. Figures 2(a) and 2(b) show an example I_t and $\mathcal{I}_t$, respectively. Notice that continuity is violated, as the tool has been displaced since the last white-light image received, thus causing "ghosting" effects.

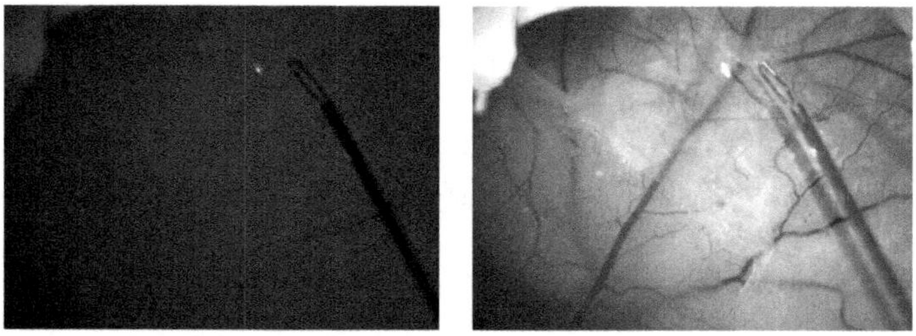

(a) (b)

Fig. 2. (a) Example of a non-white light image from our device and (b) the image rendered by the naive algorithm. Notice that simply using the G and B channels from the last white frame does not generate good color images. This is particularly the case when there is motion in the scene.

3.2 Active Scene Rendering Approach

A natural extension of the naive approach is to infer the motion observed in the image sequence and correct the associated artifacts. We present our novel color fusing algorithm: Active Scene Rendering (ASR). Here the idea is to estimate the different forms of motion which appear in the scene and take this information into account when rendering the colored images.

Here, it is still assumed that a strong temporal correlation between adjacent images is present. Furthermore, it is stipulated that a transformation, T, from image I_t to I_{t+1} can be inferred. Intuitively, T can be regarded as the motion, induced by the surgeon, which the eye undergoes during a procedure. Notice that this transformation only accounts for the eye motion and not the tool motion. Hence, to further reduce colorization errors (as those in figure 2(b)), we model the tool and its motion as well. The idea is to first detect the pose of the tool to obtain a 2D segmentation and then use this information to recolor the image correctly. We now describe how the estimation of the transformation T and the 2D tool segmentation are performed.

Image Stabilization. As previously mentioned, the surgeon is free to manipulate the eye. To compensate for this motion, a simple translation model for the motion of the retina is assumed. Although it has been shown that wide angle retinal image deformation is best modeled with a quadratic deformation [15], small motion can be approximated with pure translation when under high magnification. To estimate the translation we first extract SIFT features [16] (I_t is treated as a gray scale image for any value of L_t), find correspondences and then apply the robust ASKC method [17] to find the translation that best explains the correspondences. This permits us to find a transformation regardless of whether the tool is present in the image or not. Note that in order to present coherent image sequences, images are cropped by removing border regions.

Tool Detection. Given that the most consistent clue for the tool is its constant and known 3D shape, we use the framework proposed in [18] for simultaneous segmentation and pose estimation which exploits this information. This framework requires, as input, the 3D shape (represented as voxel occupancies) and color probability distribution (represented as a mixture of Gaussians) of the tool, and the color probability distribution for each background pixel (represented as a single Gaussian). The output of the framework is a segmentation of the tool in each frame, and also an estimate of the 3D pose of the tool in the 3D coordinate system of the camera, for each frame. The estimated 3D pose in one frame is used to initialize the segmentation and pose estimation in the following frame. Using this method guarantees finding the globally optimal 3D pose and segmentation in a computationally efficient manner.

The algorithm for ASR is similar to that of section 3.1. At $t = 1$, we let $\mathcal{I}_1 = I_1$ and set $\mathcal{M}_1 = \{G_1, B_1\}$. I_1 is then treated as the initial frame of reference, such that subsequent images are stabilized with regards to I_1. That is, for every new image I_t, we compute the transformation T_t from I_t to I_1. Then, using T_t, we translate I_t and compute a rectified image, $\tilde{I}_t$. When $L_t = 1$, we set $\mathcal{M}_t = \{\tilde{B}_t, \tilde{G}_t\}$ and $\mathcal{I}_t = \tilde{I}_t$.

If $L_t = 0$ (figure 3(a)), the 2D segmentation of the tool is determined (figure 3(b)). To do this, $\mathcal{M}_t$ and the known color model of the tool are used to initialize the detection process described above. Once the segmentation has been computed, this region is rendered using the tool color model. The rest of the image is rendered as $\mathcal{I}_t = (\tilde{R}_t, m_G, m_B)$ (figure 3(c)).

(a) (b) (c)

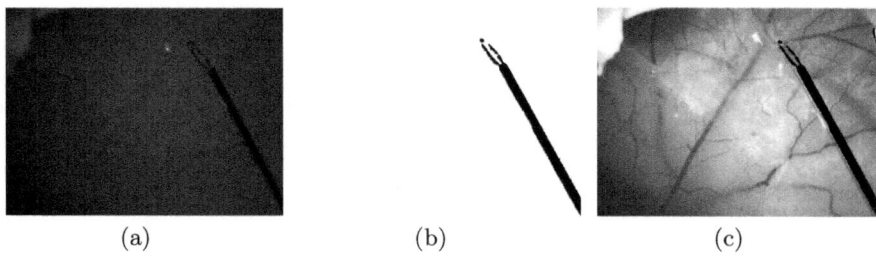

Fig. 3. (a) Example non-white light image from our device, (b) segmented tool, and (c) rendered image by ASR. Here, the tool is correctly estimated and image regions are updated in a coherent manner.

4 Experimentation

We now show how our system performs on phantom image sequences. A quantitative comparison of both methods is described in section 4.1, where it is shown that ASR surpasses the naive approach in a setting where ground truth is known. This is shown by measuring the error for different values of ϕ. Qualitative results of our system on image sequences are then provided in section 4.2.

4.1 Validation with Ground Truth

To validate both approaches described in section 3 we recorded two image sequences of membrane peeling on embryonic eggs using only white light. Doing so allows us to synthetically generate limited-spectrum images at any rate ϕ, by using only the red band of white light images. Hence, we know that the transformation F (see section 3) is known to be $F = I$. As detailed in [19, 20], this phantom setup provides a similar environment to in-vivo settings. Image sequences consist of 500 images, acquired at 20 frames per second using the system described in section 2.

Using this data, 5 image sequences are generated where $\phi = \{1/2, 1/4, 1/8, 1/16, 1/32\}$. For each sequence, both naive and ASR colorization approaches are evaluated. Since the ground truth – the original recorded white light images – is always available, an error can be computed for each frame generated by either approach. In the following experiments the L2 (or mean squared error) norm is chosen to measure the error between the ground truth and the rendered images. In addition, we also compute the error using the Bounded Variation (BV) norm, which has been used to quantify image quality during denoising tasks [21]. This provides us with a measure of image quality, taking into account both photometric and rectification errors.

Figure 4(a) shows the L2 norm error when varying ϕ for both methods. Figure 4(b) shows a similar result for the BV norm. In general, one can observe that as ϕ decreases, the error rate increases. This is expected as the assumption of similarity between frames, discussed in section 3.1, is increasingly violated. Naturally, the naive approach suffers greatly when ϕ is small, as the true color

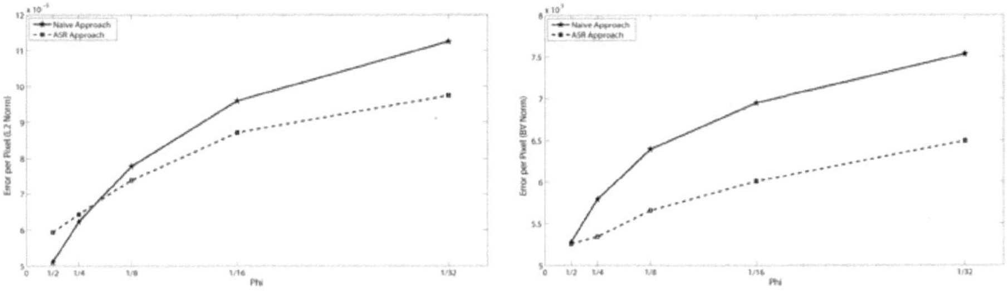

(a) (b)

Fig. 4. Evaluation of the proposed methods when varying the fraction of available white-light images, ϕ. The average error per pixel ((a) L2 norm (b) BV norm) is computed on image sequences where ground truth is known. Both error metrics indicate that ASR (dashed line) provides accuracy gains over the naive approach (solid line).

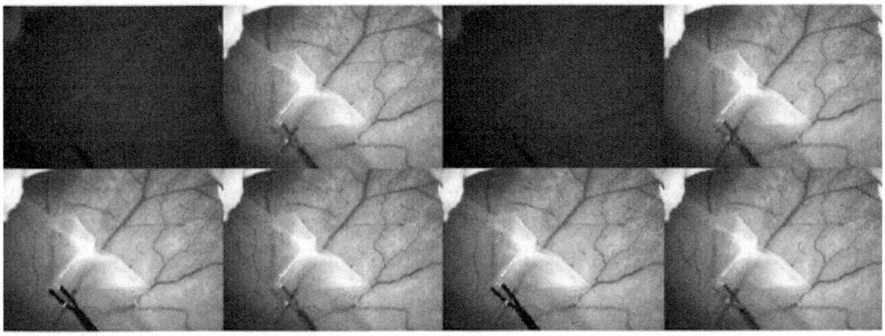

Fig. 5. (*top row*) Example image sequence from the device ($\phi = 1/2$) and corresponding rendered sequence using ASR (*bottom row*)

may differ greatly from the last observed color. ASR however suffers significantly less from small ϕ values, as it is able to maintain a more accurate color model.

4.2 Egg Peeling

Having observed that ASR provides a better way to model retinal-type scenes, we set up our system to record and display images for different values of ϕ. We record several image sequences in a similar setup as in section 4.1 and show the resulting recolored sequence. Note that the color mapping transformation F is assumed to have $R = I$, and a uniform scaling factor (determined empirically).

In figure 5 we show a typical image sequence ($\phi = 1/2$), of a chorioallatonic membrane peel from an 11 day old chicken embryo. The resulting recolored images rendered by our system are shown. The entire image sequence and recolored images can be viewed in a video included in the supplementary materials. The video shows four similar peeling sequences where each row corresponds to a different ϕ value (1/2,1/4,1/8,1/16). The first column shows the images provided by the device, while the second and third columns show how the naive and model approach, respectively, render the sequence. Since the device is being used to obtain these image sequences, no ground truth is available for quantitative comparison.

Notice that in general the model approach renders a more coherent image than the naive approach. This is particularly true at smaller ϕ values, concurring with the results of section 4.1.

5 Discussion and Conclusion

In this paper we have presented a novel system that can be used to reduce toxic light exposure in retinal microsurgeries. The system consists of a new lighting device which reduces emission of highly toxic wavelengths. In addition we have developed a novel algorithm that can be used with this device in order to render a fully colored image sequence to the user, thus avoiding visual discomfort. We have shown qualitatively and quantitatively that our method provides superior rendering over naive approaches. Even at low ϕ rates (*e.g.* 1/8 or 1/16), we showed that maintaining high color fidelity is possible, allowing for low levels of phototoxicity.

However, most retinal surgeries involve changing the structure of the retina, and hence the color of the retina (as described in [13]). As seen in our image sequences, regions of the retina which are altered by the surgeon cannot be recolored correctly until a new white light image is provided. Hence a potential improvement of this method would involve a dynamic ϕ, which could change as a function of the activity in the image sequence.

Another natural future direction of this work would consist in understanding the effect of using such a system and phototoxicity levels observed in live tissue. Determining the exact relationship would allow for a quantitative evaluation in toxicity reduction; something which currently can not be determined.

Although phototoxicity reduction in retinal surgery provided the motivating focus for this paper, our technical approach to the problem is potentially more broadly applicable. We have developed methods for actively controlling the illumination spectrum in video microscopy and endoscopy and for fusing the resulting image sequences to form continuous and coherent image sequences. These methods are applicable in many clinical applications, including neurosurgery and cancer surgery. For example, changing the illumination spectrum can be used to improve tissue contrast or discrimination or the depth of penetration of light into tissue structures. The methods proposed in this paper may be adapted to such cases while still giving the surgeon more options on the actual visualization. Exploring these options will be another direction for future work.

Acknowledgements

Funding for this research was provided in part by NIH Grant 1 R01 EB 007969-01, in part by a research subcontract from Equinox Corporation, in part by NSF Cooperative Agreement EEC9731478, and in part by Johns Hopkins University internal funds.

References

1. McDonald, H., Irvine, A.: Light-induced maculopathy from the operating microscope in extracapsular cataract extraction and intraocular lens implantation. Ophthalmology 90, 945–951 (1983)
2. Khwarg, S., Linstone, F., Daniels, S., Isenberg, S., Hanscom, T., Geoghegan, M., Straatsma, B.: Incidence, risk factors, and morphology in operating microscope light retinopathy. American Journal of Ophthalmology 103, 255–263 (1987)
3. Byrnes, G., Antoszyk, A., Mazur, D., Kao, T., Miller, S.: Photic maculopathy after extracapsular cataract surgery a prospective study. Ophthalmology 99, 731–738 (1992)
4. International Commission on Non-Ionizing Radiation Protection: Guidelines on limits of exposure to broad-band incoherent optical radiation (0.38 to 3). Health Phys. 73, 539–554 (1997)
5. van den Biesen, R., Berenschot, T., Verdaasdonk, R., van Weelden, H., van Norren, D.: Endoillumination during vitrectomy and phototoxicity thresholds. British Journal of Ophthalmology 84, 1372–1375 (2000)
6. Poliner, L., Tornambe, P.: Retinal pigment epitheliopathy after macular hole surgery. Ophthalmology 99, 1671–1677 (1992)
7. Michels, M., Lewis, H., Abrams, G., Han, D., Mieler, W., Neitz, J.: Macular phototoxicity caused by fiberoptic endoillumination during pars plana vitrectomy. American Journal of Ophthalmol. 114, 287–292 (1992)
8. Banker, A., Freeman, W., Kim, J., Munguia, D., Azen, S.: Vision-threatening complications of surgery for full-thickness macular holes. Ophthalmology 104, 1442–1453 (1997)
9. Ham, W.J., Mueller, H., Ruffolo, J.J., Guerry, D., Guerry, R.: Action spectrum for retinal injury from near-ultraviolet radiation in the aphakic monkey. American Journal of Ophthalmology 93, 299–306 (1982)
10. Museum of Broadcast Communication: Encyclopedia of Television (online), `http://www.museum.tv/archives/etv/c/htmlc/colorization/colorization.htm`
11. Skora, D., Burinek, J., Zra, J.: Unsupervised colorization of black and white cartoons. In: Int. Symp. NPAR, Annecy, pp. 121–127 (2004)
12. Yatziv, L., Sapiro, G.: Fast image and video colorization using chrominance blending. IEEE Transactions on Image Processing 15, 1120–1129 (2006)
13. Sznitman, R., Lin, H., Manaswi, G., Hager, G.: Active background modeling: Actors on a stage. In: International Conference on Computer Vision, Workshop on Visual Surveillance (2009)
14. Mallick, S., Zickler, T., Belhumeur, P., Kriegman, D.: Specularity removal in images and videos: A PDE approach. In: Leonardis, A., Bischof, H., Pinz, A. (eds.) ECCV 2006. LNCS, vol. 3951, pp. 550–563. Springer, Heidelberg (2006)
15. Stewart, C., Chia-Ling, T., Roysam, B.: The dual-bootstrap iterative closest point algorithm with application to retinal image registration. IEEE Transactions on Medical Imaging 22(11), 1379–1394 (2003)
16. Lowe, D.: Distinctive image features from scale-invariant keypoints. International Journal of Computer Vision 20, 91–110 (2003)
17. Wang, H., Mirota, D., Hager, G.: A generalized kernel consensus based robust estimator. IEEE Transactions on Pattern Analysis and Machine Intelligence 32(1), 178–184 (2010)

18. Rother, D., Sapiro, G.: Seeing 3D objects in a single 2D image. In: International Conference on Computer Vision (2009)
19. Leng, T., Miller, J., Bilbao, K., Palanker, D., Huie, P., Blumenkranz, M.: The chick chorioallantoic membrane as a model tissue for surgical retinal research and simulation. Retina 24(3), 427–434 (2004)
20. Fleming, I., Balicki, M., Koo, J., Iordachita, I., Mitchell, B., Handa, J., Hager, G., Taylor, R.: Cooperative robot assistant for retinal microsurgery. In: International Conference on Medical Image Computing and Computer Assisted Intervention, vol. 11(2), pp. 543–550 (2008)
21. Chang, Q., Chern, I.: Acceleration methods for total variation-based image denoising. SIAM Journal of Applied Mathematics 25(3), 982–994 (2003)

An Iterative Framework for Improving the Accuracy of Intraoperative Intensity-Based 2D/3D Registration for Image-Guided Orthopedic Surgery

Yoshito Otake[1], Mehran Armand[2], Ofri Sadowsky[1],
Robert S. Armiger[2], Peter Kazanzides[1], and Russell H. Taylor[1]

[1] Department of Computer Science, the Johns Hopkins University,
3400 North Charles Street, Baltimore, MD, 21218, USA
[2] The Johns Hopkins University Applied Physics Laboratory,
11100 Johns Hopkins Road, Laurel, Maryland 20723, USA
{otake,osadow,pkaz,rht}@jhu.edu,
{Mehran.Armand,Robert.Armiger}@jhuapl.edu

Abstract. We propose an iterative refinement framework that improves the accuracy of intraoperative intensity-based 2D/3D registration. The method optimizes both the extrinsic camera parameters and the object pose. The algorithm estimates the transformation between the fiducials and the patient intraoperatively using a small number of X-ray images. The proposed algorithm was validated in an experiment using a cadaveric phantom, in which the true registration was acquired from CT data. The results of 50 registration trials with randomized initial conditions on a pair of X-ray C-arm images taken at 32° angular separation showed that the iterative refinement process improved the translational error by 0.32 mm and the rotational error by 0.61 degrees when compared to the 2D/3D registration without iteration. This tool has the potential to allow routine use of image guided therapy by computing registration parameters using only two X-ray images.

Keywords: Intensity-based 2D/3D registration, Image-guided therapy.

1 Introduction

In an image-guided surgery system using external tracking devices, the process of patient registration involves calculating a transformation that maps preoperative datasets to the patient's physical anatomy. Point-based registration is performed using corresponding points between the preoperative data and the surface of target patient anatomy. This broadly adopted registration method is used in most commercial navigation systems. The intraoperative workflow for point-based registration is well established and registration error properties such as fiducial localization error (FLE), fiducial registration error (FRE) and target registration error (TRE) are extensively analyzed (e.g., [1]). Point-based methods, however, have a major disadvantage: they require physical contact with multiple points over the target anatomy using a navigated instrument. Consequently, the surgeon often needs to create a larger exposure than required for navigation-free minimally invasive surgery. Also, due to

N. Navab and P. Jannin (Eds.): IPCAI 2010, LNCS 6135, pp. 23–33, 2010.

the time involved in performing the registration, this procedure is usually conducted once at the beginning of the surgery, and the tracker reference body is carefully handled until the end of the surgery to avoid losing the registration. Ideally, the registration process should be fast enough to repeat several times during the surgery just before each procedure which requires the navigation.

In order to overcome the shortcomings of point-based registration (invasiveness and processing time), image-based registration has been investigated [2]. In image-based registration, intraoperative X-ray images and a 2D/3D registration technique are used for deriving patient position. The method has been often used for radiation therapy, usually with a fixed X-ray device capable of accurate control of the detector position [3]. Image-based registration has also been employed for orthopaedic procedures (e.g., [4]), because it requires less time and no additional surgical exposure compared to the point-based method. The tradeoff, however, is increased radiation exposure.

One of the difficulties precluding routine use of image-based registration during image-guided therapies is its relatively low accuracy and uncertain robustness. Most clinically available C-arm devices lack the position information for the acquired images, which is crucial for an accurate 2D/3D registration, due to poor physical stability of the large supported masses and no motion encoding. The pose estimation of the C-arm detector is a key technical challenge. Some researchers proposed attaching optical tracking fiducials on the detector itself [5]; however, this approach has several drawbacks in real clinical settings such as maintaining the line-of-sight of the optical tracker, remaining within the field of view of the tracker, and synchronizing the C-arm and tracker (due to the inherent physical instability of the C-arm). Our approach uses instead a previously developed fiducial [6] that is visible within the field of view and contains optical markers. Knowing the unique geometry of the fiducial, it is possible to resolve the 3D position of that fiducial relative to the detector from a 2D projection image. However, image distortion and background clutter adversely affect the registration accuracy in this approach. While some of these issues are mitigated by using lighter-weight and distortion-free flat-panel detectors, recovery of the C-arm pose and the patient pose still applies and can benefit from an iterative method for registration.

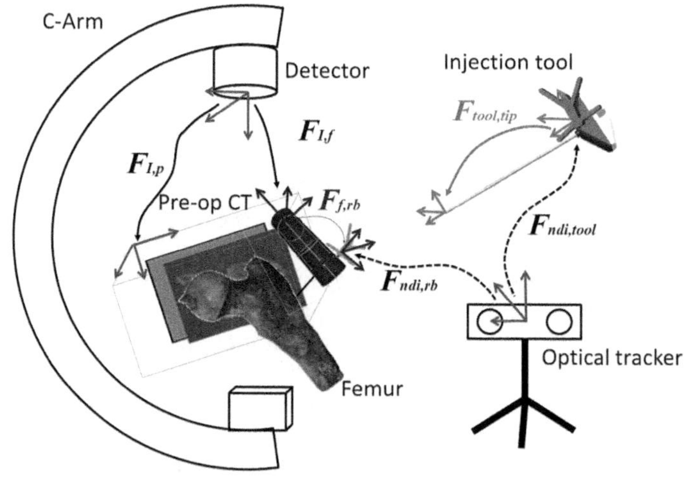

Fig. 1. An application scenario in orthopedic surgical navigation system

In this paper, we propose an iterative refinement framework for image-based registration that recovers the geometric transformations between the C-arm detector, images and CT coordinates while compensating for the error induced by image distortion and background clutter associated with intraoperative X-ray imaging. The motivation of this paper is to allow routine use of image-based 2D/3D registration in image-guided therapy, and to avoid the time-consuming point-based registration methods that require larger surgical exposures. In order to improve the accuracy and the stability of the image-based registration process given image distortion and background clutter, we propose a framework in which the C-arm pose estimation and object pose estimation are iteratively updated.

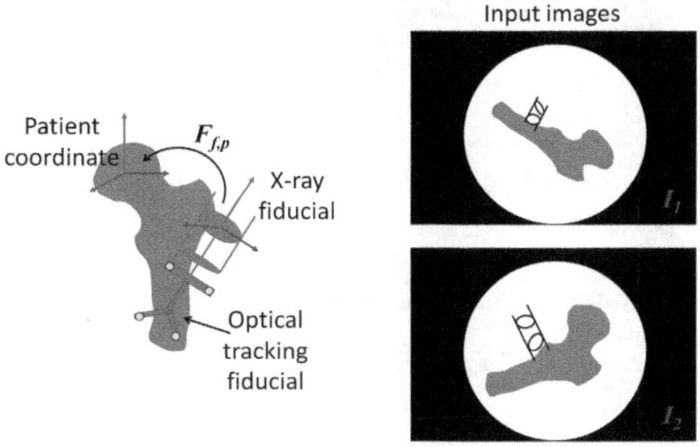

Fig. 2. Problem description of the X-ray image-based fiducial registration

2 Materials and Methods

2.1 An Application Scenario in Orthopedic Surgical Navigation System

A case-study scenario of our X-ray image-based registration algorithm is shown in Fig.1. The schematic shows an orthopedic surgical navigation system for delivering a planned amount of bone cement to the proximal femur, as a proposed method for reducing the risk of fracture in osteoporotic bones. Prior to the surgery, calibration of the intrinsic camera parameters and distortion correction are performed on a conventional C-arm using a calibrated phantom proposed by Sadowsky *et al.* [7]. A fiducial structure [6] is then attached to the patient using a bone screw. Next, between two to five X-ray images are taken from various directions. Using the preoperative CT data and the known geometry of the fiducial, the transformation between the tracking fiducial and the patient anatomy is computed. The transformation is then used to determine the pose of the surgical tools (e.g. needle, drill, etc.) relative to the patient as seen by an optical tracker.

2.2 Problem Description

The main problem in X-ray image-based registration is described in Fig. 2. Several X-ray source images (for simplicity, we consider 2 images, I_1 and I_2) are used to compute the transformation between patient and fiducial, $F_{f,p}$. (Note that we use the convention $F_{a,b}$ to describe a transformation from coordinate system a to coordinate system b throughout this paper). The registration process is divided into two parts: C-arm detector pose estimation and patient pose estimation. The following sections describe each of the two steps respectively.

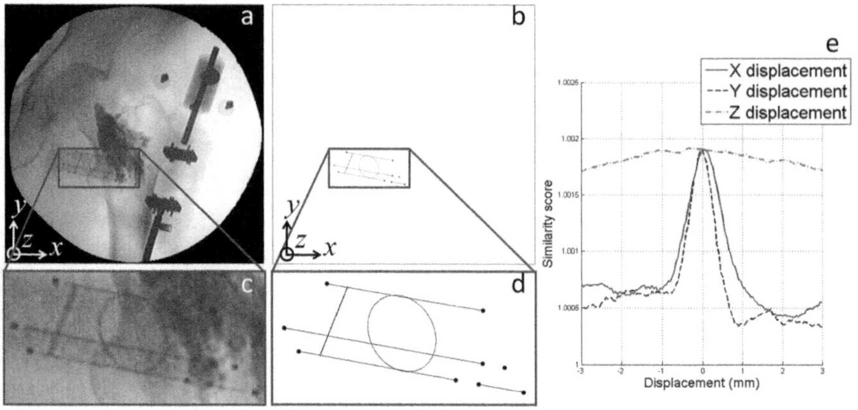

Fig. 3. C-arm detector pose estimation method. a) original fluoroscope image. b) projection image of the CAD model. c), d) magnified image of the fiducial. e) plot of the similarity score while displacing the object in x, y, and z direction.

2.3 C-arm Detector Pose Estimation

The six DOF transformation between the C-arm detector and the fiducial is computed from a 2D projection image using the custom hybrid fiducial that includes radio opaque features. The method for computing the transformation from segmented features (bead points, lines and ellipses) was described previously [6]. In clinical settings, however, due to severe background clutter, the segmentation of features is not always possible. The contributing factors to the background clutter and image noise may include patient anatomy, surgical tools and so on. Therefore we use an alternative approach to estimate the C-arm pose, eliminating the need for the segmentation process. In this approach, shown in Fig.3, first the pose is roughly estimated manually by point correspondence of the beads on the fiducial. Then a projected image of the CAD model of the fiducial is created based on the roughly estimated pose. A similarity score, mutual information [8], between the generated image and the intraoperative X-ray image is computed. A non-linear optimization method, the Nelder-Mead Downhill Simplex Algorithm [9], is applied to find the pose that yields the maximum similarity score per each image (I_1 and I_2). The pose is then used as an initial guess for our iterative framework.

2.4 Patient Pose Estimation Using Intensity-Based 2D/3D Registration Algorithm

The pose of the patient with respect to the fiducial is estimated using intensity-based 2D/3D registration, and is described in detail in our previously published work [10-11]. The 2D/3D registration algorithm makes use of a computationally fast DRR (Digitally Reconstructed Radiograph) created from CT data. To achieve this, the CT data is represented as a tetrahedral mesh model. Given any arbitrary source and detector location, a simulated radiograph is produced using the line integral of intensities. Our objective is to vary the pose parameters to maximize the similarity score between the DRRs and X-ray projection images. In the DRR generation step, the projection of the X-ray tracking fiducial is merged in the DRR in order to create an image similar to the target image (Fig. 4 p_2). The similarity measure maximization process is described as:

$$\hat{F}_{f,p} = \arg\max_{F_{f,p}} \left[\sum_{i=1}^{N} S\left(I_i, DRR^{+}\left(F_{f,p}, F_{f,I_i}\right)\right) \right] \quad (1)$$

where $S(I_1, I_2)$ denotes a similarity score, which could be implemented as any type of similarity score. As described in 2.5, we implemented gradient information. $DRR^{+}(F_{f,p}, F_{f,Ii})$ denotes the DRR image created from the CT data and the X-ray fiducial transformed into the CT coordinate system using $F_{f,p}$. The DRR projection is in the coordinate system of the *i*th image, which is the same as the C-arm detector position, with respect to the fiducial coordinate system of $F_{f,Ii}$.

2.5 Similarity Measure

Gradient information (defined in [12]) was used as a similarity measure in our algorithm (Fig. 4). First, the gradient vector is computed for each sample point in each image using a Gaussian gradient filter with kernel of scale σ. Section 4 discusses the determination of the proper σ value. The angle α and weighting function *w* between the gradient vectors is defined as:

$$\alpha_{i,j} = \arccos \frac{\nabla I_1(i,j) \cdot \nabla I_2(i,j)}{\left|\nabla I_1(i,j)\right|\left|\nabla I_2(i,j)\right|}, \quad w(i,j) = \frac{\cos\left(2\alpha_{i,j}\right) + 1}{2} \quad (2)$$

where $\nabla I(i,j)$ denotes the gradient vector of the pixel located at (i,j) in image I. In order to take into account strong gradients that appear in both images, the weighting function is multiplied by the minimum of the gradient magnitudes. Summation of the resulting product is defined as a gradient information $GI(I_1,I_2)$.

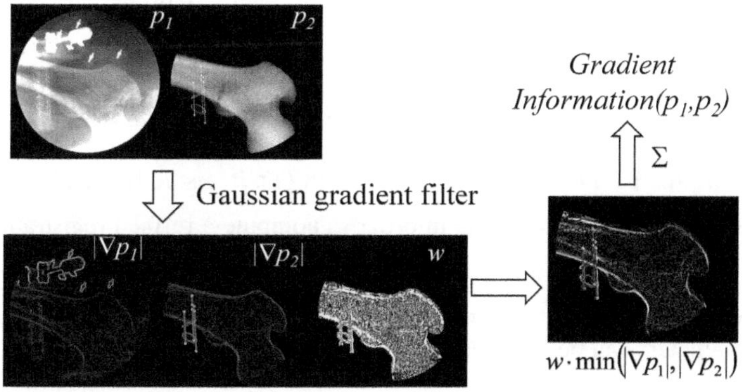

Fig. 4. Computation of the gradient-based similarity measure that is used as a cost function for the optimization

2.6 Iterative Refinement Framework

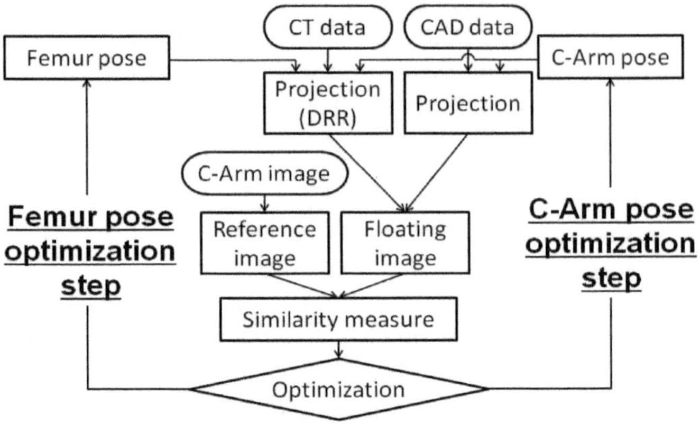

Fig. 5. Workflow of the proposed iterative refinement approach

Both C-arm and patient pose estimation algorithms suffer from the error induced by C-arm intrinsic parameter estimation error, incomplete distortion correction and background clutter in the images. These errors are most severe in the axis perpendicular to the image plane as the similarity score does not change significantly when the object is moved in this direction.
This is shown in Fig. 3(e) where the maximum of the z-displacement similarity score is not as distinct as that of the x- and y- displacement. Because of this limitation, the optimization process is less stable and may converge incorrectly to a local maximum. If the C-arm pose estimation includes error, the patient pose estimation algorithm becomes less accurate and vice versa. In order to overcome this issue, we developed an iterative refinement framework as shown in Fig. 5. In the iterative framework, both the C-arm pose and the patient pose are refined with respect to the fiducial. Note that the intrinsic parameters were assumed constant throughout the procedure. Given the estimated transformation between the fiducial and patient, ($F_{f,p}$) in equation (1), the C-arm pose for each image is refined using both patient anatomy and fiducial information as the following.

$$\hat{F}_{f,I_i} = \arg\max_{F_{f,I_i}} \left[S\left(I_i, DRR^{+}\left(F_{f,p}, F_{f,I_i} \right) \right) \right] \tag{3}$$

where the parameters are the same as in (1). $\hat{F}_{f,p}$ is computed by (1) and inserted into (3) as a dependent variable in order to compute a refined registration F_{f,I_i} denoted as $\hat{F}_{f,I_i}$. The two optimization processes (1) and (3) are iteratively repeated (Fig. 6). The intuition behind this iterative approach is that incorrectly estimated camera parameters can be adjusted by using the patient itself as a fiducial.

2.7 Experiment

We have evaluated our method on images acquired from a cadaveric specimen. The X-ray tracking fiducial was fixed to the femur bone using a bone screw (Fig. 7). CT data was acquired with a spatial resolution of 0.835× 0.835 × 0.3mm. We defined a local coordinate system for the femur bone at the center of the femoral head by fitting

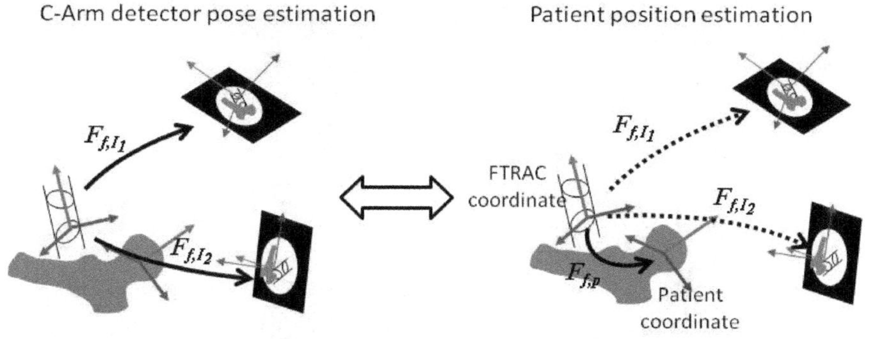

Fig. 6. Proposed iterative refinement process. C-Arm detector pose estimation and patient position estimation are iterated in order to improve the accuracy of registration between fiducial coordinates and CT coordinates ($F_{f,p}$).

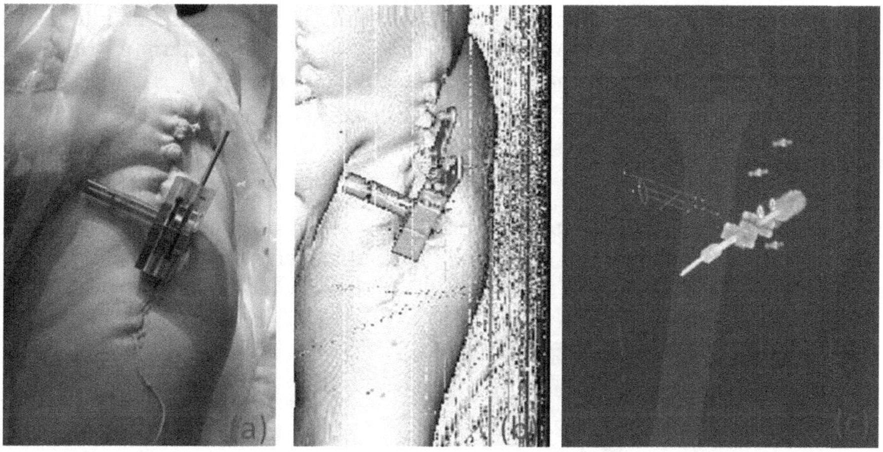

Fig. 7. Cadaver phantom used for the validation experiment. (a) specimen, (b)(c) Volume rendering and Maximum Intensity Projection images of CT data.

a sphere to a manually segmented femur surface model. Two X-ray images were acquired from two different directions (Fig. 8) with an angle of 32 degrees between the normal vectors of the two images. This relatively small angular separation between images is sub-optimal for registration accuracy, but is typical of the practical constraints often encountered intraoperatively. The ground truth registration was obtained by applying rigid-body point-based registration [13] to nine beads on the FTRAC. Fifty registration trials were performed using fifty different initial guesses in order to simulate the operator dependent error during the manual process. The initial guesses were obtained by concatenating randomly selected transformations with uniform and independently distributed translations within ±10 mm and within ±10° of the ground truth registration. The average error between the transformation estimated by the proposed algorithm and the ground truth registration was computed relative to the coordinate system of the image plane associated with the first image. The rotational part of the error was first computed as the arithmetic mean of the rotations represented as unit quarternions, then converted into Euler angle representation to give an intuittive sense on the direction of rotation. While this estimate of the mean rotation using a unit quaternion ignores the fact that rotations belong to a nonlinear manifold, it was shown previously that a linear approximation of a set of unit quaternions that spans a small area on the four-dimensional sphere is adequate [14].

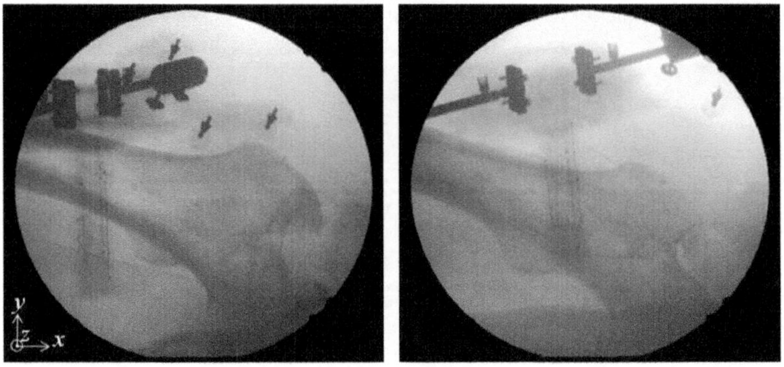

Fig. 8. C-Arm images captured for validation experiment

3 Results

The average errors and their standard deviations along each axis for 50 registration trials are shown in Table 1. We compared the results using a conventional approach to the proposed iterative method after five iterations. The directions of each axis are

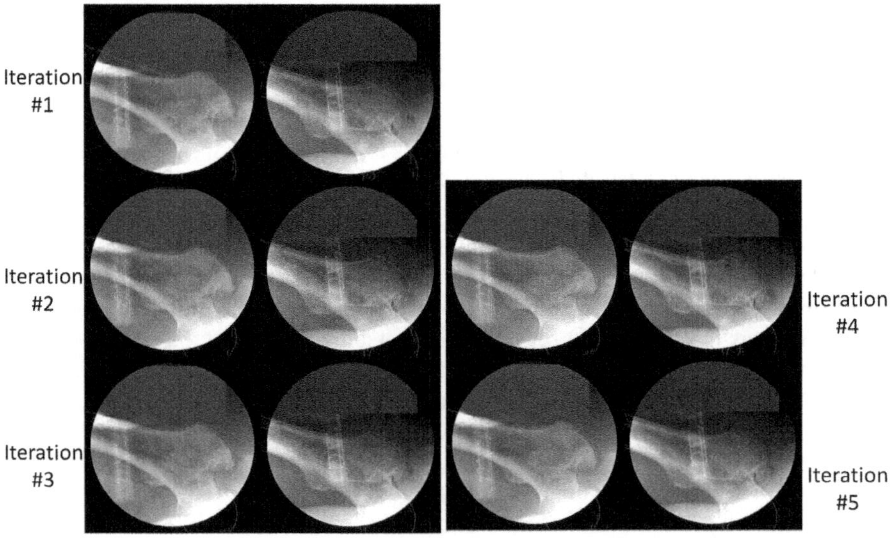

Fig. 9. Exemplar result of the iterative refinement process. Red line indicates the edge of the DRR which was generated based on the femur position estimated at the previous iteration step.

Table 1. Results of the 50 registration trials using randomly selected initial guess within ±10 mm translation and within ±10° rotation

		X	Y	Z	X-Y plane
Translation (mm)	Without iteration	1.18±0.74	1.73±1.04	3.50±2.07	2.09±0.87
	After 5 iterations	0.97±0.62	1.80±1.02	3.06±1.74	2.05±0.89
Rotation (deg)	Without iteration	1.72±2.13	2.19±3.38	1.04±2.06	
	After 5 iterations	1.36±1.82	1.77±2.65	1.00±1.99	

shown in Fig. 8(lower-left). The iterative approach improved errors for all parameters except Ty, and decreased the Euclidean translation error from 4.1 to 3.7mm. The translational error along the Z-axis, which is perpendicular to the image plane, improved 0.43mm after 5 iterations. As noted, the greatest errors are usually observed along the Z-axis. Table 1 shows that the standard deviations of the error were reduced in all axes, implying increased stability in the presence of an error in the initial guess. Fig. 9 shows an example of the iteration process. The outline of the DRR images, shown in red, was created based on the C-arm pose. Each outline was created using its prior iteration step. In the figure, the outlines are overlaid onto the original C-arm images. The results clearly show that the DRR approached to the correct registration, as the iterations continued.

4 Discussion and Conclusions

This paper has presented an iterative refinement framework for intensity-based 2D/3D registration without external tracking of the C-arm pose. Because of the cost, technical difficulties, and insufficient accuracy associated with tracking the pose of the imaging device, intensity-based 2D/3D registration is not commonly used in commercial surgical navigation systems. By using the image information for tracking the device, and by improving the accuracy and robustness of the registration technique, the proposed method increases the potential to use intensity-based 2D/3D registration routinely in image-guided therapy.

The method combines two different optimization problems: C-arm pose estimation and patient pose estimation. The experimental results show the iterative approach improves the registration accuracy along the Z-axis (normal to the image plane), which is important to accurately resolve tool position in three-dimensional space. Note that maximizing the similarity measure along the Z-axis was found to be most problematic because the global maximum is not clearly defined (see Fig. 3(e)). The actual amount of error also depends on experimental conditions including tissue quality and on the relatively narrow difference in the viewing angle of the acquired images. The images acquired in this experiment were not optimized to show the best performance of the proposed algorithm. Additional experiments to expand this initial result are planned. The key contribution of this paper is the demonstration of a novel iterative framework for reducing geometric uncertainties resulting from imperfect C-arm calibration and patient registration errors. Our framework utilizes the patient CT information not only for estimating the patient pose but also for improving the C-arm pose estimation by using the patient as a type of reference *fiducial.*

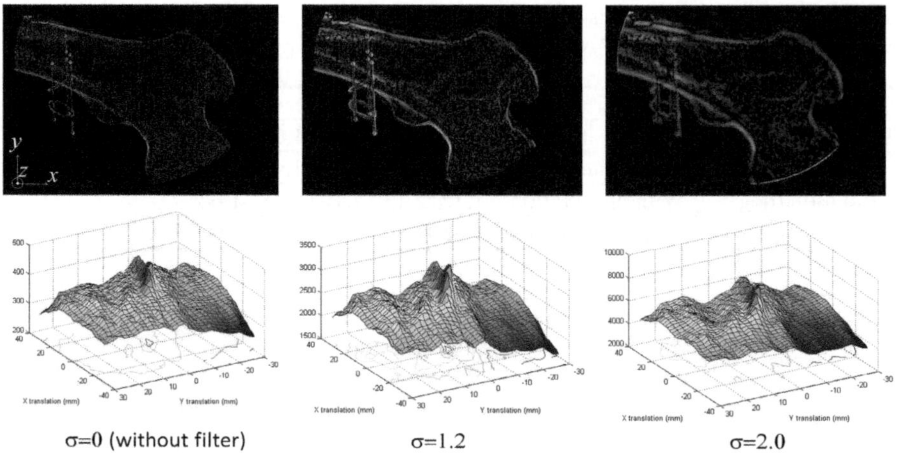

Fig. 10. Comparison of the similarity measure between different sigma values for Gaussian gradient filtering. (upper row: gradient image *w* computed by (2) was used as a cost function. lower row: Plot of the cost function, summation of the intensities of the upper row images.)

The use of a statistics-based similarity measure without considering spatial information results in an ill-defined metric that can contain local maxima in the presence of significant background clutter [12]. Therefore, instead of the mutual information which is widely used in intensity-based 3D/3D and 2D/3D registration, we used the gradient information as the similarity measure.

The scale of the kernel (σ) in the Gaussian filter has a great influence on the similarity measure computation described in 2.4. In order to have information about the preferable σ value in our application, we tested three different σ values. In this analysis, we first generated the DRR using the femur pose derived from the ground truth registration. We then translated the femur position from -30 to +30 mm along the X and Y directions. The gradient information between the DRR and the original C-arm image was computed for each pose and plotted (Fig. 10). For convergence to the global maximum, the cost function should be smooth and have a sharp peak at the center. Based on the results, we used σ=2.0 for our experiments.

The experiment described here used a C-arm device with a conventional X-ray image-intensifier, which is ubiquitous in the current operating theater. Flat-panel detector systems are emerging in operating rooms and have the advantage of less image distortion and high image contrast. Our iterative registration approach is still applicable and expected to be beneficial with these devices by resolving the ambiguity due to the errors related to the DRR generation process, C-arm intrinsic parameter calibration, and optimization of a cost function with inherent local minima. Although the cadaver experiment showed sufficient accuracy and robustness of the proposed method, we note that the movement of the fiducial with respect to the target organ after capturing the C-arm image may introduce additional errors in the actual surgery when compared to the cadaver experiments. Thus the framework would further the potential for performing minimally invasive registration using a small number of X-ray images (e.g. two to five images) during the routine image-guided orthopedic surgery. We believe that the methods reported here can apply to broader applications of image-guided therapy including plastic surgery, neurosurgery, and dentistry and so on.

We have demonstrated a unique approach for intensity-based registration that improves the accuracy compared to conventional 2D/3D registration through iterative optimization. We plan to perform additional cadaveric studies in order to investigate the effects of the number of images and different angular separation. These additional studies will produce a more comprehensive analysis of the robustness of the reported method for intensity-based 2D/3D registration.

Acknowledgements

This research has been financially supported by NIH grant 5R21EB007747-02 and a JSPS Postdoctoral Fellowships for Research Abroad grant.

References

1. Moghari, M.H., Abolmaesumi, P.: Distribution of fiducial registration error in rigid-body point-based registration. IEEE Trans. Med. Imaging 28(11), 1791–1801 (2009)
2. Gueziec, A., Kazanzides, P., Williamson, B., Taylor, R.H.: Anatomy-based registration of CT-scan and intraoperative X-ray images for guiding a surgical robot. IEEE Trans. Med. Imaging 17(5), 715–728 (1998)
3. Chen, X., Gilkeson, R.C., Fei, B.: Automatic 3D-to-2D registration for CT and dual-energy digital radiography for calcification detection. Med. Phys. 34(12), 4934–4943 (2007)
4. Scarvell, J.M., Pickering, M.R., Smith, P.N.: New registration algorithm for determining 3D knee kinematics using CT and single-plane fluoroscopy with improved out-of-plane translation accuracy. J. Orthop. Res. (October 1, 2009)
5. Livyatan, H., Yaniv, Z., Joskowicz, L.: Gradient-based 2-D/3-D rigid registration of fluoroscopic X-ray to CT. IEEE Trans. Med. Imaging 22(11), 1395–1406 (2003)
6. Jain, A., Fichtinger, G.: C-arm tracking and reconstruction without an external tracker. In: Larsen, R., Nielsen, M., Sporring, J. (eds.) MICCAI 2006, Part I. LNCS, vol. 4190, pp. 494–502. Springer, Heidelberg (2006)
7. Sadowsky, O.: Image registration and hybrid volume reconstruction of bone anatomy using a statistical shape atlas [dissertation]. The Johns Hopkins University (2008)
8. Wells III, W.M., Viola, P., Atsumi, H., Nakajima, S., Kikinis, R.: Multi-modal volume registration by maximization of mutual information. Med. Image Anal. 1(1), 35–51 (1996)
9. Nelder, J.A., Mead, R.: A simplex method for function minimization. The Computer Journal 7(4), 308–313 (1965)
10. Sadowsky, O., Cohen, J.D., Taylor, R.H.: Projected tetrahedra revisited: A barycentric formulation applied to digital radiograph reconstruction using higher-order attenuation functions. IEEE Trans. Vis. Comput. Graph. 12(4), 461–473 (2006)
11. Sadowsky, O., Chintalapani, G., Taylor, R.H.: Deformable 2D-3D registration of the pelvis with a limited field of view, using shape statistics. In: Ayache, N., Ourselin, S., Maeder, A. (eds.) MICCAI 2007, Part II. LNCS, vol. 4792, pp. 519–526. Springer, Heidelberg (2007)
12. Pluim, J.P., Maintz, J.B., Viergever, M.A.: Image registration by maximization of combined mutual information and gradient information. IEEE Trans. Med. Imaging 19(8), 809–814 (2000)
13. Horn, B.K.P.: Closed-form solution of absolute orientation using unit quaternions. J. Opt. Soc. Am. A. 4(4), 629–642 (1987)
14. Gramkow, C.: On averaging rotations. International Journal of Computer Vision 42(1), 7–16 (2001)

Automatic Phases Recognition in Pituitary Surgeries by Microscope Images Classification

Florent Lalys[1,2,3], Laurent Riffaud[4], Xavier Morandi[1,2,3,4], and Pierre Jannin[1,2,3]

[1] INSERM, U746, Faculty of Medicine CS 34317, F-35043 Rennes, France
[2] INRIA, VisAGeS Unit/Project, F-35042 Rennes, France
[3] University of Rennes I, CNRS, UMR 6074, IRISA, F-35042 Rennes, France
[4] Department of Neurosurgery, Pontchaillou University Hospital, F-35043 Rennes, France

Abstract. The segmentation of the surgical workflow might be helpful for providing context-sensitive user interfaces, or generating automatic report. Our approach focused on the automatic recognition of surgical phases by microscope image classification. Our workflow, including images features extraction, image database labelisation, Principal Component Analysis (PCA) transformation and 10-fold cross-validation studies was performed on a specific type of neurosurgical intervention, the pituitary surgery. Six phases were defined by an expert for this type of intervention. We thus assessed machine learning algorithms along with the data dimension reduction. We finally kept 40 features from the PCA and found a best correct classification rate of the surgical phases of 82% with the multiclass Support Vector Machine.

Keywords: Surgical phase, digital microscope, neurosurgery, feature extraction.

1 Introduction

With the increased number of technological tools incorporate in the OR, the need for new computer-assisted systems has emerged [1]. Moreover, surgeons have to deal with adverse events during operations, coming from the patient itself but also from the operation management. The idea is to limit and be aware of these difficulties, and to better handle risks situations as well as to relieve surgeon's responsibilities. The purpose of recent works is not to substitute medical staff in the OR but to increase medical safety and support decision making. One solution is to assist surgeries through the understanding of operating room activities, which could be introduce in current surgical management systems. It could be useful for OR management optimization, providing context-sensitive user interfaces or generating automatic reports. Thus, surgical workflow recovery as well as surgical process modelling has gained much interest during the past decade.

Neumuth et al. [2] defined Surgical Process (SP) as a set of one or more linked procedures or activities that realize a surgical objective. Surgical Process Models (SPMs) are simply defined by models of surgical interventions. A detailed SPM may help in understanding the procedure by giving specific information of the intervention course. Applications of SPMs are the evaluation of surgeons (training and learning),

N. Navab and P. Jannin (Eds.): IPCAI 2010, LNCS 6135, pp. 34–44, 2010.

system comparison, procedures documentations and surgical feedbacks. As Jannin et al. [3] mentioned, the modeling must address behavioral, anatomical, pathological aspects and surgical instruments. They also defined surgical workflow, which relates to the performance of a SP with support of a workflow management system.

Teams have understood the necessity of real-time information extraction for the creation of complex surgeries models. The difference in the level of granularity for the extraction process allows deriving complementary numeric models for workflow recovery. Thus, data extraction is performed either from a human sight or from sensor devices. In this context, different methods have been recently used for data acquisition: patient specific procedures description [2-4], interview of the surgeons [5], sensor-based methods [6-16], using fixed protocols created by expert surgeons [17], or combination between them [18].

Within sensor-based approaches, Padoy et al. [6] segmented the surgical workflow into phases based on temporal synchronization of multidimensional state vectors, using Dynamic Time Warping (DTW) and Hidden Markov Models (HMMs). These algorithms permit to recognize patterns and extract knowledge. Signals recorded were binary vectors indicating the instrument presence.

At a lower level, the force/torque signals of the laparoscopic instruments recorded during a suturing task can be learned with HMMs [7]. Close to this work, Lin et al. [8] also trained HMMs to automatically segment motion data during a suturing task perform with the Da Vinci robot. With the same robot, Voros and Hager [9] used kinematic and visual features to classify tool/tissue interactions in real-time. Their work was a first step towards intelligent intraoperative surgical system. Recent work of Ahmadi et al. [10] used accelerometers placed on the operator along with motif discovery technique to identify alphabets of surgical activity. Models of gestures relied on tools only and motions may not be well segmented with rare movements.

Using others data extraction techniques, Bhatia et al. [11] analyzed OR global view videos for better management, whereas Xiao et al. [12] implemented a system that record patient vital signs in order to situate the intervention process. James et al. [13] installed an eye-gaze tracking system on the surgeon combined with visual features to detect one important phase. Nara et al. [14] introduced an ultrasonic location aware system that continuously tracks 3-D positions of the surgical staff. Results on identifying key surgical events were presented. For the construction of a context-aware system, Speidel et al. [15] used laparoscopic videos to create a situation recognition process. In their work, they focused on risk situation for surgical assistance. Finally, Sanchez-Gonzales et al. [16] extracted useful information from videos such as 3D map to help surgeons performing operating techniques.

Our project is based on the extraction of information from digital microscope videos. It permits not only to avoid the installation of supplementary materials in the OR, but also to have a source of information that has not to be controlled by human. Computer vision techniques bring processing algorithms to transform images and videos into a new representation that can be further used for machine learning techniques (supervised or non-supervised classification). We decided in a first phase to use image from videos (called frames) in a static way without taking into account the motion. The problem is thus reduced to an image classification problem. Even with this restriction, technical possibilities remain very large. We focused on the automatic recognition of surgical phases and validated our methodology with a specific type of neurosurgical interventions.

2 Materials and Methods

We evaluated our algorithm on pituitary adenoma surgeries [19]. It's tumors that occur in the pituitary gland and which are representing around ten percent of all intracranial tumour removals. Neurosurgeons mostly use a direct transnasal approach, where an incision is made in the back wall of the nose. Rarely, a craniotomy is required. In this work all surgeries were performed according to the first approach.

2.1 Data

Our project is currently composed of 16 entire pituitary surgeries (mean time of surgeries: 50min), all performed in Rennes by three expert surgeons. Videos were recorded using the surgical microscope OPMI Pentero (Carl Zeiss). The initial video resolution was 768 x 576 pixels at 33 frames per second. Recordings were obtained from nasal incision until compress installation (corresponding to the microscope use). From these videos, we randomly extracted 400 images which were supposed to correctly represent the six phases of an usual pituitary surgery. These phases, which were validated by an expert surgeon, are: nasal incision, nose retractors installation, access to the tumor along with tumor removal, column of nose replacement, suturing and nose compress installation (Fig. 1). Each image of the database was manually labeled with its corresponding surgical phase.

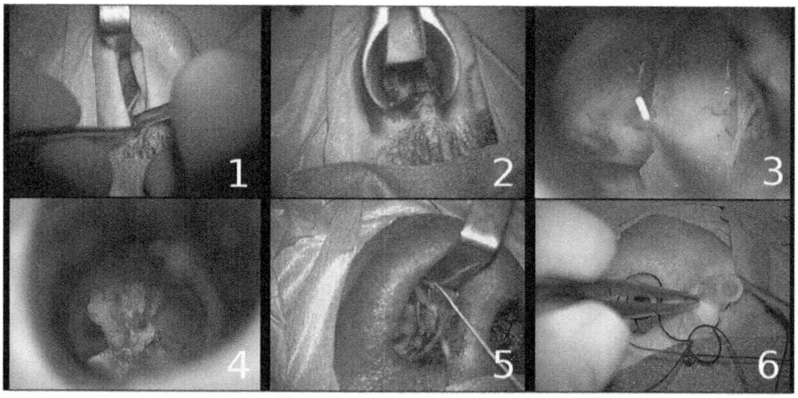

Fig. 1. Example of typical digital microscope images for the six phases: 1) nasal incision, 2) nose retractors installation, 3) access to the tumor along with tumor removal, 4) column of nose replacement, 5) suturing, 6) nose compress installation

2.2 Feature Extraction

We defined for each image a feature vector that represented a signature. Images signatures are composed of three main information that usually describe an image: the color, the texture and the form.

The color has been extracted with two complementary spaces [20]: RGB space (3 x 16 bins) along with Hue (30 bins) and Saturation (32 bins) from HSV space.

The texture has been extracted with the co-occurrence matrix along with Haralick descriptors [21]. The co-occurrence matrix is used to describe the patterns of neighboring pixels in an image I at a given distance. Mathematically, the matrix C is defined over an image n x m and an offset:

$$C_{\Delta x,\Delta y}(i,j) = \sum_{p=1}^{n} \sum_{q=1}^{m} \begin{cases} 1, if\ I(p,q) = i\ and\ I(p+\Delta x, q+\Delta y) = j \\ 0, otherwise \end{cases} \quad (1)$$

Four such matrices are needed for different orientations (horizontal, vertical and two diagonal directions). A kind of invariance was achieved by taking into account the four matrices. Haralick descriptors were then used by computing the contrast, the correlation, the angular second moment, the variance of the sum of squares, the moment of the inverse difference, the sum average, the sum variance, the sum entropy, the difference of variance, the difference of entropy, and the maximum correlation coefficient of the co-occurrence matrix.

The form was represented with spatial moments [22], which describe the spatial distribution of values. For a grayscale image the moments $M_{i,j}$ are calculated by:

$$M_{i,j} = \sum_{p=1}^{n} \sum_{q=1}^{m} p^i q^j I(p,q) \quad (2)$$

The 10 first moments were included in the signatures.

We then computed the Discrete Cosine Transform (DCT) [23] coefficients B_{pq} that reflect the compact energy of different frequencies. DCT is calculated by:

$$B_{pq} = \alpha_p \alpha_q \sum_{m=0}^{M-1} \sum_{n=0}^{N-1} A_{mn} \cos\frac{\pi(2m+1)p}{2M} \cos\frac{\pi(2n+1)q}{2N}, \quad \begin{matrix} 0 \le p \le M-1 \\ 0 \le q \le N-1 \end{matrix} \quad (3)$$

with $\alpha_p = \begin{cases} 1/\sqrt{M}, & p=0 \\ \sqrt{2/M} & 1 \le p \le M-1 \end{cases}$ and $\alpha_q = \begin{cases} 1/\sqrt{N}, & p=0 \\ \sqrt{2/N} & 1 \le p \le M-1 \end{cases}$

The B_{pq} coefficients of upper left corner represent visual information of lower intensities, whereas the higher frequency information is gathered at right lower corner of the block. Most of the energy is located in the low frequency area, that's why we took the 25 features of the upper left corner.

Each signature was finally composed of 185 complementary features.

2.3 Data Reduction

Original frames were first downsampled by a factor of 8 with a 5-by-5 Gaussian kernel (internal studies have shown that until this downsampling rate, it had no impact on the classification process). After features extraction, we performed a statistical normalization. On each feature value we subtracted the mean and divided by the variance. After normalization, data closely followed a normal distribution (mean=0 and standard deviation=1) and were more easily used for data variations comparisons.

In order to decrease the data dimension, and knowing that too many features can decrease the correct classification rate, we also performed a Principal Component Analysis (PCA) [24]. PCA is a statistical method used to decrease the data dimension while retaining as much as possible of the variation present in the data set to process the data faster and effective. Fig. 3 shows the extracted cumulative variance.

2.4 Cross-Validation

With the image data-base we are now able to train models by using machine learning techniques. We performed a study to find the most appropriate algorithm. We tested multiclass Support Vector Machine (SVM), K-Nearest Neighbors (KNN), Neural Networks (NN), decision tree and Linear Discriminant Analysis (LDA).

The goal of SVM is to find the optimal hyperplane that separates the data into two categories. The multiclass SVMs [25] extends it into a K-class problem, by constructing K binary linear SVMs. The KNN algorithm (used with the Euclidean distance) is the simplest method for classification. Each point in the space is assigned to the class C if it is the most frequent class label among the k-nearest training samples. NN [26] are non-linear statistical methods based on biological neural networks. They are often used to model complex relationships between inputs and outputs. We used it in a supervised way with a back-propagation neural network. The decision tree is a quick classification algorithm where each internal node tests an attribute. It is specially used when data are noised and classes are discrete. Finally, the LDA is based on a Fisher analysis. It is a linear combination of features that best separate two or more classes.

Algorithms were evaluated with a random 10-fold cross-validation study [27]. The data-set was divided into 10 random subsets. Nine were used for training while the prediction is made on the 10th subset. This procedure was repeated 10 times and correct classification rates were averaged. In addition, the cross-validation study allows computing the sensitivity and the specificity. The specificity is defined by: $Spe = \frac{TN}{TN + FP}$ and the sensitivity is defined by $Sen = \frac{TP}{TP + FN}$, where FP is False Positive, TP is True Positive, FN is false Negative and TN is True Negative.

The cross-validation was computed for each algorithm but also for each number of principal components used in order to keep the best classification algorithm and to decide how many principal components we had to take.

3 Results

Fig. 2 shows the cross-validation study. Multiclass SVMs and LDA give best results. For both algorithms the correct classification rate increase until 40 principal components and then LDA decreases while SVMs stays at a higher recognition rate.

From 30 principal components, correct classification rates of the NN and KNN are almost unchanging, but their best scores are significantly lower than for SVM and LDA. Finally, the decision tree gives the worst results compare to other classifiers.

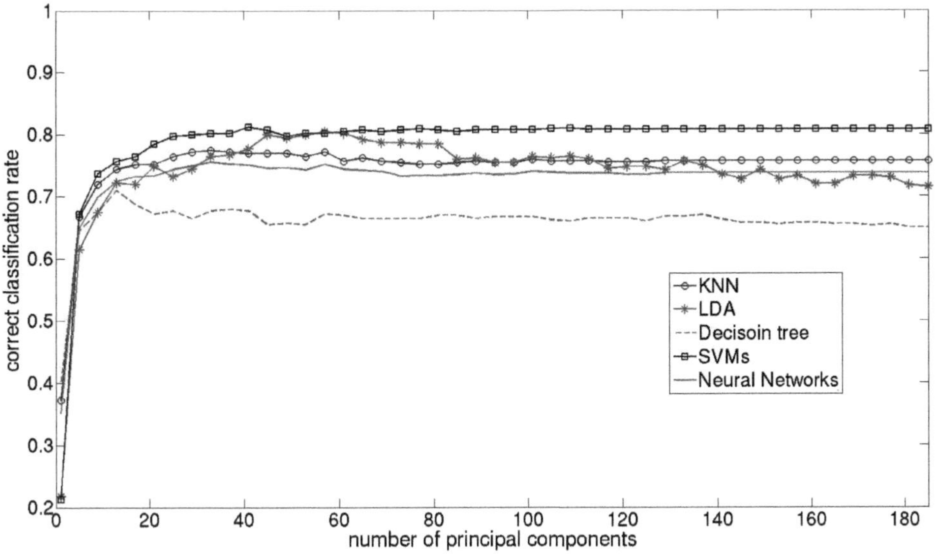

Fig. 2. Correct classification rate of the surgical phases with five different algorithms, according to the number of principal components

We decided to keep 40 principal components, which represent 91.5% of the energy of all the data set (Fig. 3). With these features we obtained accurate statistical results:

Table 1. Correct classification rate (accuracy), sensitivity and specificity of classification algorithms. Image signatures are composed of the 40 first principal components

Algorithms	Accuracy	Sensitivity	Specificity
Multiclass SVMs	82.2%	78.7%	98.1%
KNN	74.7%	66.0%	95.4%
Neural Network	71.3%	65.1%	92.8%
Decision tree	66.2%	52.3%	94.0%
LDA	81.5%	77.0%	97.6%

We can see from Tab. 1 that specificity is always upper than sensitivity for all algorithms. Not surprisingly, multiclass SVMs obtained best sensitivity (78.7%) and specificity (98.1%) whereas the decision tree shows its limits (specificity: 52.3%).

The computation time of the classification process of one image (feature extraction + data transformation + classification) was less than 0.5s. We didn't take into account the computation time of the learning database, considering that it was done off-line.

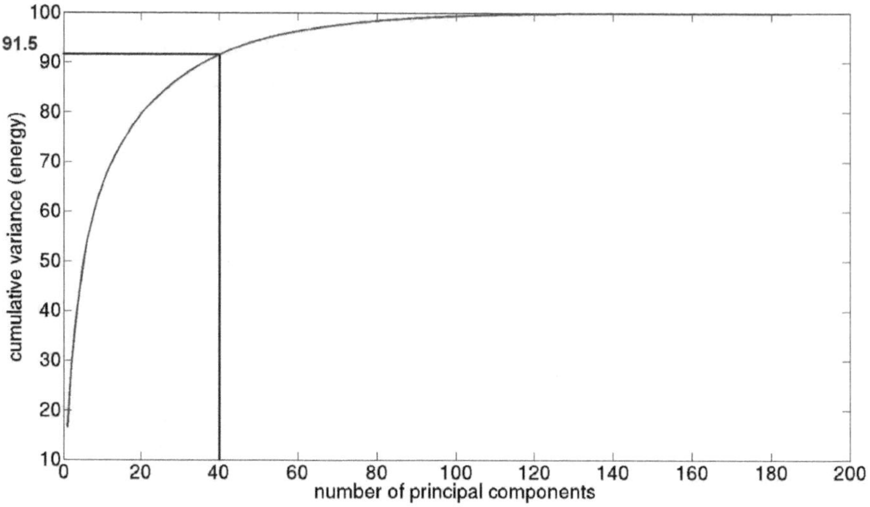

Fig. 3. Cumulative variance of the Principal Component Analysis

4 Discussion

Our global workflow, including image database labelisation, features extraction, PCA, and cross-validation studies make possible the extraction of discriminant image features for each phase. After experiments, we finally kept 40 principal components for a best correct classification rate of the surgical phases of 82% with SVMs.

4.1 Images Database

The performance is strongly linked to the diversity and the power of discrimination of the database. We can easily imagine that accuracy may sorely decrease if images are not efficiently representing all phases or all scene possibilities within phases.

There are other limitations to this type of study. The image database may not be adaptable to other neurosurgery departments, due to the difference of materials and equipment in each department. For instance, the color of surgical tissue in Rennes may be different elsewhere and the corresponding features would completely affect the training process. The solution would be to train specific image databases for each department which would be well adapted to the surgical environment. The idea would also be to have several databases for each type of procedure with specific phases. For other departments and/or surgeries, discriminant images features may differ, which would require adapting the feature extraction process by launching identical studies. Other factors of variability within the data-set can affect the recognition. For instance, differences can be found in the way that surgeons are working or in patient specific surgery. Ideally, one database should be created for each department, associated with each type of surgery and each surgeon.

4.2 Explanation of Classification Errors

We decided to fuse the initial possible phases "access to the tumor" and "tumor removal" because for this type of surgical procedure it's currently hard to distinguish them only with image features. The transition between both is not clearly defined due to similar tools and same microscope zooms used while performing these tasks.

The correct classification rate includes the results of the cross-validation study for the six phases. From these results, we noticed frequent confusions mainly between phase n°3 and n°4, and also between n°1 and n°5. These errors are explained by the very close image features of these phases. Same microscope zooms, along with similar colors and same surgical instruments make the recognition task very difficult. One solution of this issue would be to integrate one other signal: the surgery time. This information would for instance permit to correctly recognize an image originally identified as part of phase n°5 or part of phase n°1. On the other hand it would still be hard to separate consecutive phases.

4.3 Classification Algorithms

In this study (Fig. 2), multiclass SVMs and LDA gave the best correct classification rates. SVMs have been used in a linear way and are known to have good generalization properties that permit to outperform classical algorithms. LDA, used as a classifier, is like many others optimal when the features have a normal distribution (true in our case after normalization). On the opposite, the decision tree, NN and KNN gave worse results. Decision trees are often instable, especially with small changes in the training samples. Our data-set was probably too variable (in color, texture...) and not enough discriminant to train accurate models with decision trees. While KNN is generally outperformed by other classifiers, it may be well interesting because of its simplicity and flexibility. Nevertheless, our results showed that it was not suitable for our data-set. Concerning NNs, it was quite surprising regarding their capabilities to improve their performances when the amount of data increases. Non-linear algorithms are generally more suitable for complex systems, which is not the case here. On the opposite, linear ones are more straightforward and easy to use, that's why it seems that they are more adaptable for our system.

The correct classification rates for SVMs, KNN and NN are almost constant until 185 features, whereas accuracy of the decision tree and especially LDA decrease. This is due to the high dimension of inputs which usually decreases results of classifiers. It's also the reason why we only kept 40 features for images signatures. If PCA would not have been performed, we would only have obtained an accuracy of 78% (with KNN), which demonstrated the usefulness of this step in our workflow.

According to Tab. 1, most of the difference between classifiers is made by sensitivities, which are lower than specificities. A high specificity is due to the absence of FP (image belonging to phase x not identified as part of phase x), whereas a low sensitivity is due to a high FN rate (image not belonging to phase x identified as part of phase x). Thus the challenge in the future would be to increase FN rates.

In presence of unexpected events, such as bleeding or brutal microscope move, the specificity sensibly decreases and thus affects global accuracy. Such situations, as being unpredictable, are a high limitation to the classification from static images only.

One solution of this issue, not implemented yet, would be to detect such images (containing features that are very different from the others, and therefore easily detectable) and to take into account the recognized phase of the precedent image.

4.4 Applications

The idea is to assist surgeries through the understanding of operating room activities. This work could be integrated in an intelligent architecture that extracts microscope images and transform it in a decision making process. The purpose would be to bring a plus-value to the OR management (as in [10]) and to the surgery (as in [14]). For now, even with a low on-line computation time (< 0.5s), the best obtained correct classification rate is certainly not accurate enough to be included in such systems. For intra-operative clinical applications, accuracy must definitively be higher than our results before establishing on-line surgical phases detection.

However, with the present methodology, the system could be introduced in the surgical routine as an help for post-operative indexation of videos. Surgical videos are very useful for learning and teaching purposes, but surgeons often don't use them because of the huge amount of surgical videos, the lack of data organization and storage. The created video data-base would contain relevant surgical phases of each procedure for easy browsing. Moreover, we could imagine the creation of post-operative reports, automatically pre-filled by recognized events that will have to be further completed by surgeons themselves. For such clinical applications, even with few errors, the automatic indexation would be relevant, as there is no need of perfect detection and it has no impact on the surgery itself.

We deliberately remain at a high level of granularity with the recognition of global phases. The recognition of lower level information, such as surgical gestures, is very difficult (almost impossible) only with images. Other computer vision techniques (such as tracking) or specific video processing methods (such as spatio-temporal features extraction) will have to be inserted and mixed for dynamic information extraction.

5 Conclusion

With this large labeled images database, we are now able to recognize surgical phases of every unknown image, by computing his signature and then simulating with machine learning techniques. We have validated our methodology with a specific type of neurosurgery, but it can easily be extended to other type of interventions. With this recognition process, it's a first step toward the construction of a context-aware surgical system. Currently this work could be used for post-operative video indexation as a help for surgeons. Image features will have to be mixed with other type of information to generate a more robust and accurate recognition system. Other methods usually used by the computer vision community (segmentation, tracking) could also be integrated in future works in order to bring complementary features.

Acknowledgments. The authors would like to acknowledge the financial support of Carl Zeiss Surgical GmbH.

References

1. Cleary, K., Chung, H.Y., Mun, S.K.: OR 2020: The operating room of the future. Laparoendoscopic and Advanced Surgical Techniques 15(5), 495–500 (2005)
2. Neumuth, T., Jannin, P., Strauss, G., Meixensberger, J., Burgert, O.: Validation of Knowledge Acquisition for Surgical Process Models. J. Am. Med. Inform. Assoc. 16(1), 72–82 (2008)
3. Jannin, P., Morandi, X.: Surgical models for computer-assisted neurosurgery. Neuroimage 37(3), 783–791 (2007)
4. Jannin, P., Raimbault, M., Morandi, X., Riffaud, L., Gibaud, B.: Model of surgical procedures for multimodal image-guided neurosurgery. Computer Aided surgery 8(2), 98–106 (2003)
5. Morineau, T., Morandi, X., Le Moëllic, N., Diabira, S., Haegelen, C., Hénaux, P.L., Jannin, P.: Decision making during preoperative surgical planning. Human factors 51(1), 66–77 (2009)
6. Padoy, N., Blum, T., Essa, I., Feussner, H., Berger, M., Navab, N.: A boosted segmentation method for Surgical Workflow Analysis. In: Ayache, N., Ourselin, S., Maeder, A. (eds.) MICCAI 2007, Part I. LNCS, vol. 4791, pp. 102–109. Springer, Heidelberg (2007)
7. Rosen, J., Solazzo, M., Hannaford, B., Sinanan, M.: Task decomposition of laparoscopic surgery for objective evaluation of surgical residents' learning curve using hidden markov model. Comput. Aided Surg. 7(1), 49–61 (2002)
8. Lin, H.C., Shafran, I., Yuh, D., Hager, G.D.: Towards automatic skill evaluation: Detection and segmentation of robot-assisted surgical motions. Computer Aided Surgery 11(5), 220–230 (2006)
9. Voros, S., Hager, G.D.: Towards "real-time" tool-tissue interaction detection in robotically asisted laparoscopy. Biomed. Robotics and Biomechatronics, 562–567 (2008)
10. Ahmadi, S.A., Padoy, N., Rybachuk, K., Feussner, H., Heinin, S.M., Navab, N.: Motif discovery in OR sensor data with application to surgical workflow analysis and activity detection. In: M2CAI workshop, MICCAI, London (2009)
11. Bhatia, B., Oates, T., Xiao, Y., Hu, P.: Real-time identification of operating room state from video. In: AAAI, pp. 1761–1766 (2007)
12. Xiao, Y., Hu, P., Hu, H., Ho, D., Dexter, F., Mackenzie, C.F., Seagull, F.J.: An algorithm for processing vital sign monitoring data to remotely identify operating room occupancy in real-time. Anesth. Analg. 101(3), 823–832 (2005)
13. James, A., Vieira, D., Lo, B.P.L., Darzi, A., Yang, G.-Z.: Eye-gaze driven surgical workflow segmentation. In: Ayache, N., Ourselin, S., Maeder, A. (eds.) MICCAI 2007, Part II. LNCS, vol. 4792, pp. 110–117. Springer, Heidelberg (2007)
14. Nara, A., Izumi, K., Iseki, H., Suzuki, T., Nambu, K., Sakurai, Y.: Surgical workflow analysis based on staff's trajectory patterns. In: M2CAI workshop, MICCAI, London (2009)
15. Speidel, S., Sudra, G., Senemaud, J., Drentschew, M., Müller-stich, B.P., Gun, C., Dillmann, R.: Situation modelling and situation recognition for a context-aware augmented reality system. Progression in biomedical optics and imaging 9(1), 35 (2008)
16. Sanchez-Gonzales, P., Gaya, F., Cano, A.M., Gomez, E.J.: Segmentation and 3D reconstruction approaches for the design of laparoscopic augmented reality. In: Bello, F., Edwards, E. (eds.) ISBMS 2008. LNCS, vol. 5104, pp. 127–134. Springer, Heidelberg (2008)
17. MacKenzie, C.L., Ibbotson, A.J., Cao, C.G.L., Lomax, A.: Hierarchical decomposition of laparoscopic surgery: a human factors approach to investigating the operating room environment. Min. Invas. Ther. All. Technol. 10(3), 121–128 (2001)
18. Neumuth, T., Czygan, M., Goldstein, D., Strauss, G., Meixensberger, J., Burgert, O.: Computer assisted acquisition of surgical process models with a sensors-driven ontology. In: M2CAI workshop, MICCAI, London (2009)

19. Ezzat, S., Asa, S.L., Couldwell, W.T., Barr, C.E., Dodge, W.E., Vance, M.L., McCutcheon, I.E.: The prevalence of pituitary adenomas: a systematic review. Cancer 101(3), 613–622 (2004)
20. Smeulders, A.W., Worrin, M., Santini, S., Gupta, A., Jain, R.: Content-based image retrieval at the end of the early years. IEEE Trans. on pattern analysis and machine learning intelligence 22(12), 1349–1380 (2000)
21. Haralick, R.M., Shanmugam, K., Dinstein, I.: Textural features for image classification. IEEE Trans. on Systems, Man, and Cybernetics 3(6), 610–621 (1973)
22. Hu, M.K.: Visual pattern recognition by moment invariants. IRE Trans. on Information Theory 8(2), 179–187 (1962)
23. Ahmed, N., Natarajan, T., Rao, K.R.: Discrete Cosine Transform. IEEE Trans. Comp., 90–93 (1974)
24. Jolliffe, T.: Principal component analysis. Springer, New York (1986)
25. Crammer, K., Singer, Y.: On the Algorithmic Implementation of Multi-class SVMs. JMLR (2001)
26. Haykin, S.: Neural Networks and Learning Machines, 3rd edn., Hardcover (2008)
27. Duda, R., Hart, P., Stork, D.: Pattern Classification. Wiley-Interscience, New York (2001)

C-arm Tracking by Intensity-Based Registration of a Fiducial in Prostate Brachytherapy

Pascal Fallavollita[1], Clif Burdette[2], Danny Y. Song[3], Purang Abolmaesumi[4], and Gabor Fichtinger[1]

[1] Queen's University, Canada
[2] Acoustic MedSystems Inc, Illinois
[3] Johns Hopkins Hospital, Baltimore
[4] University of British Columbia, Canada

Abstract. Motivation: In prostate brachytherapy, intra-operative dosimetry optimization can be achieved through reconstruction of the implanted seeds from multiple C-arm fluoroscopy images. This process requires tracking of the C-arm poses. Methodology: We compute the pose of the C-arm relative to a stationary radiographic fiducial of known geometry. The fiducial was precisely fabricated. We register the 2D fluoroscopy image of the fiducial to a projected digitally reconstructed radiograph of the fiducial. The novelty of this approach is using image intensity alone without prior segmentation of the fluoroscopy image. Experiments and Results: Ground truth pose was established for each C-arm image using a published and clinically tested segmentation-based method. Using 111 clinical C-arm images and ±10° and ±10 mm random perturbation around the ground-truth pose, the average rotation and translation errors were 0.62° (std=0.31°) and 0.73 mm (std= 0.55mm), respectively. Conclusion: Fully automated segmentation-free C-arm pose estimation was found to be clinically adequate on human patient data.

1 Introduction

Prostate cancer is the second most common cancer in men, diagnosed in 250,000 new patients each year in North America [1]. Brachytherapy is a definitive treatment of early stage prostate cancer, chosen by over 50,000 men each year with excellent long-term disease-free survival [2]. The procedure entails permanent implantation of small radioactive isotope capsules (a.k.a. seeds) into the prostate to kill the cancer with radiation. Success hinges on precise placement of the implants to provide the needed dose distribution. Unfortunately, primarily due to tissue motion, organ deformation, and needle deflection, implants never turn out to be as planned. Dynamic dosimetry optimization during the procedure would allow the physician to account for deviations from the plan and thus tailor the dose to cancer without harming surrounding healthy tissues. This requires localization of the prostate and the implanted seeds; a much coveted function that is not available today [3]. Prostate brachytherapy is performed with transrectal ultrasound guidance that provides adequate real-time visualization of the prostate but not of the implanted seeds. At the same time, C-arm fluoroscopy is

N. Navab and P. Jannin (Eds.): IPCAI 2010, LNCS 6135, pp. 45–55, 2010.

widely used for visual assessment and 3D reconstruction of the implanted seeds (Figure 1, left), but it cannot show the prostate and other relevant structures. Fusion of these two complementary modalities would enable dynamic dosimetry. A variety of fluoroscopic implant reconstruction and fusion techniques have been investigated [4-7]. These methods share one common requirement: the relative poses of the fluoroscopy images must be known prior to reconstruction.

Pose recovery on C-arm machines is a major technical problem that presently does not have a clinically practical solution in many areas of application. The relative poses of fluoroscopy images are determined in one of following three ways: (i) electronic joint encoders, (ii) optical or electromagnetic tracker, and (iii) radiographic fiducials. Fully encoded C-arms are very expensive and thus virtually non-existent in brachytherapy. External trackers are also impractical for various reasons and also add costs. Optical tracking[1,2] requires line of sight which imparts alterations in clinical setup and workflow. Electromagnetic tracking[3] overcomes these issues, but it is susceptible to field distortion from metal objects, such as the C-arm itself, and thus compromise on accuracy. Several researchers have explored fiducial-based radiographic tracking [8-11]. In an effort of making fiducials better integrated in the clinical setup, compact fiducials have been explored. Unfortunately, decreasing the size of the fiducial fixture also decreases tracking accuracy. In fiducial structures made up of beads, the typical number of beads was between 6 and 28. With these structures, researchers achieved 1-3 mm translation accuracy and 1°–2° orientation accuracy in tracking the C-arm [9-11]. Accuracy was primarily governed by bead configuration [9] and implementation [10] choices. In all, the best accuracy that bead-shape fiducials can achieve is about 1 mm error in translation and 1° error in rotation.

For prostate brachytherapy Jain *et al.* developed a fluoroscope tracking (FTRAC) fiducial [12] and validated the device clinically [7]. In addition to spherical beads, they used straight lines and ellipses that are invariant to projection, in that they project as straight lines and ellipses (Figure 1, center). Such parametric curves segment accurately and constrain the optimization during pose recovery, allowing for a mean accuracy of 0.56 ± 0.33mm in translations and 0.33°± 0.21° in rotations [12]. The FTRAC design has small dimensions (3x3x5cm), no special proximity requirements to the anatomy, and is relatively inexpensive. They mounted the FTRAC fiducial over the seed insertion needle template using a mechanical connector (Figure 1, right) [7]. After semi-automatic segmentation of the FTRAC fiducial in all C-arm images, the implanted seeds were reconstructed in 3D, registered with transrectal ultrasound space and sent back to the treatment planning system for dosimetric evaluation. In this process, the single point of failure is segmentation of the FTRAC. Sequential semi-automated segmentation of different features of the FTRAC was found to be fragile in actual field practice [7].

In essence, Jain *et al.* computed a registration between the 3D geometrical model of their tracking fiducial and its 2D projection pre-segmented in the C-arm image: i.e. they performed a 2D/3D registration. Prior work in 2D/3D registration algorithms can be divided into two major categories: feature-based and intensity-based methods. The

---

[1] VectorVision® Navigation System, "Brainlab, Inc., Heimstetten, Germany.
[2] StealtStation®, Medtronic Surgical Navigation Technologies, Louisville, CO, USA.
[3] OEC 9800 FluoroTrak™, GE Healthcare, Waukesha, WI, USA.

former, such as [15-17], use distance between corresponding point pairs or surfaces as a measure to be optimized. Establishing point correspondences and minimizing the distance between them is alternated and repeated iteratively until convergence. Consequently, prior segmentation of the image data is required. Many researchers in computer vision have tried to recover pose based on point features. For calibrated cameras the so called five-point algorithm has been used extensively [18]. This method can cope with planar scenes, but in case of more than five points it computes multiple solutions. Minimal solvers are of importance for algorithms like random consensus sampling [19] to establish unknown correspondences between the features across images. Intensity-based methods compare the 2D image with a digitally reconstructed radiograph (DRR) created from the 3D volume. One can compare the imprints of anatomical structures obtained from either gradient information or voxel intensity [20-22].

We propose computing the relative pose of C-arm images by the registration of fluoroscopy image to a radiographic fiducial, without segmentation, with an accuracy that is sufficient for subsequent reconstruction of brachytherapy seeds. While all computational components used have been previously described by others, this should not belie the investment of creative effort required for devising a clinically practical approach and testable embodiment. We present methodology, implementation, and performance analysis on clinical patient data.

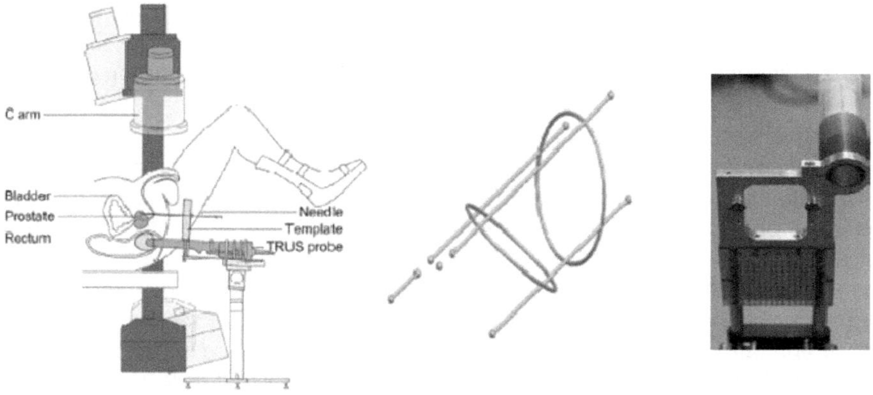

Fig. 1. *Left*: Prostate brachytherapy setup using transrectal ultrasound imaging to visualize the prostate and C-arm fluoroscopy to assess seed positions. *Center*: Sketch of the FTRAC fluoroscope tracking fiducial. *Right:* The fiducial is mounted and affixed to the needle insertion template during the procedure.

2 Methodology

2.1 Hypothesis

Our hypothesis is that the C-arm pose can be recovered adequately using a 2D/3D intensity-based registration algorithm between the fiducial's C-arm image and the fiducial's known geometrical model. For proving the concept, we used the aforementioned FTRAC fiducial introduced by Jain *et al.* [12] (Figure 1, right). The proposed 2D/3D registration scheme, depicted in Figure 2, follows several steps. (1) Calibrate the C-arm explicitly or assume a sufficiently accurate model of it. (2) Filter the fluoroscopy image to simultaneously enhance FTRAC features and to suppress neighboring structures. (3) Take an initial guess for pose of the C-arm relative to FTRAC. (4) Compute a DRR of the FTRAC. (5) Apply blurring operator on the lines/features in the DRR. (6) Run 2D/3D optimization to compute the pose using a normalized cross correlation metric and an Evolution Strategy with Covariance Matrix Adaptation (CMA-ES) optimizer. Adjust the C-arm pose and step back to (4) until convergence is achieved or failure to converge is detected.

2.2 C-arm Image Filtering

C-arm images are characterized by a low signal-to-noise ratio inducing image artifacts such as motion blur (i.e. object are blurred or smeared along the direction of relative motion). A three-step filter is used to diminish the negative effects of artifacts. All filter parameter definitions are listed in Table 1 and explained below.

2.2.1 Morphological Filtering

Morphological filtering is applied in grayscale to suppress the background of the C-arm image and enhance the FTRAC features. The structuring element chosen was in the shape of a disk of small radius, since the ball bearing and ellipse perimeter making up the FTRAC can be modeled as disk elements of small size. The morphological operator has only one filter parameter, which is the size of the structuring element.

2.2.2 Homomorphic Filtering

A homomorphic filter is used to de-noise the C-arm image. It sharpens features and flattens lighting variations in the image. The illumination component of an image is generally characterized by slow spatial variation while the reflectance component of an image tends to vary abruptly. These characteristics lead to associating the low frequencies of the Fourier transform of the natural log of an image with illumination and high frequencies with reflectance. Kovesi [23] provides excellent insights to the use of homomorphic filter. Even though these assumptions are approximation at best, a good deal of control can be gained over the illumination and reflectance components with a homomorphic filter. For the homomorphic filter to be effective, it needs to affect the low- and high-frequency components of the Fourier transform differently. To compress the dynamic range of an image, the low frequency components need to be attenuated to some degree. At the same time, in order to enhance the contrast, the high frequency components of the Fourier transform needs to be magnified. Thus Butterworth low and high pass filters are implemented and the image histograms are truncated accordingly.

2.2.3 Complex Shock Filtering

Gilboa *et al.* [24] have developed a filter coupling shock and linear diffusion in the discrete domain. The shock filter's main properties are the following: (i) shocks develop at inflection points (i.e. second derivative zero-crossings), (ii) local extrema remain unchanged in time, (iii) the scheme is total variation preserving, (iv) the steady state (weak) solution is piece-wise constant, and finally (v) the process approximates deconvolution. Unfortunately, noise in the blurred signal will also be enhanced. Robustness to noise can be improved by convolving the signal's second derivative with a Laplacian of Gaussian filter. This, however, is generally not sufficient to overcome the noise problem entirely, because convolving the signal with a Gaussian of moderate width in many cases will not cancel the inflection points produced by noise [24]. In order to alleviate this problem, a more complex approach is suggested: smoother parts are denoised while edges are enhanced and sharpened. The complex shock filter is hereby given by:

$$I_{t=}-\frac{2}{\pi}\arctan\left(aIm\left(\frac{I}{\theta}\right)\right)|\nabla I|+\lambda I_{\eta\eta}+\tilde{\lambda}I_{\xi\xi} \tag{1}$$

where a is a parameter that controls the sharpness of the slope, $\lambda = re^{i\theta}$ is a complex scalar, $\tilde{\lambda}$ is a real scalar, ξ is the direction perpendicular to the gradient and η is the direction of the gradient. In this way the inflection points are not of equal weight anymore; regions near edges with a large magnitude of second derivative near the zero crossing will be sharpened much faster than relatively smooth regions [24].

Table 1. Three step filter parameter definitions and assigned values, (parameter units in parenthesis)

	Filter Definitions	Value
I.	**Morphology filter**	
	- Structuring element size (radius in pixels)	2
II.	**Homomorphic filter**	
	- boost ratio of high frequency relative to low frequency	2
	- cutoff frequency of the filter	0.05
	- order for low and high pass Butterworth filters	3
	- truncation of the lower end of the image histogram	5
	- truncation of the higher end of the image histogram	0.01
III.	**Complex Shock Filter**	
	- number of iteration	10
	- time step size	1
	- grid step size	0.1
	- magnitude of the complex diffusion in the gradient direction	0.1
	- amount of diffusion in the level set direction	0.5
	- slope of the arctangent	0.3
	- phase angle of the complex term (in radians)	π/1000

2.3 Single-View Registration

We apply 2D/3D registration considering the DRR as the moving image and the C-arm image as the fixed image. We used MATLAB R2008a for implementation purposes.

As we only use one C-arm image at a time, to estimate the pose for that image, we termed this single-view registration, explained by the flowchart in Figure 2.

Metric: We implemented the normalized cross correlation metric that considers all pixel values in the images during registration. Fixed image pixels and their positions are mapped to the moving image. The correlation is normalized by the autocorrelations of both the fixed and moving images. The normalized cross correlation metric minimizes a cost function and the registration parameters will be optimal when minimum cost is reached.

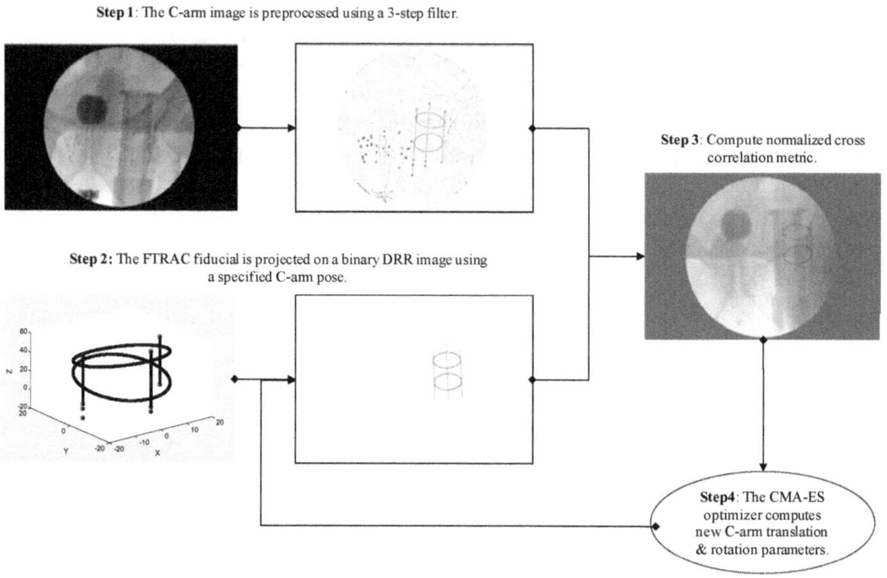

Fig. 2. C-arm pose recovery algorithm flowchart. (1) C-arm image is filtered by the 3-step filter to enhance FTRAC features while suppressing background structures. (2) FTRAC projected as a binary DRR image at a specified C-arm pose. (3) A normalized cross correlation metric computed. (4) CMA-ES optimizer computes new pose, process steps back to (2), until convergence or failure to convergence.

Transform: As the FTRAC is a rigid mechanical structure, rigid registration suffices. We implemented a transformation of six parameters, with three for Euler angles and three for translation.

Initial Guess: In the operating room, we have a consistently good initial guess for the registration. Standard patient positioning allows for aligning the main axes of the FTRAC, transrectal ultrasound and C-arm, enabling us to compute a gross registration in the anterior-posterior pose of the C-arm. Additional C-arm images are acquired according to a set protocol at 15° increments.

DRR Generation: The FTRAC fiducial is projected on a two dimensional binary image and blurred using a Gaussian filter. The filter parameters that need to be considered during implementation are the kernel size, kernel, and the sigma (σ) used for the Gaussian kernel.

Optimizer: The CMA-ES is an evolutionary algorithm for difficult non-linear non-convex optimization problems in continuous domain. In contrast to quasi-Newton methods, the CMA-ES does not use or approximate gradients and does not even presume or require their existence. This makes the method applicable to non-smooth and even non-continuous problems, as well as to multimodal and/or noisy problems [25]. The CMA-ES has several invariance properties. Two of them, inherited from the plain evolution strategy, are (i) invariance to order preserving (i.e. strictly monotonic) transformations of the objective function value and (ii) invariance to angle preserving (rigid) transformations of the search space (including rotation, reflection, and translation), if the initial search point is transformed accordingly. The CMA-ES does not require a tedious parameter tuning for its application. With the exception of population size, tuning of the internal parameters is not left to the user [25].

3 Results and Discussion

3.1 Registration Evaluation

We recall the primary objective of this work: provide an estimation of the C-arm fluoroscope poses for subsequent brachytherapy implant reconstruction. The implant reconstruction of Jain *et al.* requires curtailing the pose estimation error to ±4° in rotation and to ±2 mm in lateral translation [13]. In 2D/3D registration, the cost metric usually has difficulties with properly "driving" the depth component of the pose. In C-arm reconstruction, however, the exact same effect is working for our advantage, because the reconstruction metric is similarly insensitive to the depth component of the C-arm pose. Jain *et al.* found that "reconstruction error is insensitive to miscalibration in origin and focal length errors of up to 50 mm", inferring that even large depth errors are permissible if all image poses shift together [14]. What follows is that if the prostate is kept near the isocenter, projection and reconstruction are both insensitive to depth.

The registration error was evaluated against the C-arm pose obtained from ground truth (i.e. average errors of 0.56mm and 0.33° obtained by the FTRAC fiducial). In this paper, the values for mean registration error and standard deviations were calculated as the difference obtained from the ground truth and the registration, respectively. Capture range was defined as the range within which the algorithm is more likely to converge to the correct optimum. We applied random misalignment of maximum ±10 mm translation and ±10 degree rotation to ground truth obtained by segmenting the FTRAC and recovering pose. This capture range, especially for rotation, is larger than the error of the initial guess one can achieve clinically. We set the number of iterations for the optimizer to 30 and the population size at 65, resulting in 98.5% algorithm convergence. Using a total of 13 patient datasets, we performed the registration 25 times for each of the 111 clinical C-arm patient images, acquired under ethics board approval.

3.2 Results

The filter parameters were determined empirically by using a subsample of 10 C-arm images, with varying initial contrast, and fine-tuning the values so that the FTRAC features are always enhanced with respect to their neighborhood. Values for the proposed 3-Step filter are listed in Table 1. For the DRR binary image Gaussian smoothing, the sigma value was set to σ=1.5 pixels.

The performance of our proposed filter is presented in Figure 3. First, we observe that image contrast differs between patients. However, the chosen filter parameters improved the robustness and performance of our proposed filter; the pelvic bone and other neighboring structures were suppressed successfully while both the FTRAC fiducial and implanted seeds were enhanced. The filtered C-arm image was given as input to our intensity-based registration algorithm.

Five of the six degrees of freedom parameters were consistently below 0.5 mm and 1°. Using 111 clinical C-arm images and ±10° and ±10 mm random perturbation, the average rotation and translation errors were 0.62° (std=0.31°) and 0.73 mm (std= 0.55mm), respectively. As expected, the single view registration process did not recover the depth robustly (T_z parameter), yet on average the value is below clinical requirement of 2 mm.

Table 2. Final single-view registration results for 111 C-arm images

±10 mm and ±10° perturbation			
Tx (mm)	Ty (mm)	Tz (mm)	Rotations (degree)
0.14±0.08	0.11±0.16	1.9±1.4	0.6±0.3

3.3 Discussion

Of the 2775 trials, only 36 showed failure in registration convergence. Approximately half of the failures were due to the FTRAC fiducial being positioned near the black circular mask of the C-arm images (Figure 3, right), meaning that some features such as the top ball bearings and part of the top ellipse were not visible in the image. Also, since we started the registration from random initial guess, some runs were launched from an initial guess that projected the FTRAC outside the fluoroscopy image into the black mask where there was no feature guide the optimization into the image. We did not rerun registration with new initial guess since the purpose of the study was to show the true viability and robustness of our registration algorithm in a single run. Nevertheless, we expect the reported results in Table 2 to improve with restarting the registration process and/or with launching from an initial guess that projects the FTRAC within the C-arm image.

For the un-optimized MATLAB prototype implementation, a typical registration took about 170 seconds per image with Intel Core2, 2.4 GHz, dual-core computer. Figure 4 shows images after registration of binary FTRAC and C-arm images. A useful byproduct of our registration scheme is implicit and automatic segmentation of the radiographic fiducial, allowing the clinical user to visually approve the result of registration.

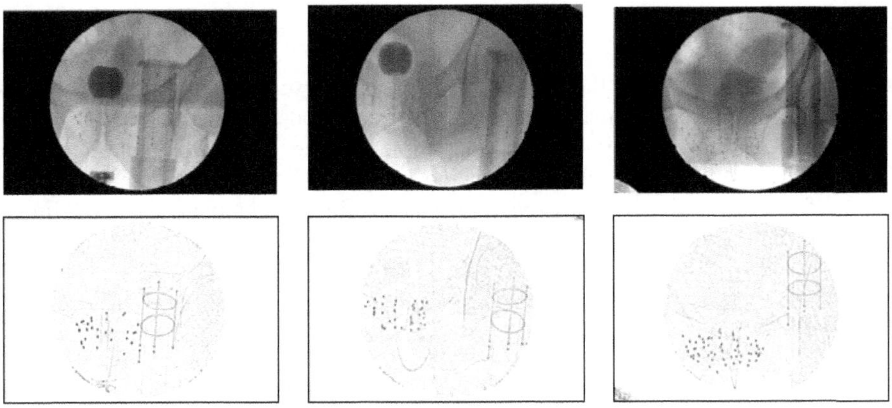

Fig. 3. C-arm image filtering. Here, three sample clinical images from three different patients with varying contrast. The morphology, homomorphic and shock filters smooth the image and enhance both the implanted seeds and FTRAC features while suppressing neighboring structures.

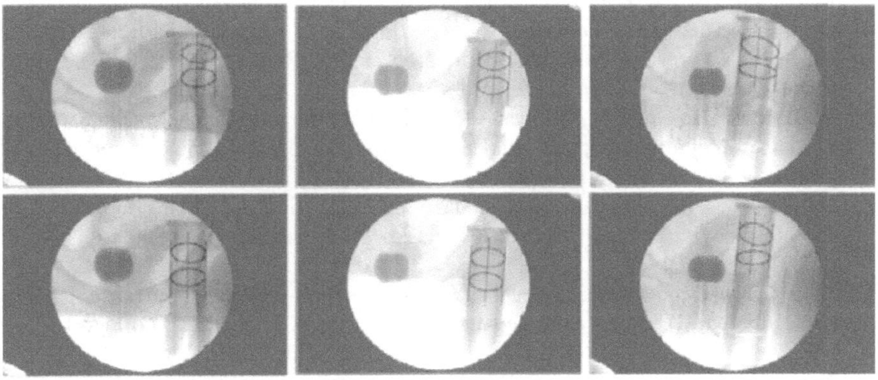

Fig. 4. Sample results before and after registration. With respect to original FTRAC size, initial perturbations had the same scale (*left*), smaller scale (*center*), and larger scale (*right*). The final overlay shows accurate superposition of the FTRAC fiducials. We note the 1 cm error in translations as initial perturbation for the left image.

Follow-up work will focus on adaptive filtering to compensate for varying C-arm image quality. Ideally, adaptive filter will analyze the image histograms and select optimal filter parameters accordingly. As of now, the parameters were empirically chosen and were found to be adequately robust in processing all available images. In order to test this approach prospectively in clinical trial, running time must be reduced below 1 minute per pose. As C-arm images are acquired by a well-defined protocol, we always know in which area of the C-arm the fiducial will appear, which in turn enables us to crop the C-arm image and thus reduce computation time. Additional speedup will be obtained from recoding the registration in C++.

4 Conclusion

In summary, we presented the first report of C-arm pose recovery by intensity-based registration of projected images of a geometrical model of a fluoroscope tracking fiducial and its C-arm images. Fluoroscopy images were pre-treated with a three-step filter that was found to be robust to varying image quality experienced in 111 C-arm images from 13 patients. Retrospective analysis of patient data showed clinically sufficient accuracy.

References

[1] Jemal, A., Siegel, R., Ward, E., et al.: Cancer Statistics. CA Cancer J. Clin. 59(4), 225–249 (2009)

[2] Zelefsky, M.J., Kuban, D.A., Levy, L.B., et al.: Multi-institutional analysis of long-term outcome for stages T1-T2 prostate cancer treated with permanent seed implantation. Int. J. Radiat. Oncol. Biol. Phys. 67(2), 327–333 (2007)

[3] Nag, S., Ciezki, J.P., Cormack, R., et al.: Intraoperative planning and evaluation of permanent prostate brachytherapy: report of the American Brachytherapy Society. Int. J. Radiat. Oncol. Biol. Phys. 51(5), 1422–1430 (2001)

[4] Orio, P.F., Tutar, I.B., Narayanan, S., et al.: Intraoperative ultrasound-fluoroscopy fusion can enhance prostate brachytherapy quality. Int. J. Radiat. Oncol. Biol. Phys. 69(1), 302–327 (2007)

[5] Westendorp, H., Hoekstra, C.J., van't Riet, A., et al.: Intraoperative adaptive brachytherapy of iodine-125 prostate implants guided by C-arm cone-beam computed tomography-based dosimetry. Brachytherapy 6(4), 231–237 (2007)

[6] Su, Y., Davis, B.J., Furutani, K.M., et al.: Seed localization and TRUS- fluoroscopy fusion for intraoperative prostate brachytherapy dosimetry. Computer Aided Surgery 12(1), 25–34 (2007)

[7] Jain, A.K., Deguet, A., Iordachita, I., et al.: Intra-operative Guidance in Prostate Brachytherapy Using an Average Carm. In: Ayache, N., Ourselin, S., Maeder, A. (eds.) MICCAI 2007, Part II. LNCS, vol. 4792, pp. 9–16. Springer, Heidelberg (2007)

[8] Yao, J., Taylor, R.H., Goldberg, R.P., et al.: A C-arm fluoroscopy-guided progressive cut refinement strategy using a surgical robot. Comput. Aided Surg. 5, 373–390 (2000)

[9] Zhang, M., Zaider, M., Worman, M., Cohen, G.: On the question of 3d seed reconstruction in prostate brachytherapy: the determination of x-ray source and film locations. Phys. Med. Biol. 49, 335–345 (2004)

[10] Yaniv, Z., Joskowicz, L.: Precise robot-assisted guide positioning for distal locking of intramedullary nails. IEEE Trans. Med. Imaging 24, 624–635 (2005)

[11] Tang, T.S.Y., MacIntyre, N.J., Gill, H.S., et al.: Accurate assessment of patellar tracking using fiducial and intensity-based fluoroscopic techniques. Med. Image Anal. 8, 343–351 (2004)

[12] Jain, A.K., Mustufa, T., Zhou, Y., et al.: FTRAC–a robust fluoroscope tracking fiducial. Medical physics 32(10), 3185–3198 (2005)

[13] Jain, A., Fichtinger, G.: C-arm Tracking and Reconstruction without an External Tracker. In: Larsen, R., Nielsen, M., Sporring, J. (eds.) MICCAI 2006, Part I. LNCS, vol. 4190, pp. 494–502. Springer, Heidelberg (2006)

[14] Jain, A., Kon, R., Zhou, Y., et al.: C-arm calibration - is it really necessary? In: Duncan, J.S., Gerig, G. (eds.) MICCAI 2005. LNCS, vol. 3749, pp. 639–646. Springer, Heidelberg (2005)
[15] Gueziec, A., Wu, K., Kalvin, A., et al.: Providing visual information to validate 2-d to 3-d registration. Medical Image Analysis 4, 357–374 (2000)
[16] Zuffi, S., Leardini, A., Catani, F., et al.: A model-based method for the reconstruction of total knee replacement kinematics. IEEE Trans. Med. Imag. 18(10), 981–991 (1999)
[17] Yamazaki, T., Watanabe, T., Nakajima, Y., et al.: Improvement of depth position in 2d/3d registration of knee implants using single-plane fluoroscopy. IEEE Trans. on Medical Imaging 23(5), 602–612 (2004)
[18] Nister, D.: An efficient solution to the five-point relative pose problem. IEEE Trans. on Pattern Analysis and Machine Intelligence 26(6), 756–770 (2004)
[19] Fischler, M., Bolles, R.: Random sample consensus: A paradigm for model fitting with applications to image analysis and automated cartography. Comm. Assoc. Comp. Mach. 24(6), 381–395 (1981)
[20] Livyatan, H., Yaniv, Z., Joskowicz, L.: Gradient-based 2-D/3-D rigid registration of fluoroscopic X-ray to CT. IEEE Trans. Med. Imaging 22, 1395–1406 (2003)
[21] Mahfouz, M., Hoff, W., Komistek, R., Dennis, D.: A robust method for registration of three-dimensional knee implant models to two-dimensional fluoroscopy images. IEEE Transactions on Medical Imaging 22, 1561–1574 (2003)
[22] Lau, K., Chung, A.: A global optimization strategy for 3d-2d registration of vascular images. In: Proceedings of 17th British Machine Vision Conference, pp. 489–498 (2006)
[23] Kovesi, P.: Functions for Computer Vision and Image Processing (2009), `http://www.csse.uwa.edu.au/~pk/research/matlabfns/`
[24] Gilboa, G., Sochen, N., Zeevi, Y.: Regularized shock filters and complex diffusion. In: Heyden, A., Sparr, G., Nielsen, M., Johansen, P. (eds.) ECCV 2002. LNCS, vol. 2350, pp. 399–413. Springer, Heidelberg (2002)
[25] Hansen, N.: The CMA Evolution Strategy: A Comparing Review. Studies in fuzziness and soft computing 192, 75–102 (2006)

First Animal Cadaver Study for Interlocking of Intramedullary Nails under Camera Augmented Mobile C-arm

A Surgical Workflow Based Preclinical Evaluation

Lejing Wang[1], Juergen Landes[2], Simon Weidert[2], Tobias Blum[1], Anna von der Heide[2], Ekkehard Euler[2], and Nassir Navab[1]

[1] Chair for Computer Aided Medical Procedures (CAMP), TU Munich, Germany
[2] Trauma Surgery Department, Klinikum Innenstadt, LMU Munich, Germany

Abstract. The Camera Augmented Mobile C-arm (CamC) system that augments a regular mobile C-arm by a video camera provides an overlay image of X-ray and video. This technology is expected to reduce radiation exposure during surgery without introducing major changes to the standard surgical workflow. Whereas many experiments were conducted to evaluate the technical characteristics of the CamC system, its clinical performance has not been investigated in detail. In this work, a workflow based method is proposed and applied to evaluate the clinical impact of the CamC system by comparing its performance with a conventional system, i.e. standard mobile C-arm. Interlocking of intramedullary nails on animal cadaver is chosen as a simulated clinical model for the evaluation study. Analyzing single workflow steps not only reveals individual strengths and weaknesses related to each step, but also allows surgeons and developers to be involved intuitively to evaluate and have an insight into the clinical impact of the system. The results from a total of 20 pair cases, i.e. 40 procedures, performed by 5 surgeons show that it takes significantly less radiation exposure whereas operation time for the whole interlocking procedure and quality of the drilling result are similar, using the CamC system compared to using the standard mobile C-arm. Moreover, the workflow based evaluation reveals in which surgical steps the CamC system has its main impact.

1 Introduction

Many image guided surgery (IGS) systems have been introduced in the last decades, e.g. systems using external camera tracking for navigation or augmented reality visualization. All of them provide various promising solutions to either simplify surgery or improve patient treatment. However, very few IGS systems have succeeded to become clinically accepted and even a small number of them were integrated into daily clinical routine. Development of novel IGS systems involves a long and complicated process from the initial idea until their acceptance and use for clinical applications. This process includes the phases of

N. Navab and P. Jannin (Eds.): IPCAI 2010, LNCS 6135, pp. 56–66, 2010.

clinical problem investigation and analysis, problem modeling, system and algorithm design, system implementation and verification, and finally evaluating the system in terms of its clinical outcome. The practicability, efficiency and clinical suitability of a system are mostly confirmed within the clinical evaluation phase.

The assessment of IGS systems has been discussed in detail by Jannin and Korb [1]. They proposed an assessment framework with six levels ranging from technical system properties to social and legal impacts. These six levels are classified according to the progress of the clinical acceptance.

Mobile C-arms are a common tool to acquire X-ray images in the operating room during trauma and orthopedic surgery. The Camera Augmented Mobile C-arm (CamC) system that augments a regular mobile C-arm by a video camera was proposed by Navab et al. [2] for X-ray and video image overlay (see figure 1). Thanks to the mirror construction and one time calibration of the device, the acquired X-ray images are co-registered with the video images without any further calibration or registration during the intervention. This technology is expected to reduce radiation exposure during surgery without introducing major changes to the standard surgical workflow. Many works were conducted to quantify and qualify the CamC system regarding to the overlay accuracy [3] and absorbed and scattered radiation of the mirror [4], which can be categorized into the level of technical system properties and reliability [1]. The clinical performance of the CamC system has not yet been investigated in detail. Traub et al. [5] performed a reference based assessment, comparing the workflow when using the CamC system to the one of using CT for vertebroplasty on a simulated procedure using five spine phantoms. This interesting initial study involved only one surgeon and a very small number of samples, and could therefore not show significant results. It however showed that one way of estimating clinical impacts of the CamC system on trauma and orthopedic surgery is to evaluate it in a simulated clinical scenario. Interlocking of intramedullary nails has been recognized as a challenging surgical task, for which several ingenious methods and devices were developed, e.g. miniature robot based guide positioning [6] and optical tracking with using two non-constrained X-ray images [7]. Suhm et al. peformed a clinical comparison study of interlocking using a surgical navigation system versus a standard C-arm system [8]. In this work, our objective is not to compare the robotics or external tracking based interlocking solution to that of using the CamC system for guidance. Here we focus on the evaluation of the CamC system versus conventional C-arm solutions. This surgical procedure was chosen because of its various different tasks that allow a good workflow oriented evaluation of the new image-guided surgery. In this paper, a proposed workflow and reference based evaluation method is applied to evaluate the CamC system and to predict some of its possible clinical impacts. Carrying out an animal cadaver study, we compare the interlocking of intramedullary nails using the CamC system vs. a standard C-arm in order to evaluate and predict the clinical impact of this new IGS alternative. Five surgeons participated in this study. The results are presented and discussed in sections 3.5 and 4.

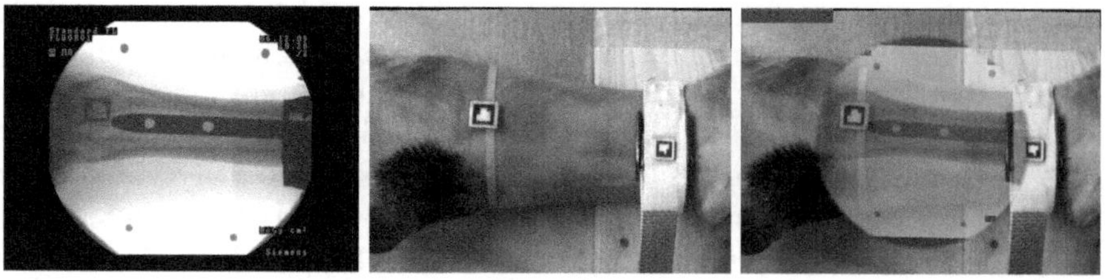

Fig. 1. Thanks to a joint construction and calibration, the CamC system register the X-ray image (left) onto the video image (middle) to provide an X-ray and video image overlay (right)

2 Surgical Workflow Based Evaluation for Image Guided Surgery Systems

In order to evaluate the clinical performance of a new IGS system and easily identify its advantages and disadvantages, we propose a workflow based comparison of the new system with a reference, i.e. conventional method. Assessment criteria, like patient outcome and radiation dose, are defined to compare the new method to the reference method. Instead of using only criteria for the whole procedure our workflow based method differentiates between single workflow steps. This has several advantages. Novel systems may introduce changes to the overall workflow or change the strategy within a single workflow step. While a system might have advantages in some steps of the procedure, it might also have disadvantages in other steps. Therefore, sometimes we may need to combine the functions of the novel solution and the traditional solution for the best result. A workflow based evaluation allows analyzing these aspects in more detail. Also the advantages and problems can be identified more clearly when estimating the impact on single steps instead of only investigating the impact on the whole procedure. For systems that can be used in different procedures it is usually not possible to deduce the possible impact on other procedures from the results of one procedure. Using a workflow based assessment it is easier to generalize results for single workflow steps that are common to several procedures. Moreover, workflow analysis plays a role of a connection between technical researchers and surgeons. This provides a way to involve surgeons intuitively to evaluate impacts of the system.

The workflow based assessment evaluation consists of the following steps:

a. **Initial formulation of assessment objective.** It includes a description of the motivation, the system, surgical context, assessment level and a hypothesis of the anticipated result [1].
b. **Modeling the workflows of the reference and the IGS based procedure.** First the workflow of the conventional method is modeled. Depending on the assessment objective and level a suitable workflow model has to be chosen. This can range from simple models, consisting only of few subsequent workflow steps, to more detailed methods [9]. Based on the reference

workflow and the anticipated use of the IGS, the new workflow is designed. This is done jointly by surgeons and technical researchers which facilitates a common understanding of technical and medical advantages and challenges. In this step, the hypothesis might be refined for each workflow step.

c. **Definition of evaluation criteria for each workflow step.** Based on the assessment objective, evaluation criteria for comparing the new system to the conventional one are first defined for each workflow step. In order to quantify the comparison, measurement parameters must be chosen, such that they represent the evaluation criteria. Then, measures of statistics are defined, e.g. mean value or standard deviation, and hypotheses for these measures are made.
d. **Experiments and acquisition of measurement parameters.** A protocol for recording the measurement parameters must be established. This can be data done using e.g. video or live observations [10] or data that is captured from medical devices. When introducing a novel system, it often cannot be used on real patients. So the procedure can be performed in a simulated setup. To avoid a bias, also the conventional system has to be used in the simulated setup.
e. **Comparison of values from reference and IGS based procedure.** A statistical comparison of the measured parameters is performed for each workflow step in order to obtain quantitative results.

3 Animal Cadaver Study of Interlocking of Intramedullary Nails: CamC vs. Mobile C-arm

Intramedullary nailing is a common surgical operation method that can be used mostly in fracture reduction of the tibial and femoral shaft. After implanting successfully a nail into the medullary canal, the nail must be fixed inside the bone by inserting locking screws through locking holes in the nail in order to avoid unwanted rotation and movement of the bone. This procedure is called interlocking of intramedullary nails and is performed in a minimally invasive way. Thus, intra-operative X-ray images are required for targeting and drilling the locking holes through the patient's skin. Currently, the clinical procedure for interlocking is generally performed with using mobile C-arms that can offer continuous intra-operative guidance based on a huge amount of X-ray images. Furthermore, interlocking of intramedullary nails involves various common surgical tasks, e.g. X-ray positioning, targeting, instrument alignment, and drilling. Therefore, interlocking is chosen in order to evaluate the clinical impact of the CamC system. The study design was approved by the veterinary public health office at the institution of our medical partners.

3.1 Assessment Objective

We evaluate the system at the level of surgical strategy and performance and we expect a reduction of x-ray images. Motivation, system and clinical context have been discussed above and in section 1.

3.2 Surgical Workflow for Interlocking of Intramedullary Nails

In this evaluation study, a single interlocking procedure starts after successfully implanting the long nail into the medullary canal, and ends in successfully inserting one locking screw. Based on the principle of the workflow-based evaluation presented in section 2, the workflow of interlocking is constructed manually in a close collaboration between scientists, engineers and surgeons. All the steps in the workflow are fundamental surgical tasks, and some of them, e.g. X-ray positioning, skin incision, and drilling, are also necessary steps in other surgical procedures. Thus, the results of the workflow-based evaluation for each single step of interlocking become very valuable and meaningful for understanding clinical impacts of the CamC system beyond this particular study. The general workflow for using CamC and normal C-arm is the same and includes seven steps:

i. **X-ray positioning.** Position the C-arm from outside of the operation field into the operation workspace. It ends after the C-arm is moved to the desired position confirmed by an X-ray image showing the desired operation area.
ii. **Adjustment of hole.** Turn the nail until the locking hole appears as a circle in the X-ray image in order to allow for orthogonal drilling.
iii. **Skin incision.** Find the incision position and cut the skin. The correct incision position is confirmed by an X-ray image when using the standard mobile C-arm, or by the X-ray and video image overlay when using the CamC system.
iv. **Center punch.** Align the sharp tip of a nail to the target hole. Then, form a small dimple on the bone surface in which the tip of the drill will fit with the help of a hammer.
v. **Alignment of the tip of the drill.** Align the tip of the drill to the target hole. It ends after one X-ray image shows that the projection of the tip is located inside the circle of the target hole.
vi. **Drilling.** Drill the bone and the drill bit must pass through the locking hole of the nail. It ends after a successful drilling is confirmed by an X-ray image.
vii. **Locking screw insertion.** Insert a locking screw into the hole. One X-ray image is required to confirm the success of locking screw insertion, which indicates the end of the procedure for interlocking.

3.3 Evaluation Criteria

Modern trauma and orthopedic surgical procedures use X-ray images during surgery as intervention guidance, especially in minimally invasive surgery. This increases radiation exposure for both patient and surgical team. Radiation exposure should be reduced as much as possible, since the effects of exposure to radiation have been reported to increase the risk of fatal cancer [11,12] and genetic defects [13]. As demonstrated in the work of [3], employing the X-ray and video image overlays from the CamC system as image guidance has huge potential to reduce radiation exposure compared to just using a conventional mobile C-arm. Thus, the first evaluation criterion is to compare the amount of applied radiation exposure using the CamC system to the standard mobile C-arm. Through the whole comparison study, we fix the tube voltage and radiation time to a setting we found was ideal for imaging the cow bone structures in order to produce constant radiation doses for each shot on the level of the x-ray tube. The number of X-ray shots can therefore be used to compare the radiation exposure. It is claimed that employing the CamC system for interventional procedures does not complicate the surgical procedure compared to using the standard mobile [3]. Thus, we record the parameters of operation time and quality of drilling.

The authors hypothesized that it takes less number of X-ray shots by using the CamC system than using the standard C-arm for the whole procedure, particularly in step 1, 3, and 6. We also expect both systems to have similar results with regard to operation time and drilling quality for the whole procedure.

3.4 Materials and Experiments

In this pre-clinical study, we use forelegs of cow cadavers (see figure 2), all of which have similar shape and size. We use the same medical instruments, e.g. long nail, locking screw and drill, as used in real surgeries. In the experiments, the cow leg is placed on a carbon table that is designed for medical experiments on animals. Different from the situation of real patients, our cow forelegs are too short to be held by operation assistants. Thus, we fix them roughly to a $30 \times 15cm^2$ wooden board to make the cow leg more stable (see figure 2), while not being totally fixed. So, some minor movements of the cow leg during our study are inevitable, which sometimes requires surgeons to hold it by themselves. This setup of leg is very close to the real clinical situation.

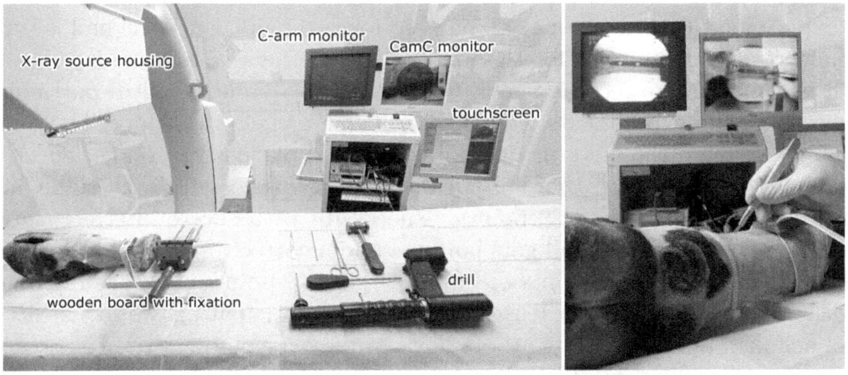

Fig. 2. The experimental setup for interlocking of intramedullary nails on a cow bone is shown in the left image. The right image demonstrates the system configuration for the procedure using the CamC system. In the system configuration for the procedure using the standard mobile C-arm, the CamC monitor is turned off.

The CamC system used in our study is built by attaching a video camera and mirror construction, covered by a X-ray source housing, to a mobile C-arm. The proposed one time calibration of [2] is used to calibrate the CamC system. An LCD monitor mounted on the top of the C-arm cart displays the live video overlaid by the X-ray image, and a touch screen monitor mounted on the side of the C-arm cart provides a user interface (see figure 2).

If the cow leg moves away from the initial position where the X-ray image was acquired, X-ray and video image overlay have a misalignment. For this reason, a visual square marker tracking method [14] is employed to track square markers that are rigidly attached to the cow leg surface. For visually informing surgeons about misalignments, the initial positions of markers are drawn as green quadrilaterals and their positions in the current video image are drawn as red quadrilaterals in the video images. Moreover, a gradient color bar is shown on the right side of the video images, whose length indicates the pixel-difference between the marker's initial and current positions (see figure 3).

For the interlocking procedure by using the standard C-arm, we employ the CamC system as a standard C-arm with the same setup except for turning off the CamC monitor of the X-ray and video image overlay (see figure 2), in order to reduce the bias from handling different C-arm systems.

Participated surgeons are selected such that they cover all following three groups, young surgeons with less than 20 surgical cases, experienced surgeons with 20-100 surgical cases, and expert surgeons with more than 100 surgical cases. Five surgeons participate in the study, i.e. two young surgeons, one experienced surgeon, and two expert surgeons. The study covers 20 pair cases (i.e. 40 procedures), 10 performed by expert, 6 by intermediate and 4 by young surgeons. Each pair carried out by the same surgeon consists of one interlocking using the CamC system and one using the standard C-arm system. The sequence of two procedures within one pair is randomized by coin flipping. The inserted nail has two distal locking holes inside the cow bone, and both of which are used for one pair experiment. One cow bone can be used for two pairs, since the nail is turned to another side of the bone for the interlocking of the second pair.

All parameters are recorded by a team of medical and technical participants by observing the experiments, which is verified by video recording. The quality of drilling through the holes in the nail is assessed by the surgeon as "successful without interference with the nail" given 1 point, "successful with slight interference with the nail" given 2 points, "successful with severe interference with the nail" (in this case the drill gets jammed and a correction of drilling angle has to be performed) given 3 points or "failure" given 5 points. The drilling quality level is determined as a consensus reached by participating surgeons directly after each drilling. In [8], the authors have employed a similar criterion to assess the quality of drilling in interlocking of intramedullary nails.

3.5 Results and Comparison

In order to obtain statistical results with regard to the number of X-ray shots, operation time and drilling quality, we calculate their mean and standard deviation

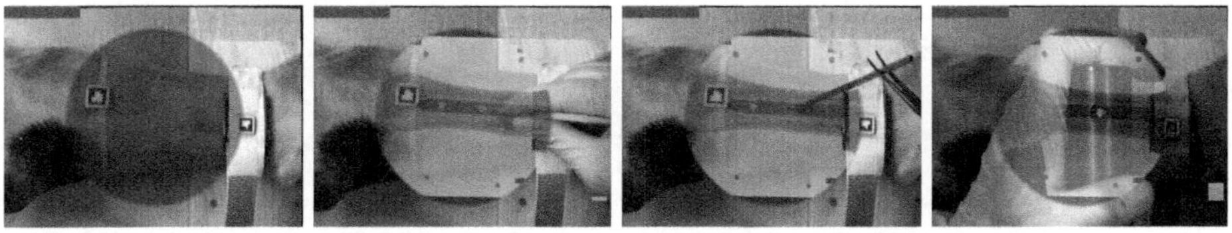

(a) Xray Positioning (b) Skin Incision (c) Center Punch (d) Drill

Fig. 3. The CamC system provides X-ray and video image overlays, which can give intuitive advanced optics-Xray image guidance for many surgical tasks, e.g. X-ray positioning (a), skin incision (b), instrument alignment in center punch (c), and axis control of drilling (d)

(STD). Moreover, we apply paired t-test to find out the level of significant difference, i.e. p-value, for all three evaluation parameters between the two groups of CamC and C-arm, i.e. interlocking procedures performed by using the CamC system and using the standard mobile C-arm. Table 1 shows the mean, STD, and p-value of the number of X-ray shots and operation time for the whole interlocking procedure, as well as for each surgical step, in the two groups. The results of drilling quality are 1.80 ± 0.70 for the CamC group and 2.20 ± 0.77 for the C-arm group.

For the whole interlocking procedure, significantly less X-ray shots are needed in the CamC group compared to the C-arm group ($p < 0.0001$). The CamC group needs longer operation time, while demonstrating better drilling quality in our study. However, there are no significant differences in operation time ($p = 0.55$) and drilling quality ($p = 0.12$) between these two groups.

In the step of X-ray positioning, The CamC group performs better with significantly less X-ray shots ($p = 0.028$). The reason is that the live video with an overlaid X-ray image circle (like an aiming circle) provides an intuitive video-based guidance for moving C-arm to the desired position (see figure 3(a)). The CamC group takes significantly less X-ray shots ($p < 0.0001$) and significantly less operation time ($p = 0.026$) than the C-arm group in the step of skin incision, since surgeons can quickly find the target place for skin incision using the guidance of the video with an aligned X-ray image (see figure 3(b)). In the step of center punch, the number of required X-ray shots is significantly smaller in the CamC group than in the C-arm group ($p = 0.0066$), since surgeons can identify the location for center punch based on the guidance of overlay (see figure 3(c)). For aligning the tip of the drill, a smaller number of X-ray shots is needed, which, however, does not reach a level of significance ($p = 0.069$). In the step of drilling, the overlay of X-ray and video image can support the control of drilling axis (see figure 3(d)), and thus the CamC group needs significantly smaller number of X-ray shots ($p = 0.028$) than the C-arm group. Operation time seems to be the same ($p = 0.98$). The steps of adjustment of hole and screw insertion do not provide any signs of significant differences between the two groups.

Table 1. The mean, standard deviation (STD), and p-value of the number of X-ray shots and operation time (seconds) for the whole interlocking procedure, as well as for each surgical step, in CamC group and C-arm

	X-ray positioning	Adjustment of hole	Skin incision	Center punch	Alignment of the tip of the drill	Drilling	Locking screw insertion	Overall
The number of X-ray shots (mean±*STD*)								
CamC Group	**1.05** ±*0.22*	**2.65** ±*1.09*	**0.05** ±*0.22*	**2.15** ±*1.50*	**1.65** ±*1.27*	**1.30** ±*0.73*	**1** ±*0*	**9.85** ±*3.10*
C-arm Group	**1.45** ±*0.76*	**2.80** ±*1.40*	**2.65** ±*1.09*	**4.05** ±*2.28*	**2.20** ±*1.47*	**2.90** ±*2.90*	**1** ±*0*	**17.05** ±*4.61*
p-value	**0.028**	0.65	**<0.0001**	**0.0066**	0.069	**0.028**	1.00	**<0.0001**
Operation time (mean±*STD*)								
CamC Group (seconds)	**21.95** ±*5.93*	**23.70** ±*18.88*	**19.30** ±*5.58*	**55.15** ±*22.02*	**26.55** ±*19.01*	**161.00** ±*115.40*	**59.65** ±*54.25*	**367.30** ±*173.70*
C-arm Group (seconds)	**25.05** ±*9.90*	**19.35** ±*10.73*	**28.75** ±*10.78*	**52.30** ±*26.19*	**22.85** ±*9.77*	**160.40** ±*91.28*	**39.75** ±*17.34*	**348.45** ±*114.07*
p-value	0.17	0.40	**0.0026**	0.73	0.27	0.98	0.05	0.55

In our study, the CamC group has smaller STD values for the number of X-ray shots in the whole procedure, as well as in each surgical step, than the C-arm group, whereas for operation time, the CamC group has smaller STD values in step 1 and step 3, but larger STD values in other steps and the whole procedure.

4 Discussion and Conclusion

The technical characteristics of the CamC system, e.g. overlay accuracy, have already been well studied. In this work, the proposed workflow based method was applied to evaluate the clinical impact of the CamC system for Interlocking of intramedullary nails. We compared the performance of the CamC system with the standard mobile C-arm. Interlocking of intramedullary nails on cow forelegs was chosen as a simulated clinical model for our evaluation study. This study covered a total of 40 procedures and involved 5 surgeons with three different skill levels.

Surgeons performed surgical tasks more confidently when using an X-ray image augmented by a live video than a pure X-ray image. This reduced the number of unnecessary X-ray shots that depends on the experience and skill of the surgeon. This point was confirmed by all participating surgeons. The CamC group not only required less radiation exposure, but also showed relatively low variations, i.e. smaller STD, in number of taken X-ray shots. From our point of view, this could be a sign of enhanced reliability and stability on the surgeon's side. The last step of screw insertion took much longer in the CamC group than in the C-arm group. The reason is that the surgeons tend to check the overlay image to find the hole to put the screw in, although they could definitely find it even faster without any image based guidance, since the hole is visible and easy to feel. This point was agreed by all participating surgeons. Due to the learning curve of the new system, the variation of operation time is higher in the CamC group than in the C-arm group for the whole procedure. The cow leg moved quite often in the steps of center punch and drilling. This resulted in a misalignment of X-ray and video image. Informing surgeons about such a misalignment is compulsory, especially for real surgery. In our approach, we employed the visual marker tracking in order to visually inform surgeons about any misalignment in the overlay image. As the visual markers were attached on the skin surface and skin sometimes has a minor movement relative to the bone, there could be misinterpretations of the image alignment. However, this did not introduce any major problem during the study due to the fact that this movement was very small and skin generally moves back to its original position.

The results of our evaluation study show that the CamC group required significantly less radiation exposure but needed similar operation time, and also achieved a similar drilling quality for the whole interlocking procedure compared to the C-arm group. The workflow based evaluation reveals that the CamC system has its main positive impact in the steps of X-ray positioning, skin incision, center punch, and drilling. Due to the fact that X-ray positioning and skin incision are the necessary steps in many other surgical procedures, our results are also valuable and useful for predicting the clinical impact of the CamC system beyond this particular application. We are planning to use our proposed workflow based method to also evaluate the clinical performance of the CamC system on real patients in the near future.

References

1. Jannin, P., Korb, W.: Image-Guided Interventions - Technology and Applications, ch. 18. Springer, Heidelberg (2008)
2. Navab, N., Mitschke, M., Bani-Hashemi, A.: Merging visible and invisible: Two camera-augmented mobile C-arm (CAMC) applications. In: Proc. IEEE and ACM Int'l. Workshop on Augmented Reality, San Francisco, CA, USA, pp. 134–141 (1999)
3. Navab, N., Heining, S.M., Traub, J.: Camera augmented mobile c-arm (camc): Calibration, accuracy study and clinical applications. IEEE Transactions on Medical Imaging (to appear, 2010)
4. Wang, L., Weidert, S., Traub, J., Heining, S.M., Riquarts, C., Euler, E., Navab, N.: Camera augmented mobile c-arm: Towards real patient study. In: Proceedings of Bildverarbeitung fuer die Medizin (BVM 2009), Heidelberg, Germany (2009)
5. Traub, J., Ahmadi, S.A., Padoy, N., Wang, L., Heining, S.M., Euler, E., Jannin, P., Navab, N.: Workflow based assessment of the camera augmented mobile c-arm system. In: AMIARCS, New York, NY, USA. MICCAI Society (2008)
6. Yaniv, Z., Joskowicz, L.: Precise robot-assisted guide positioning for distal locking of intramedullary nails. IEEE Transactions on Medical Imaging 24, 624–635 (2005)
7. Leloup, T., El Kazzi, W., Schuind, F., Warzee, N.: A novel technique for distal locking of intramedullary nail based on two non-constrained fluoroscopic images and navigation. IEEE Transactions on Medical Imaging 27, 1202–1212 (2008)
8. Suhm, N., Messmer, P., Zuna, I., Jacob, L.A., Regazzoni, P.: Fluoroscopic guidance versus surgical navigation for distal locking of intramedullary implants: A prospective, controlled clinical study. Injury 35, 567–574 (2004)
9. Neumuth, T., Durstewitz, N., Fischer, M., Strauss, G., Dietz, A., Meixensberger, J., Jannin, P., Cleary, K., Lemke, H., Burgert, O.: Structured recording of intraoperative surgical workflows. In: SPIE Medical Imaging 2006 (2006)

10. Neumuth, T., Jannin, P., Strauss, G., Meixensberger, J., Burgert, O.: Validation of Knowledge Acquisition for Surgical Process Models. Journal of the American Medical Informatics Association 16(1), 72–80 (2009)
11. National Research Council: Health Effects of Exposure to Low Levels of Ionizing Radiation: BEIR V (1990)
12. National Radiological Protection Board: Estimates of Radiation Detriment in a UK Population, NRPB Report 260 (1994)
13. International Commission on Radiological Protection: Recommendations of the International Commission on Radiological Protection. ICRP Publication 60 (1990)
14. Zhang, X., Fronz, S., Navab, N.: Visual marker detection and decoding in ar systems: A comparative study. In: ISMAR 2002 (2002)

Robot-Assisted Laparoscopic Ultrasound

Caitlin M. Schneider, Gregory W. Dachs II, Christopher J. Hasser,
Michael A. Choti, Simon P. DiMaio, and Russell H. Taylor

Department of Computer Science, Johns Hopkins University
Department of Surgery, Johns Hopkins Medicine
Intuitive Surgical Inc.
rht@jhu.edu

Abstract. Novel tools for existing robotic surgical systems present opportunities for exploring improved techniques in minimally invasive surgery. Specifically, intraoperative ultrasonography is a tool that is being used with increased frequency, yet has limitations with existing laparoscopic systems. The purpose of this study was to develop and to evaluate a new ultrasound system with the *da Vinci*® Surgical System (Intuitive Surgical Inc., Sunnyvale CA) for laparoscopic visualization. The system consists of a prototype dexterous laparoscopic ultrasound instrument for use with the *da Vinci* surgical system, an integrated image display, and navigation tools. The system was evaluated by surgeons during pertinent activities, including phantom lesion detection and needle biopsy tasks, as well as in vivo porcine visualization and manipulation tasks. The system was found to be highly dexterous, clinically desirable, and advantageous over traditional laparoscopic systems. This device promises to improve performance of complex minimally-invasive surgical procedures.

1 Introduction

Systems such as Intuitive Surgical's *da Vinci*® combine high dexterity telerobotic control of laparoscopic instruments and high fidelity 3D visualization to give surgeons the ability to manipulate patients' anatomy in a minimally-invasive manner while still preserving many of the advantages of open surgery, including natural hand-eye coordination and improved visual appreciation of the surgical field. In many cases, these systems have been shown to enable surgeons to achieve outcomes equivalent to or better than those of open surgery while still gaining the low morbidity and other advantages of minimally-invasive surgery (MIS) [1, 2]. Although such systems are widely deployed, opportunities exist to improve their capabilities in order to further expand clinical utility and patient safety. In recent years, a number of research groups—including our own—have begun to explore means for more fully exploiting the potential of computers to augment or extend surgeons' capabilities for MIS. These efforts have included preoperative image registration [3, 4], haptic feedback or palpation capabilities [5, 6], "virtual fixtures" to improve accuracy or safety of surgical maneuvers [7-9], and software "toolkits" or environments to promote system integration [10].

Intraoperative ultrasonography (IOUS) is a valuable tool in a wide variety of surgical procedures, including hepatobiliary, urologic, gynecologic, and gastrointestinal surgery.

N. Navab and P. Jannin (Eds.): IPCAI 2010, LNCS 6135, pp. 67–80, 2010.

Unlike other modalities of imaging, IOUS provides easily attained real-time anatomical information for operative assessment, staging, and real-time guidance for biopsy and ablative procedures. IOUS is being increasingly used with minimally invasive procedures as well. With the loss of tactile information, laparoscopic IOUS provides particular advantages when evaluating solid organs such as the liver or kidney. While the minimally-invasive approach of IOUS offers significant advantages over open ultrasound, constraints exist that limit its efficacy and utility. These include lack of probe mobility, flexibility, maneuverability, and image co-viewing with the endoscopic video. The *da Vinci* platform provides a unique opportunity to develop a useful image-guidance tool for minimally-invasive surgery, yet offer the advantages of dexterity and image quality that could otherwise only be achieved with open surgical approaches.

This paper reports the development of a high dexterity robotic laparoscopic ultrasound (RLUS) tool for the *da Vinci* and its integration into our open-source research software environment, together with initial user experiments. Tasks were created and evaluated based on clinically relevant procedures, including liver scanning and staging, lesion detection, and biopsy.

Hepatic (liver) surgery was the focusing application for this work. Liver cancer surgery is being performed with increasing frequency. Primary liver cancer is the fifth most common malignancy worldwide, accounting for over 500,000 new cases per year [11]. Secondary or metastatic cancer to the liver, originating in the colon, pancreas, breast, lung, among others, is also extremely common. IOUS is a critical component of all liver surgery, used for staging, planning resection, and guiding tumor biopsy and ablation [12]. It is the most accurate method for detecting liver metastases, with accuracy rates above 90 percent [13]. Currently, resection of liver tumors is most commonly performed using open or laparoscopic surgery, with IOUS performed by the direct placement of the ultrasound probe on the liver surface. Liver biopsies and tumor ablations are commonly performed using transcutaneous ultrasound guidance to guide percutaneous needle placement. Although percutaneous approaches have potential advantages of lower morbidity compared to open or laparoscopic surgery, there are also advantages for performing biopsy or ablation in an open laparotomy or laparoscopic environment. Placing the ultrasound probe directly on the liver provides improved imaging compared to transcutaneous ultrasound. Moreover, it allows advanced techniques such as elastography to be employed [14, 15], further improving the surgeon's ability to locate and target structures within this solid organ. Surgical approaches also permit the identification of both hepatic and extrahepatic disease that may not be seen on preoperative imaging, as well as providing better access to difficult-to-reach tumors. In the case of multiple tumors, surgical resection can be combined with ablation. Finally, some studies have suggested that operative surgical ablation may result in better outcomes compared to percutaneous ablation [16].

Several investigators have active programs in robotically-assisted ultrasonography. Fenster, et al. have reported using tracked and robotically-manipulated 2D US probes to produce 3D US images [17]. Several groups have described ultrasound targeting for robotically-assisted needle placement procedures [17-21] while others have developed robotically-manipulated extracorporeal ultrasound systems [22-26]. None of these systems involve laparoscopic ultrasound (LUS) or integrate US into an interventional procedure. Dupont *et al.* have reported work using 3D ultrasound to help guide robotically-manipulated endoscopic instruments, and one experimental system for remote LUS probe manipulation [18] was reported part of a 1998 EU telemedicine initiative. The use of a *da Vinci* robot to manipulate drop-in ultrasound probes has also been reported (e.g., [19]). Many groups have reported use of navigational tracking devices for extracorporeal and laparoscopic ultrasound.

In earlier work [20], we reported on preliminary efforts to produce an integrated IOUS imaging capability for the *da Vinci*, in which we used a simple rigid (i.e., non-articulated) IOUS tool that could be attached to one of the *da Vinci*'s instrument interfaces and manipulated under control of the surgeon's master manipulator. Although experience with this tool was encouraging, it had many limitations. In particular, the lack of a "wrist" made it extremely difficult (in come cases, impossible) for the surgeon to obtain the view desired, especially for tasks such as placing a biopsy needle or ablation probe. Even simply accommodating the probe to the external surface of the organ was difficult to achieve. For these reasons, we undertook development of the more advanced system reported here, in which a wristed (i.e., articulated) IOUS tool is manipulated by the surgeon much as any other *da Vinci* instrument. Our main goals in this study were: i) to demonstrate that such a tool could be integrated and that it could be used effectively by surgeons; and ii) to obtain further feedback to guide further development.

2 Materials and Methods

2.1 System Overview

The schematic shown in Figure 1 illustrates the integration of a prototype articulated RLUS instrument, as well as enhanced image visualization capabilities, with the *da Vinci* surgical robot. The purpose of this system is to allow the surgeon to manipulate a laparoscopic ultrasound probe directly from the *da Vinci*'s surgical console, just as he/she would manipulate a surgical instrument, while observing ultrasound images and associated guidance information within the stereo display of the console.

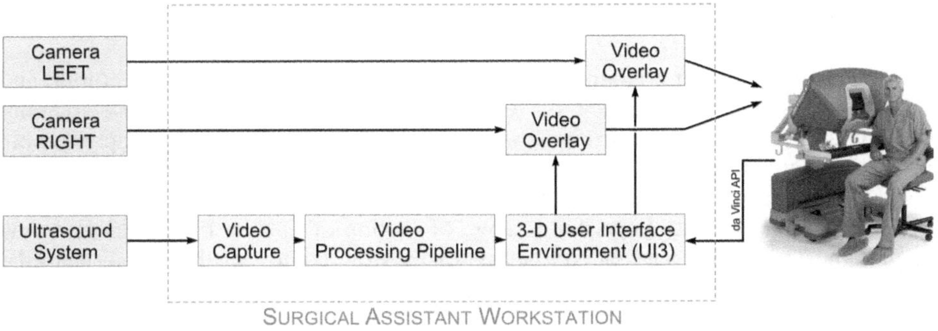

Fig. 1. A high-level system schematic illustrating the use of the Surgical Assistant Workstation (SAW) for video processing, 3-D user interface, and display within the *da Vinci* console. SAW is an open-source medical robotics software framework.

The ultrasound probe, user interface and visualization components are integrated by means of the Surgical Assistant Workstation (SAW) [10]. The SAW is an open-source software framework that has been developed to support medical robotics research. The remainder of this section describes the design and specifications of the RLUS instrument, as well as methods for the visualizing ultrasound images and other guidance information.

2.2 Ultrasound Instrument Design

A prototype *da Vinci* laparoscopic ultrasound instrument was developed based on the 5mm EndoWrist instrument architecture, but scaled to a diameter of 10mm in order to accommodate an off-the-shelf linear laparoscopic transducer (Gore Tetrad, Colorado, U.S.A.). The 5mm wrist is based on a cable-driven multi-link snake architecture that—when scaled to 10mm—is able to accommodate the coaxial cable bundle that is routed through the center of the instrument shaft from the transducer to the system cable interface at the rear of the instrument (shown in Figure 2b).

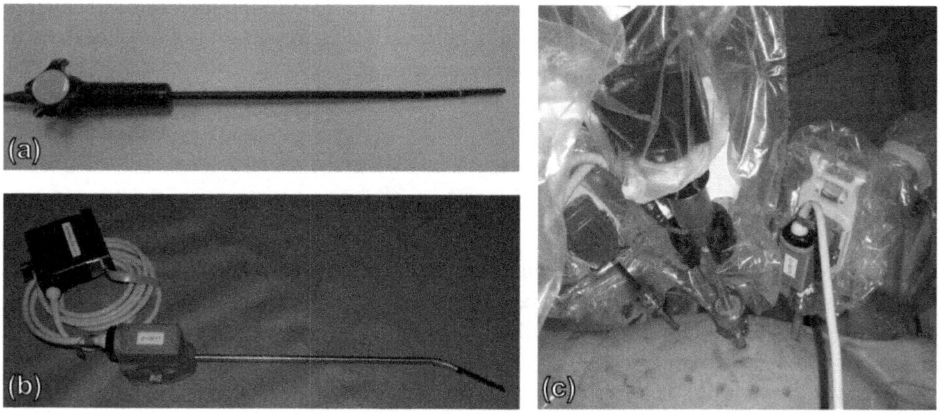

Fig. 2. (a) A hand-held laparoscopic ultrasound probe (Aloka UST-5536-7.5). (b) The prototype *da Vinci* ultrasound instrument. (c) The ultrasound instrument manipulated by a *da Vinci* robotic manipulator.

The linear transducer contains 128 elements, has a total array length of 46mm, and operates at a center frequency of 7.5MHz. In terms of geometry and imaging performance, the RLUS instrument is similar to standard hand-held laparoscopic probes that are in use today, such as the Aloka UST-5536-7.5 shown in Figure 2a (Aloka America, Connecticut, U.S.A.).

The articulated wrist allows for a range of motion of ±80° in both pitch and yaw angles, thus giving the surgeon six-degree-of-freedom control of the probe, from the master tool manipulators of the surgical console.

2.3 Image Visualization and User Interface

An open-source software framework has been used to display ultrasound images, probe status and guidance information in the stereo display of the *da Vinci* surgical console. B-Mode ultrasound images can be displayed in a variety of ways, including:

1 A split screen display mode in which the surgeon sees the endoscopic and ultrasound views side by side (Figure 3a).

2 A picture-in-picture display mode that insets the ultrasound image into the endoscopic view (Figure 3b). In this configuration, the surgeon is able to select the position and size of the inset image by manipulating the master tool manipulators within the console—this is a user interface feature that is provided by a 3D user interface module implemented within the software library.

3 A "flashlight" display mode in which the ultrasound image is overlaid onto a three dimensional representation of the imaging plane in the stereo view of the console. The effect of this mode is to display the ultrasound image in the plane in which it is physically acquired by the transducer, such that the image is co-located with the view of the tissue that is being imaged in the surgical field. This third display mode is illustrated in Figure 3c. Issues of automatic calibration and image-probe registration were addressed in our prior work with a non-articulated probe [20].

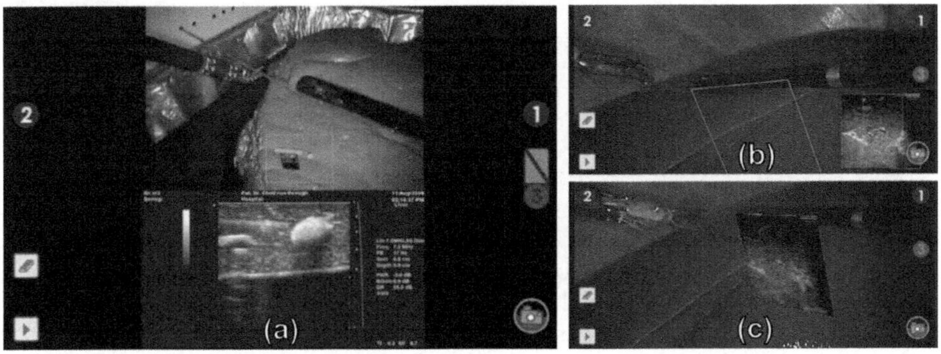

Fig. 3. (a) A split-screen display that shows the endoscopic view and the ultrasound image adjacent to one another in the surgical console. (b) A picture-in-picture view of the ultrasound image. (c) The ultrasound "flashlight" overlay.

In addition to the image overlay, the system displays a graphical representation of the probe, imaging plane, and wrist configuration at the lower margin of the endoscopic view, as shown in Figure 4a. This graphical widget provides the user with cues for orienting the imaging plane of the probe, as well as for avoiding wrist range of motion limits, particularly when the ultrasound probe fills the field of view of the endoscope and the wrist is not visible.

An interesting feature of the *da Vinci* probe is that its location and motion within the surgical field can be tracked by the robotic instrument manipulator. We have implemented two tools that take advantage of this spatial information. The first is a measurement tool that allows the user to measure point-to-point motions of the probe in order to estimate the perpendicular distance between two image planes. This can be used to estimate the out-of-plane width of a lesion without having to re-orient the probe.

A second tool allows the user to map the relative locations of features of interest within the surgical field, such as the locations of lesions or anatomical landmarks. The map shows the current location and orientation of the probe as a graphical "cursor", as well as the locations of markers that have been dropped as "bread crumbs" during the course of a procedure. This is shown in Figure 4b. By moving the probe cursor to align with the markers, the user is able to return to and re-examine ultrasound views of interest.

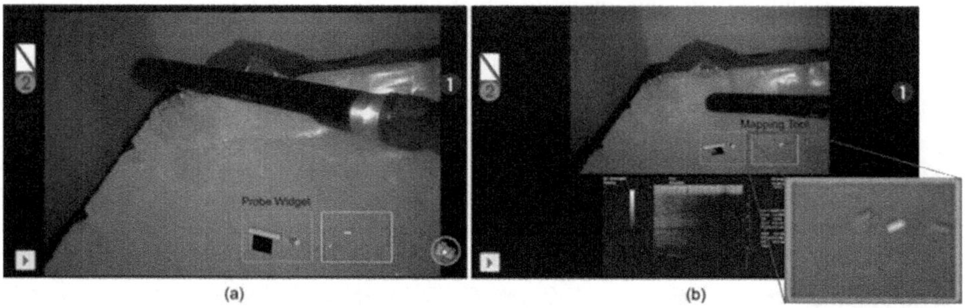

Fig. 4. (a) The graphical probe widget indicates the transducer and image plane orientation as well as wrist configuration. (b) A mapping tool indicates the current probe position and orientation (white cursor), as well as "bread crumbs" (green markers).

2.4 User Studies

A user study was conducted in order to evaluate the performance of the robotic ultrasound probe, as well as to compare its capabilities against a standard hand-held laparoscopic probe. This section describes these experiments and preliminary results.

Each task discussed below was completed with both the robotic system described above, and a standard laparoscopic ultrasound instrument (Aloka UST-5536-7.5, as shown in Figure 2a). Surgeons experienced with laparoscopy and IOUS were recruited to participate in the user study, following protocol approval by the Johns Hopkins University Institutional Review Board. A total of ten subjects participated in the study; seven completed the full protocol, while three subjects completed only the lesion finding or biopsy tasks. All subjects' results and questionnaire responses were used where appropriate. The subjects came from a wide variety of backgrounds and specialties, although we focused on subjects with some laparoscopic, robotic and ultrasound experience. Figure 5 shows the experience of the subjects in each of these main

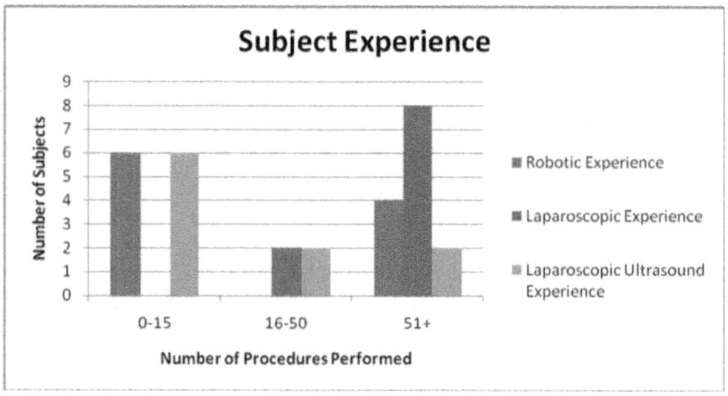

Fig. 5. The experience levels of the 10 study subjects. Each subject reported their experience as the number of procedures they had performed in several relevant areas.

areas. All subjects were scored equally, despite their level of experience in a particular area.

Specific tasks were designed based on surgical relevance and difficulty with traditional laparoscopic techniques. Both *in vivo* and *ex vivo* models were implemented, using the liver as the target organ for study. These tasks included: (1) liver surface manipulation and imaging volume capability, (2) detection and imaging quality of intrahepatic structures, (3) lesion detection and (4) needle biopsy guidance. The time to complete each task was recorded, in addition to other specific measures related to the successful completion. A short period of practice was allowed for each task. The task was explained in detail before beginning and all questions from the subjects were answered at this time. The order of the tasks was randomized in order to minimize learning effects. Upon completion of the tasks, a questionnaire was administered to each subject to query their satisfaction and clinical usefulness of the system. The results from this survey are shown in Figure 6.

The first two tasks mimic exploration of a solid organ, as might be done during the assessment of liver during hepatic surgery. First, the subjects were asked to scan of the anterior surface of an *in vivo* porcine liver, contacting as much of the liver surface and scanning as much of the liver volume as possible. Videos were recorded and blindly scored after completion, based on the amount of surface reached and the quality and consistency of the ultrasound image produced. The subjects were then asked to identify and image specific structures within the liver: gallbladder, portal veins, hepatic veins, and the inferior vena cava. They were asked to capture US images in both transverse and sagittal planes. Video and still images were then blindly scored based on the quality of ultrasound images and the ability of the surgeon to manipulate the probe into the proper orientation. Each image was scored on a scale from 1-4, 4 being outstanding and 1 being poor. A total of 44 points were awarded for the *in vivo* tasks. Subjects were scored from 1-4 on their ability to scan as much of the liver surface as possible. Points were awarded based on the percentage of each liver lobe that was covered. Each of the eight images of the four anatomical features was worth up to 4 points and additional scores were given based on image quality and the subjects' ability to manipulate the probe.

The third task mimicked lesion detection in a solid organ. For this, phantoms were constructed from polyvinyl chloride (PVC) plastic, similar to material described in [21]. Both hyper- and hypo-echoic lesions were created using different proportions of an acoustic scattering material (glass microspheres). These phantoms measured approximately 20cm × 10cm × 5cm. Lesions varied in conspicuity (echogenicity), depth, and size (5-15mm diameter). All lesions were spheroid in shape. Subjects were provided a phantom containing 1-8 lesions, the actual number being unknown to them. They were asked to identify and measure all lesions as accurately and rapidly as possible and declare when completed. The percentage of lesions correctly identified was recorded and scored, as well as the overall measurement accuracy (in estimating lesion volume). The score for this task was a combination of the percentage of lesions found within the phantom, the total percent volume error in the measurement of the lesions, and the subjects' confidence that they had found all of the possible lesions. Each of these scoring metrics was given a total of 12 points, so that the maximum score achievable in this task was 36 points.

The fourth task determined the capability of the subject to perform accurate ultrasound-guided needle core biopsy using the RLUS system. For these studies, phantoms were created from *ex vivo* bovine liver. Target *1*cm lesions were made using fast-setting dental alginate polymer and inserted at least *3*cm within the liver parenchyma. The alginate material polymerizes as a semi-firm material similar in consistency to human liver and can be biopsied using a needle core biopsy device. In addition, the polymerized material is white in color, enabling easy identification of a successful biopsy. The liver phantom was placed within an opaque torso model and subjects were allowed to practice and shown the location and US appearance of the target. They were then asked to robotically guide the biopsy needle to the target lesion using the RLUS system. The biopsy device was stabilized and deployed by an assistant from the outside when told by the subject. The success of the task was determined by the presence of the white polymer material in the extracted biopsy core. The number of times the subject punctured the surface of the liver was recorded. This is important in a clinical environment where excessive bleeding and tissue damage can be caused by repeated punctures through the surface of the organ. An overall score was determined as a combination of the positive biopsies, the number of liver punctures and the time that was required to acquire the biopsy, yielding a maximum possible score of 36 points for this task.

Average and standard deviation for each task was calculated and scoring scale was used to in order to provide each section of the task a weighted point value. All points are combined in order to produce a final score for each subject. In order to gain insight into each task that was completed, each mean and standard deviation are displayed independently and grouped by task.

Scores for each task were determined either by the evaluation of video, by comparing the values reported by the subject with known values and configurations of a phantom, or by visual confirmation. These scores were then summed for each task and summed for the entire experiment. These results are shown as percents of the maximum score in Table 1.

The robotic portion of this experiment also incorporated the image visualizations and user interfaced discussed in the previous section. To simplify the experiments and avoid confusing the subjects, the interface additions were displayed when it was believed to be most useful to the subjects. The graphical representation of the ultrasound tool, as seen in Figure 3a and Figure 4 was used during all tasks. The mapping tool (Figure 4) and the measuring tool were used during the lesion finding task. This allowed the subjects to determine if a lesion had been previously identified, and allowed an accurate measurement of out of plane motion.

The user interface illustrated in Figure 3a was used to facilitate the study described in the remainder of this paper. Early surgeon feedback indicated some discomfort with the "flashlight" display mode shown in Figure 3c, primarily due to regions of interest within the surgical field being obscured from view by the ultrasound image overlay. Surgeons much preferred a split screen or picture-in-picture display, with the probe widget and mapping feature inset for guidance. A simple manual calibration of the ultrasound-to-image transform was used to render the probe widget, as this tool was intended to indicate approximate probe orientation and wrist configuration only. While only an approximate ultrasound image calibration was required to evaluate the feasibility of the "flashlight" image overlay, one can implement a more accurate automatic calibration similar to that described in [20].

2.5 Results

Although the study subjects came from varied backgrounds and had a wide range of experience levels, experience level did not correlate to a significant change in the final score of the subjects. Table 1 shows the mean and standard deviation of the scores for each of the tasks and subtasks. The scores are shown as a percentage of the total attainable point score. The mean combined score for *in vivo* tasks completed with the robotic instrument was 80.2% ± 7.3%.

Table 1. Results from a selection of experiment tasks, as well as combined scores. All scores are shown as a percentage of the total possible points available, except in the case of the average number of punctures during biopsy. The weighting of each task represents the total possible points that are available for that particular task or subtask. Please note that not every subtask is listed in the table.

Task	*da Vinci* Mean ±σ [%]	Weighting	Scoring Method
Lesions Found	72±16.4	12	Compared to known phantom
Lesion Volume Error	27.8±11.3	12	Compared to known phantom
Confidence in Lesion Identification	72.5±15.3	12	Subject questionnaire
Overall Lesion Task Score	62.5±16.2	36	Weighted average of lesion scores
Positive Biopsy	50±35.6	12	Visual confirmation of pseudo
Average number of Punctures	2.66±2.1	12	Scored from video
Overall Biopsy task Score	56.6±20.35	36	Weighted average of biopsy scores
Liver Surface exploration	84.5 ± 8.9	12	Expert evaluation
Anatomy Identification	76.2±14.4	24	Expert evaluation
Tool Manipulation	78.6 ± 9.4	4	Expert evaluation
Combined In vivo task score	80.2 ± 7.3	44	Weighted average of expert scores
Total Combined score	**64.0 ± 13.1**	**116**	**Weighted average of all scores**

During the lesion finding task, each subject was presented with a phantom that included anywhere from 1 – 8 lesions. The average percentage of the number of lesions found with the *da Vinci* ultrasound instrument was 72%. The total error for this task was relatively low at about 30% and the overall score of this task was 62.5%.

The biopsy task presented the greatest challenge to all subjects and the results are shown in Table 1. Most of the subjects had very little experience in this area, and this was the most difficult of the 3 tasks. Out of a total of 3 biopsy attempts, the subjects were successful in, on average, 50% of the attempts with the robotic tools. A positive biopsy was verified visually by examining the core of tissue from the biopsy needle. The maximum number of punctures varied widely, from a maximum of 10 in one case to a minimum of a single puncture. There was no obvious correlation between the number of punctures and a successful outcome. All the subjects were combined and the mean and standard deviation are reported in Table 1.

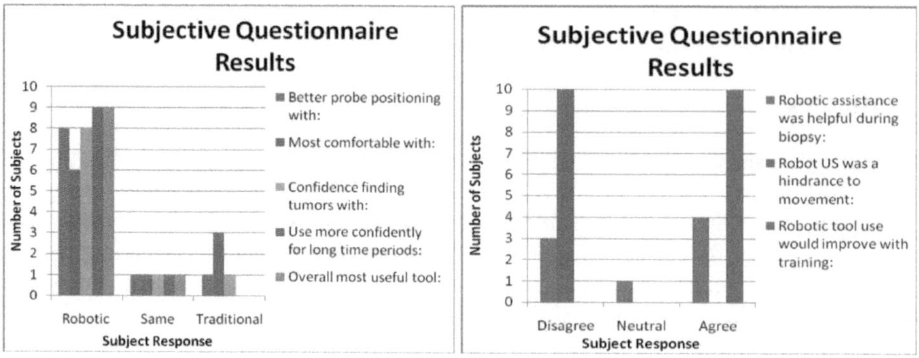

Fig. 6. The results from the subjective questionnaire, which asked subjects to agree or disagree with several statements, and compare the robotic ultrasound instrument against their experience with traditional hand-held laparoscopic probes.

A selection of results from the subjective questionnaires is presented in Figure 6. The subjective questions allowed us to assess how the subjects felt about the tasks and tools and compare there experiences during the study to their experiences with traditional handheld laparoscopic ultrasound tools. Most notable among the responses was to the question: "Which instrument did you find most useful over all?" In this case, 9 of the 10 subjects replied that the robotic instrument was most useful. The one subject that replied that they felt both tools were equally useful was only able to complete the lesion finding task. Every subject also disagreed that the robotic tool was a hindrance to their freedom of motion.

Many of the subjects expressed their enthusiasm for the user interface additions. They appreciated the additional information that was provided to them, even if they did not take full advantage of that information. The measurement tool and the mapping tool were used extensively by the subjects during the lesion identification task. This interface was used to help with lesion dimension measurements, and to avoid measuring the same lesion multiple times. The probe representation (Figure 4a) was most beneficial during the *in vivo* anatomy identification and the simulated biopsy. In both of these tasks, it was necessary to know, with some accuracy, in which direction the US beam was facing. In the first case, it was used to determine to the location of liver structures, and in the second case to align the imaging plane with the incoming needle.

3 Discussion

The robotic laparoscopic ultrasound system presented here has the potential to overcome many of the limitations found with our current technologies. We have shown that high-quality operative ultrasound imaging can be achieved using the minimally-invasive *da Vinci* robotic platform. These studies demonstrate the RLUS probe to be capable of covering a large amount of the liver surface, generating imaging comparable to that of open IOUS. The high level of dexterity and image quality documented in these studies validate the potential usefulness of our RLUS system for improving the performance of complex surgical tasks though a minimally invasive approach. Interestingly, we found that the additional features that were integrated into the system markedly contributed to user satisfaction. These included a variety of image display options (e.g., split-screen, picture-in-picture, flashlight overlay), measurement tools, probe status widget, and a landmark mapping capability.

The subjects were able to complete all the tasks to a satisfactory level, and their overall performance indicates that the system provides an effective environment for IOUS even in its current prototypical state. Qualitatively, the subjects' feedback, as drawn from responses to the study questionnaire, was very positive, both with respect to the effectiveness of the articulated *da Vinci* IOUS tool and in comparison with traditional hand-held articulated laparoscopic probe. A detailed quantitative comparison of surgeon performance between the *da Vinci* IOUS tool and a hand-held probe is beyond the scope of this paper, and will be taken in future work. Despite the small sample size and the need for rigorous statistical analyses, however, preliminary indications are that performance with the *da Vinci* IOUS tool is at least comparable to that with traditional instruments. Further, one significant advantage of the integrated *da Vinci* approach is that the surgeon has much better interactive control over the probe to obtain the image that he or she wants while doing the surgery, rather than having to coordinate with an assistant to control the imaging at the patient side.

The experience of the subjects participating in this study varied widely, from those who had almost no robotic experience to those who were very experienced robotic surgeons. Their experience with porcine anatomy and the general use of laparoscopic ultrasound also varied significantly. Nevertheless, the results of the subjective questionnaire are interesting when subject experience is taken into consideration. Whereas most subjects had more traditional laparoscopic experience than robotic, they were still likely to agree that they were better able to position the probe, and that they were more confident and less fatigued when using the robotic ultrasound instrument. In all cases, the subjects agreed that they believed their performance would improve with additional training time.

4 Conclusions and Future Work

This paper has reported the development and initial user evaluation of a dexterous laparoscopic ultrasound tool and supporting augmented reality software for the *da Vinci* surgical robot. This combination provides surgeons with an effective and natural means of using intraoperative LUS, providing much of the "feel" of open intraoperative ultrasound imaging within a *da Vinci* telerobotic environment. Our main goals in developing this system were to gain experience with an articulated IOUS tool for the *da Vinci,* to determine whether such a system could indeed provide an effective IOUS capability for a surgeon, and to obtain feedback for future study. Our initial experiences with the system are encouraging, and the response from surgeon users has been positive. The qualitative feedback from our very small preliminary study indicates that the system offers significant advantages in probe positioning and confidence in finding tumors, compared to subjects' experience with traditional freehand articulated LUS probes. A careful statistical analysis of relative quantitative task performance measures is planned for future work.

Although our initial phantom and *in vivo* studies used liver surgery as a focusing application, the system is readily applicable to other surgical procedures, including kidney and prostate surgery, pancreatectomy, and gynecologic procedures. One near-term target is laparoscopic partial nephrectomies. Concurrently, we are beginning to explore enhancements to our software environment to further exploit the potential of *da Vinci* LUS. Topics include: incorporation of "virtual fixtures" to assist surgeons in acquiring LUS images and 3-D volumes; palpation behaviors for assisting in acquisition of LUS elastography images; registration of LUS B-mode and elastography images to preoperative cross-sectional imaging and surgical plans; 3D augmented reality displays of this information within the *da Vinci* console; and improved tools and software virtual fixtures for assisting in LUS-guided biopsies and other needle placement procedures. Further study of the user interface and display methods illustrated in Figure 3 would also be interesting. In particular, a follow-on comparative study of the ultrasound image display modes, using the same tasks described in the present study, may provide guidance for further taking advantage of the robotic system for enhanced image guidance and navigation.

Application of IOUS to the *da Vinci* system provides many additional benefits above and beyond that of even open surgical imaging. The high quality stereo endoscopic visualization and control of secondary grasping and manipulating tools provided with robot further improves IOUS. Moreover, integration of IOUS into this robotic platform will allow for future improvements in the system, including robot-assisted integrated tool guidance and image registration. In order to continue expanding the indications and improving outcomes of robotic surgery, development of image-guidance tools such as these are important. Systems such as these will allow for expanded use of minimally invasive techniques for complex surgical procedures not otherwise amenable to this approach. Moreover, developments such as these have the potential to improve patient safety and reduce health care costs through more cost-effective use of robotic systems.

Acknowledgements

The research reported in this paper was supported in part by NIH STTR Grant R42RR019159 and NSF cooperative agreement EEC9731748, respectively, as well as by internal funds from our institutions. The authors also wish to acknowledge Dr. Emad Boctor for his assistance during the development of this work.

References

[1] Patel, V.R., Palmer, K.J., Coughlin, G., Samavedi, S.: Robot-assisted laparoscopic radical prostatectomy: perioperative outcomes of 1500 cases. J. Endourol. 22, 2299–2305 (2008)

[2] Drouin, S.J., Vaessen, C., Hupertan, V., Comperat, E., Misrai, V., Haertig, A., Bitker, M.O., Chartier-Kastler, E., Richard, F., Roupret, M.: Comparison of mid-term carcinologic control obtained after open, laparoscopic, and robot-assisted radical prostatectomy for localized prostate cancer. World J. Urol. 27, 599–605 (2009)

[3] Ukimura, O., Nakamoto, M., Desai, M., Herts, B., Aron, M., Haber, G.-P., Kaouk, J., Miki, T., Sato, Y., Hashizume, M., Gill, I.: Augmented Reality Visualization During Laparoscopic Urologic Surgery: the Initial Clinical Experience. In: The 102nd American Urological Association (AUA 2007) Annual Meeting, Anaheim, p. V1052 (2007)

[4] Su, L.-M., Vagvolgyi, B.P., Agarwal, R., Reiley, C.E., Taylor, R.H., Hager, G.D.: Augmented Reality During Robot-assisted Laparoscopic Partial Nephrectomy: Toward Real-Time 3D-CT to Stereoscopic Video Registration. Urology 73, 896–900 (2009)

[5] Wagner, C.R., Stylopoulos, N., Jackson, P.G., Howe, R.D.: The Benefit of Force Feedback in Surgery: Examination of Blunt Dissection. Presence: Teleoperators and Virtual Environments (2007)

[6] Okamura, A.M.: Methods for Haptic Feedback in Teleoperated Robot-Assisted Surgery. Industrial Robot 31, 499–508 (2004)

[7] Kapoor, A., Taylor, R.: A Constrained Optimization Approach to Virtual Fixtures for Multi-Handed Tasks. In: IEEE International Conference on Robotics and Automation (ICRA), Pasadena, pp. 3401–3406 (2008)

[8] Marayong, P., Bettini, A., Okamura, A.: Effect of Virtual Fixture Compliance on Human-Machine Cooperative Manipulation. In: EEE/RSJ International Conference on Intelligent Robots and Systems, pp. 1089–1095 (2002)

[9] Park, S., Howe, R.D., Torchiana, D.F.: Virtual Fixtures for Robotic Cardiac Surgery. In: Niessen, W.J., Viergever, M.A. (eds.) MICCAI 2001. LNCS, vol. 2208. Springer, Heidelberg (2001)

[10] Kazanzides, P., Hata, N., Ibanez, L.: Systems and Architectures for Computer Assisted Interventions (MICCAI 2008 Workshop) – Issue of Insight Journal, New York (2008)

[11] Bosch, F., Ribes, J., Cléries, R., Díaz, M.: Epidemiology of hepatocellular carcinoma. Clin. Liver Dis. 9, 191–211 (2005)

[12] Kane, R.A.: Intraoperative Ultrasonography, History, Current State of the Art, and Future Directions. J. Ultrasound Med. 23, 1407–1420 (2004)

[13] Zacherl, J., Scheuba, C., Imhof, M., Zacherl, M., Langle, F., Pokieser, P., Wrba, F., Wenzl, E., Muhlbacher, F., Jakesz, R., Steininger, R.: Current value of intraoperative sonography during surgery for hepatic neoplasms. World J. Surg. 26, 550–554 (2002)

[14] Fleming, I.N., Rivaz, H., Macura, K., Su, L.-M., Hamper, U., Lotan, T., Lagoda, G., Burnett, A., Taylor, R.H., Hager, G.D., Boctor, E.M.: Ultrasound elastography: enabling technology for image guided laparoscopic prostatectomy. In: SPIE Medical Imaging 2009: Visualization, Image-guided Procedures and Modeling, Orlando, Florida, vol. 7261, pp. 72612I–72612I-12 (2009)

[15] Salcudean, S., Wen, X.u., Mahdavi, S., Moradi, M., Morris, J.W., Spadinger, I.: Ultrasound elastography – an image guidance tool for prostate brachytherapy. Brachytherapy 8, 125–126 (2009)

[16] Wood, T., Rose, D., Chung, M., Allegra, D., Foshag, L., Bilchik, A.: Radiofrequency ablation of 231 unre-sectable hepatic tumors: indications, limitations, and complications. Ann. Surg. Oncol. 7, 593–600 (2000)

[17] Fenster, A., Downey, D.B., Cardinal, H.N.: Three-dimensional ultrasound imaging. Phys. Med. Biol. 46, R67–R99 (2001)

[18] Cunha, D.d., Gravez, P., Leroy, C., Maillard, E., Jouan, J., Varley, P., Jones, M., Halliwell, M., Hawkes, D., Wells, P.N.T., Angelini, L.: The MIDSTEP System for Ultrasound guided Remote Telesurgery. In: IEEE EMBS, pp. 1266–1269 (1998)

[19] Budde, R.P.J., Dessing, T.C., Meijer, R., Bakker, P.F.A., Borst, C., Gründeman, P.F.: Robot-assisted 13 MHz epicardial ultrasound for endoscopic quality assessment of coronary anastomoses. Interactive Cardiovascular and Thoracic Surgery 3 (2004)
[20] Leven, J., Burschka, D., Kumar, R., Zhang, G., Blumenkranz, S.J., Dai, X., Awad, M., Hager, G., Marohn, M., Choti, M., Hasser, C., Taylor, R.H.: DaVinci Canvas: A Telerobotic Surgical System with Integrated, Robot-Assisted, Laparoscopic Ultrasound Capability. In: Duncan, J.S., Gerig, G. (eds.) MICCAI 2005. LNCS, vol. 3749, pp. 811–818. Springer, Heidelberg (2005)
[21] Mansy, H.A., Grahe, J.R., Sandler, R.H.: Elastic properties of synthetic materials for soft tissue modeling. Phys. Med. Biol. 53, 2115–2130 (2008)

New Kinematic Metric for Quantifying Surgical Skill for Flexible Instrument Manipulation*

Jagadeesan Jayender[1,2], Raúl San Jośe Estépar[1], and Kirby G.Vosburgh[1,2]

[1] Department of Radiology, Harvard Medical School, Brigham and Women's Hospital, Boston, MA, USA
{jayender,rjosest,kirby}@bwh.harvard.edu
[2] CIMIT Image Guidance Laboratory, Boston, MA, USA

Abstract. Colonoscopy is a minimally invasive endoscopic procedure to survey, diagnose and treat possible disease in the colon. Clinicians are trained to manipulate a colonoscope while minimizing the force exerted on the colon walls to reduce the danger of luminal perforation and discomfort to the patient. Here, we propose and evaluate a metric, called Global Isotropy Index (GII), to quantify the expertise of the clinician. The colonoscope is modeled as a continuum robot with multiple bending sections. The Jacobian operator, which relates the proximal forces applied by the clinician to the distal forces, provides a basis to compute the GII. Experimental results in a colon model (CM-1, Olympus, Tokyo, Japan) are shown to compare the efficacy of this metric in characterizing operator performance compared to standard metrics such as elapsed time, path length, and kinematics factors. The GII values for experts are significantly different from those of novices; our initial studies show that it can be as much as 1.45 times greater for the experts.

1 Introduction

Historically, the performance of gastroenterologists, surgeons, and related practitioners has been assessed subjectively by senior physicians in both training and operating environments. Increasing concern regarding poor surgical dexterity [1] and the broader use of minimally invasive interventions promoted efforts to better characterize operator performance [2] and improve the effectiveness and efficacy of training [3]. Electronic instrument tracking systems provide precise measures of instrument position and movement, enabling the characterization of performance in a range of venues, including task trainers [4], electronically simulated work environments [5],[6], animal models, and robotic systems [7]. Analytical approaches, such as task partitioning [8], kinematics analysis [9], off-line "data mining" to train hidden Markov models [10] or support vector machines [11], and many others have been developed. These techniques may now be used

* This work has been funded by NIH/NCI under award 2 R42 CA115112-02A2 and the Center for Integration of Medicine and Innovative Technology (CIMIT), Boston, MA.

N. Navab and P. Jannin (Eds.): IPCAI 2010, LNCS 6135, pp. 81–90, 2010.

to measure the potential value of new interventional systems, for example determining the value of augmented reality displays to assist an endoscopist or surgeon in performing procedures [12],[13] and to elucidate features which are most "helpful" to guide the development of system capabilities. These activities may be best advanced by use of broadly accepted and widely applicable performance measures, which, in practice, should be simple to compute and both sensitive and robust.

We consider here the development of a composite metric to better differentiate classes of operators; that is, to separate "novice" from "experienced" from "expert" classes. This will enable training to proceed with more confidence, and also characterize the possible benefits of proposed enhancements of the information presented to the operator during the procedure. In this paper, we have utilized the Global Isotropy Index (GII) to quantify the expertise of the operator. GII was first proposed in [14] to quantify the isotropy of a robot's Jacobian based on which a globally optimum architecture for a planar haptic interface has been designed. In [15], a 3-DOF twin pantograph has been designed to ensure static force isotropy by optimizing the GII. A variation of GII has also been employed to analyze the isotropy of a wheeled omnidirectional mobile robot [16]. In [17], GII has been employed to evaluate the optimal port of insertion of surgical tools for performing minimally invasive coronary artery bypass graft surgery. In [18], the optimal transseptal puncture location for performing left atrial catheter ablation has been evaluated by optimizing the GII. To the best of the authors' knowledge, this is the first paper to employ the GII to quantify the surgical skill involved in manipulating a highly flexible surgical instrument.

2 Modeling of Colonoscope

The colonoscope is assumed to be comprised of infinitesimal rigid links along a backbone curve. The backbone curve is defined in terms of the Frenet-Serret frame, which is represented in the parametric form, $\bar{x} = \bar{x}(s,t)$, where s is the parameter which represents the curve length and t is the time. The Frenet-Serret

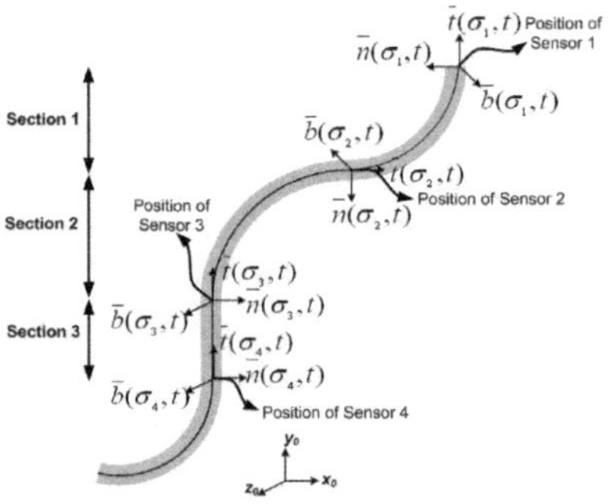

Fig. 1. Model for the Colonoscope

frame is defined at each point $\sigma(s,t)$ along the backbone curve and consists of the tangent $\bar{t}(s,t)$, normal $\bar{n}(s,t)$ and binormal $\bar{b}(s,t)$ vector at point $\sigma(s,t)$, as shown in Figure 1. At any point σ along the curve $\bar{x}(s,t)$, the local frame ${}^0\Phi(\sigma,t)$ can be defined with respect to the local frame as ${}^0\Phi(0)$ as

$$ {}^0\Phi(\sigma,t) = \begin{bmatrix} \cos(\sigma\varsigma)\cos(\sigma\tau) & -\sin(\sigma\varsigma) & \cos(\sigma\varsigma)\sin(\sigma\tau) \\ \sin(\sigma\varsigma)\cos(\sigma\tau) & \cos(\sigma\varsigma) & \sin(\sigma\varsigma)\sin(\sigma\tau) \\ -\sin(\sigma\tau) & 0 & \cos(\sigma\tau) \end{bmatrix} \tag{1} $$

where ς is the curvature and τ is the torsion of the scope. The position vector $\bar{p}(\sigma,t)$ of a point σ on the curve relative to the origin $\bar{p}(0)$ can be computed by integrating infinitesimal curve lengths along the tangent vector. In other words, ${}^0\bar{p}(\sigma)$, which represents the position of a point σ on the curve as viewed in the base frame ${}^0\Phi(0)$ is given by

$$ {}^0\bar{p}(\sigma,t) = \int_0^\sigma {}^0\Phi(\eta,t)d\eta \tag{2} $$

where $\hat{e_x} = [1\ 0\ 0]^T$. Each segment of the colonoscope can be considered to consist of two rotational joints and a prismatic joint. The joint angle vector can be written as $\bar{\theta} = [0\ \varsigma\ \tau]^t$ and the translational vector can be written as $\bar{d} = [l_x\ 0\ 0]^t$ The linear ${}^0v(\sigma)$ and rotational velocity ${}^0\omega(\sigma)$ for a joint in the local Frenet-Serret frame with respect to the base frame can be written in a compact form as

$$ \begin{bmatrix} {}^0v(\sigma) \\ {}^0\omega(\sigma) \end{bmatrix} = \int_0^\sigma \begin{bmatrix} {}^\sigma\Phi(\nu,t) & [(p(\nu,t)-p(\sigma,t))\times]\Phi(\nu,t) \\ 0 & \Phi(\nu,t) \end{bmatrix} \bar{A} \begin{bmatrix} \dot{d} \\ \dot{\varsigma} \\ \dot{\tau} \end{bmatrix} d\nu \tag{3} $$

where

$$ \bar{A} = \begin{bmatrix} 1\,0\,0\,0\,0\,0 \\ 0\,0\,0\,0\,0\,1 \\ 0\,0\,0\,0\,1\,0 \end{bmatrix}^T \quad \text{and}[a\times] \triangleq \begin{bmatrix} 0 & -a_z & a_y \\ a_z & 0 & -a_x \\ -a_y & a_x & 0 \end{bmatrix} \tag{4} $$

Using the standard robotics terminology, the Jacobian operator can be defined as

$$ \mathcal{J}(\sigma,t) = \int_0^\sigma \begin{bmatrix} {}^\sigma\Phi(\nu,t) & [p(\nu,t)-p(\sigma,t)\times]\Phi(\nu,t) \\ 0 & \Phi(\nu,t) \end{bmatrix} \bar{A}(.)d\nu \tag{5} $$

The colonoscope is considered to consist of three segments, defined in practice by four electromagnetic sensors placed along the colonoscope, which measure the position and orientation of their points of attachment. From (2), we can estimate the position of the colonoscope with respect to the base coordinates for a given configuration of the scope. However, for each segment of the scope, we assume that the consecutive sensors represent the base and end-effector coordinates of the segment and solve the inverse kinematics problem to evaluate the configuration $q = (s, \varsigma, \tau)$ of the scope.

We solve the inverse kinematics problem to determine the configuration of the scope for a given set of base and end-effector coordinates. The problem is formulated as a dynamical problem requiring only the computation of the forward kinematics, as determined by (2). Let us represent the solution of the inverse kinematics problem as $\hat{q}(t)$ corresponding to a trajectory $\hat{x}(t)$ which satisfies the forward kinematics given by (2). Let $e(t)$ represent the error between the desired Cartesian position $\hat{x}(t)$ and the actual Cartesian position obtained from the state variable q of the iteration algorithm. The error dynamics can be written as

$$\dot{e}(t) = \dot{\hat{x}}(t) - \dot{x}(t) = \dot{\hat{x}}(t) - \mathcal{J}\dot{q} \tag{6}$$

We choose a purely proportional control law to solve for $\dot{q}$ as given by

$$\dot{q} = \alpha \mathcal{J}^T e \tag{7}$$

It has been shown [19] that by choosing a control law as given by (7), the error e is bounded and can be made small with an appropriate choice of α, with the added benefit of less computational complexity. The algorithm consists of the following steps:

- `Choose the initial value of` q_0.
  Begin Loop:
- `From forward kinematics, compute the Cartesian position` x_k `for corresponding joint variable` q_k
- `Calculate the error vector` $e_k = \|\hat{x} - x_k\|$
- `If` e_k `< tol(=` $1e^{-12}$`), exit loop`
- `Calculate` $q_{k+1} = q_k + \alpha \mathcal{J}^T e_k$
- `Go to Begin Loop`
  `End Loop`
- `Inverse kinematics solution is` q_n

3 Global Isotropy Index

The Jacobian matrix relates the end-effector frame forces f to the corresponding joint torques τ, as given by the following equations

$$\tau = \mathcal{J}^T f \tag{8}$$

Condition number κ of the Jacobian $\mathcal{J}$ can be considered as the error amplification factor from the joint space to the Cartesian space. Taking the norm on both sides of (8), we obtain

$$\frac{\|\delta\tau\|}{\|\tau\|} \leq \|\mathcal{J}^{-T}\|\|\mathcal{J}^T\|\frac{\|\delta f\|}{\|f\|} \tag{9}$$

Since $\|\mathcal{J}^T\|$ is equal to $\|\mathcal{J}\|$, the condition number κ is, therefore, defined as [20]

$$\kappa(J) = \|\mathcal{J}^{-1}\|\|\mathcal{J}\| = \frac{\overline{\sigma}(J(q))}{\underline{\sigma}(J(q))} \tag{10}$$

where $\overline{\sigma}$ and $\underline{\sigma}$ represent the maximum and minimum singular values of $\mathcal{J}$. In [14], [15] the Global Isotropy Index (GII) has been proposed to define the force isotropy throughout the workspace. The GII is used in this paper to define a global metric for evaluating the expertise of the clinician in actuating the distal end of the scope from the proximal end. The GII is defined as

$$GII = \frac{\min\limits_{t_0 \leq T} \underline{\sigma}(\mathcal{J}_{t_0})}{\max\limits_{t_1 \leq T} \overline{\sigma}(\mathcal{J}_{t_1})} \tag{11}$$

where T is the duration of the procedure, t_0 and t_1 are two instants during the procedure. GII is a global variable which determines the isotropy or the uniformity of the force transmitted to the distal end from the proximal end. Since the goal of colonoscopy is to uniformly transmit forces to the distal end of the scope, GII is also a metric to define the expertise in manipulating the distal end of the scope while minimizing the amount of flexing caused due to excessive curvature in the scope.

4 Experimental Methods

The experimental setup, shown in Figure 2, consists of a colon model (CM-1, Olympus, Tokyo, Japan), which closely mimics the human colon and includes the ascending, descending and transverse colon. The model is loosely tethered to the back support, thereby allowing it to flex and stretch, as observed in an actual procedure. The entire model is draped with a cloth to prevent the user from observing the location of the scope tip inside the model. A pediatric colonoscope (PCF-Q180AL, Olympus, Tokyo, Japan) is mounted with four electromagnetic 6-DOF position sensors (Microbird sensors from Ascension Technologies Inc. (ATI), Burlington, VT). The sensors are placed at 0cm, 10cm, 30cm and 55cm from the distal end. Sensor 1 and sensor 2 are placed to record the angulation of the distal end of the scope in 2-DOF about the y and z-axis. The position of sensors 3 and 4 are chosen such that these sensors are approximately in the

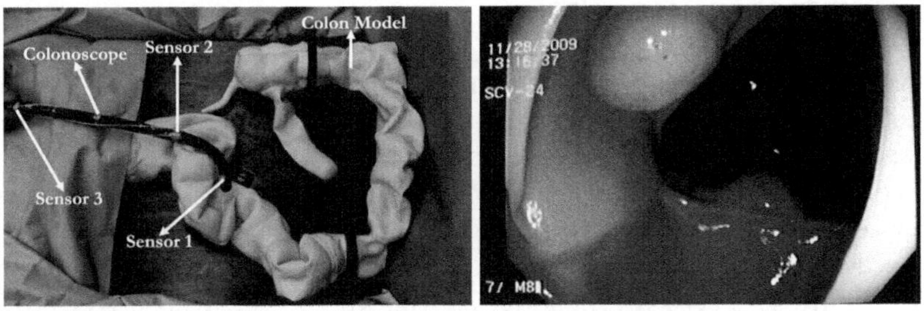

Fig. 2. (a) Colon model and colonoscope showing the position of sensor 1, 2 and 3. Sensor 4 is out of the field. (b) Inner view of the model showing a realistic modeling of the human colon.

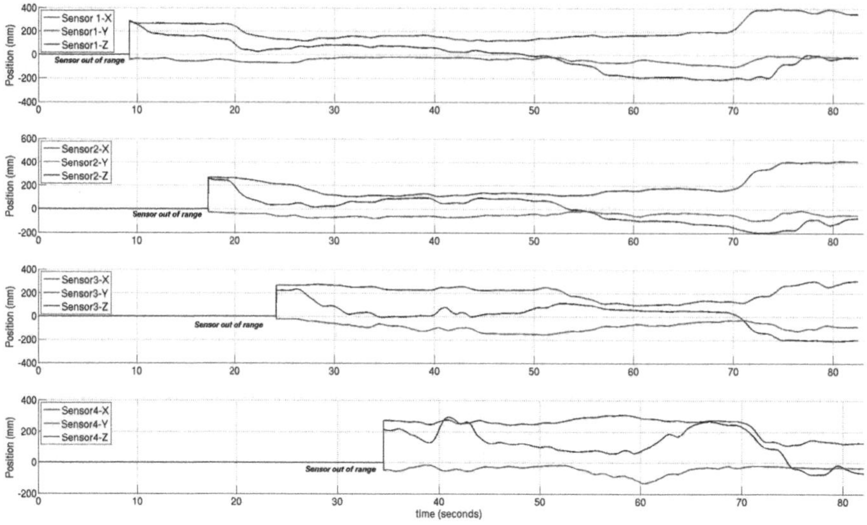

Fig. 3. Trajectory of the four electromagnetic sensors

recto-sigmoid junction when the distal end of the scope is in the traverse colon region, thereby allowing for the detection of flexing and looping of the scope. The ATI electromagnetic system is interfaced to an Intel Quad Core 2GHz computer with 4GB RAM. The position readings are logged at a sampling rate of 67 Hz using MATLAB Simulink.

Four attending endoscopists who have performed more than 2000 colonoscopies and 9 gastroenterology fellows (3 first-year, 3 second-year, 3 third-year) who have performed less than 500 colonoscopies were selected to perform a colonoscopy. Kinematics data consisting of the position and orientation of the four sensors, and time were recorded from the instant of insertion of the scope into the anus to the instant when the terminal ileum was intubated.

5 Experimental Results

Thirteen GI endoscopists performed colonoscopy in the colon model. The time taken to reach the terminal ileum from the anus ranged from 82 seconds to 1065 seconds. The position measurements from the four electromagnetic sensors were logged continuously, as shown in Figure 3. From the position measurements of the four sensors, the velocity and acceleration were calculated as the first and second order time-derivatives of the position measurements, as shown for Sensor 1 in Figure 4. These are denoted as Vel. and Accel. respectively in Table 1. In addition, the path lengths traversed by the four sensors were calculated by integrating the differential position measurements of the sensors over time

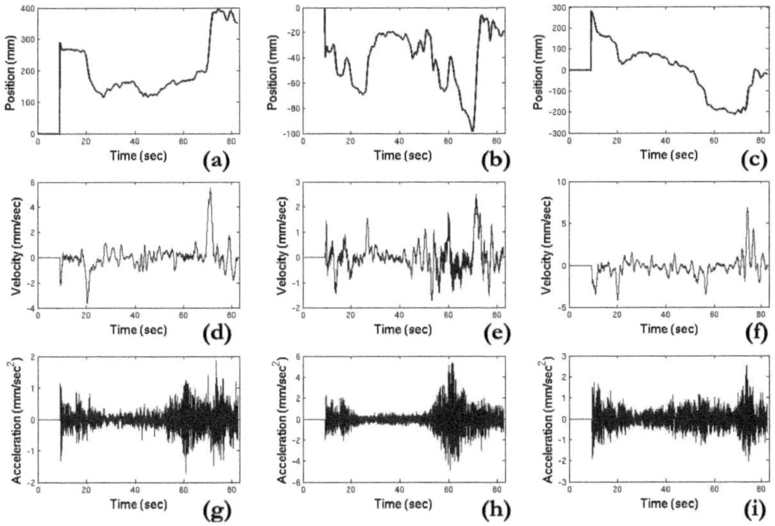

Fig. 4. Sensor 1 measurements: (a),(b),(c) represent the position trajectories in x, y and z directions respectively. (d),(e),(f) represent the velocity trajectories in x, y and z directions respectively. (g),(h),(i) represent the acceleration trajectories in x, y and z directions respectively.

(denoted as Pathlen in Table 1). A parameter called "flexing", computed as the difference in the path length of sensor 4 and sensor 2, has also been derived for different users. The rationale for calculating this parameter is that due to flexing of the scope, sensor 4, which is closer to the proximal end of the scope traverses a longer path than sensor 2, which is closer to the distal end. From the orientation measurements of sensor 1 and sensor 2, the angulation of the distal end of the scope is calculated in 2-DOF (denoted as Ang.Y and Ang.Z in Table 1), as shown in Figure 5 (a). In addition, the roll of the scope is calculated by measuring the roll of the local frame of the sensor at any time point with respect to the initial frame of reference (denoted Roll in Table 1), as shown in Figure 5 (b).

At every time point, the position readings of the four sensors are also input to the continuum robot module, which calculates the configuration (s, ς, τ) of the three segments of the colonoscope using the four sensor readings, as described in Sections 2 and 3. Based on the configuration of the scope, the Jacobian of the scope and the minimum and maximum singular values are evaluated at each time point. A search algorithm obtains the minimum and maximum singular values of the Jacobian for the duration of the experiment, based on which the GII is calculated. The experimental results are shown in Table 1. The table shows the median of the metric values for each category of users. Also the table shows the variance of the GII, represented as GII Var.

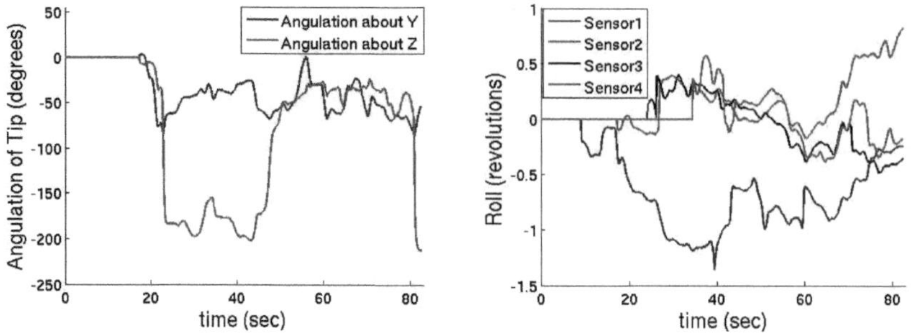

Fig. 5. (a) Graph showing the angulation of the distal end of the scope (b) Graph showing the roll of the four sensors

Table 1. Metrics for evaluating clinician's performance

	Time sec	Pathlen m	Flexing m	Av.Vel. mm/sec	Av.Accel. mm/sec^2	Av.Ang.Y degrees	Av.Ang.Z degrees	Av.Roll rev.	GII $\times 10^{-4}$	GII Var. $\times 10^{-7}$
1st Yr	715.4	10.92	5.33	0.83	0.65	39.7	95.7	0.21	3.45	0.30
2nd Yr	288.2	7.56	3.17	0.98	0.91	44.4	105.8	0.26	4.41	2.08
3rd Yr	274.9	5.16	1.53	1.15	0.63	40.5	96.8	0.16	4.60	0.32
Expert	150.1	3.31	1.75	1.29	0.99	42.0	95.3	0.22	5.01	2.03

6 Discussion

We conclude from Table 1 that the time taken for completion of the procedure is far less for an expert clinician than for the fellows. In addition, the average path length of the four sensors for the expert group is less compared with that of the first, second and third year fellows. We note that typically the length of the scope inserted into the colon model when the distal end reaches the terminal illeum is approximately 1m. The average path length traversed is much larger since the scope is repeatedly inserted and retracted to advance the scope forward. An expert clinician, therefore, appears to minimize the amount of back-and-forth motion of the scope and advances the distal end with relative ease as compared to the fellows. It can also be observed that the average velocity of the four sensors is greater for the expert group as compared to novices. However, none of the simple kinematics parameters (other than GII) shows a significant difference among the four groups of users.

We recognize that path length and time are not ideal kinematics parameters since in an actual colonoscopy procedure, the operator could take time or move the scope locally to study a particular feature or lesion. That is, path length and time are not only a function of the expertise of the clinician but also of the complexity of the procedure.

GII is an indication of isotropy or uniformity of control of the forces on the distal end of the colonoscope. GII shows a clear variation among the four groups of users. The median value of GII for the expert group is nearly a factor of 1.45 greater than that of novices. From (11), it can be seen that a larger value of GII implies that the minimum singular values of the Jacobian are further away from 0, implying that the scope is away from a singular configuration. This results in greater forces transmitted to the distal end of the scope, resulting in smoother insertion of the scope into the colon. In turn, this also results in higher velocities of the distal end, as validated by the kinematics data.

7 Conclusion

We have utilized the GII, which has been developed in the robotics literature to design isotropic robots, to quantify the skill of a clinician. We have shown that the use of position and orientation trackers can provide useful information on the performance of a colonoscope operator of a range of skills. However, simple kinematics parameters do not distinguish the performance of operators of varying skill levels. We have modeled the colonoscope as three segments of continuum robots and derived the Jacobian operator. By computing the minimum and maximum singular values of the Jacobian throughout the duration of the procedure, we have derived the GII. The GII provides a robust metric for characterizing operator skill. The GII for an expert clinician is measured to be nearly 1.45 times that of a first year fellow. This implies that the expert clinician maneuvers the colonoscope so that the force transmitted to the distal end is more uniform and results in minimal flexing while advancing the tip smoothly into the colon. Further work is underway in validating the results of this work in human colonoscopy.

References

1. Darzi, A., Smith, S., Taffinder, N.: Assessing operative skill: Need to become more objective. British Medical Journal 318, 887–888 (1999)
2. Satava, R., Cuschieri, A., Hamdorf, J.: Metrics for objective assessment: Preliminary results of the surgical skills workshop. Surgical Endoscopy 17, 220–226 (2003)
3. Peters, J., Fried, G., Swanstrom, L., Soper, N., Silin, L., Schirmer, B., Hoffman, K., et al.: Development and validation of a comprehensive program of education and assessment of the basic fundamentals of laparoscopic surgery. Surgery 135, 21–27 (2004)
4. Van Sickle, K., McClusky, D., Gallagher, A., Smith, C.: Validation of the promis simulator using a novel laparoscopic suturing task. Surgical Endoscopy 19, 1227–1231 (2005)
5. Gunther, S., Rosen, J., Hannaford, B., Sinanan, M.: The red dragon: A multi-modality system for simulation and training in minimally invasive surgery. Stud. Health Tech. and Info. 125, 149–154 (2007)
6. Neary, P., Boyle, E., Delaney, C., Senagore, A., Keane, F., Gallagher, A.: Construct validation of a novel hybrid virtual-reality simulator for training and assessing laparoscopic colectomy; results for the first course for experienced laparoscopoic surgeons. Surgical Endoscopy 22, 2301–2309 (2008)

7. Aggarwal, R., Grrantcharov, R., Murthy, K., Milland, T., Papasavas, P., Dosis, A., Bello, F., Darzi, A.: An evaluation of the feasibility, validity, and reliability of laparoscopic skills assessment in the operating room. Annals of Surgery 245, 992–999 (2007)
8. Heinrichs, W., Srivastava, S., Montgomery, K., Dev, P.: The fundamental manipulations of surgery: A structured vocabulary for designing surgical curricula and simulators. J. Amer. Assoc. of Gynecologic Laparoscopists 11, 450–456 (2004)
9. Dosis, D., Aggarwal, R., Bello, F., Moorthy, K., Munz, Y., Gillies, D., Darzi, A.: Synchronized video and motion analysis of the assessment of procedures in the oeprating theater. Arch. Surg. 140, 293–299 (2005)
10. Megali, G., Sinigaglia, S., Tonet, O., Dario, P.: Modelling and evaluation of surgical performance using hidden markov models. IEEE Transactions on BioMedical Engineering 53, 1911–1919 (2006)
11. Allen, B., Nistor, V., Dutson, E., Carman, G., Lewis, C., Faloutsos, P.: Support vector machines improve the accuracy of performance evaluation of laparoscopic training tasks. Surgical Endoscopy, 1–14 (2009)
12. Stylopoulos, N., Vosburgh, K.: Assessing technical skill in surgery and endoscopy: A set of metrics and an algorithm (C-PASS) to assess skills in surgical and endoscopic procedures. Surgical Innovation 14 (2007)
13. Vosburgh, K., Stylopoulos, N., San Jose Estepar, R., Ellis, R., Samset, E., Thompson, C.: EUS and CT improve efficiency and structure identification over conventional EUS. Gastrointestinal Endoscopy 65, 866–870 (2007)
14. Stocco, L., Salcudean, S.E., Sassani, F.: Fast constrained global minimax optimization of robot parameters. Robotica 16, 595–605 (1998)
15. Salcudean, S.E., Stocco, L.: Isotropy and actuator optimization in haptic interface design. In: IEEE International Conference on Robotics and Automation, pp. 763–769 (2000)
16. Kim, S., Jeong, I., Lee, S.: Systematic isotropy analysis of a mobile robot with three active caster wheels. In: Huang, D.-S., Heutte, L., Loog, M. (eds.) ICIC 2007. LNCS, vol. 4681, pp. 587–597. Springer, Heidelberg (2007)
17. Trejos, A.L., Patel, R.V., Ross, I., Kiaii, B.: Optimizing port placement for robot-assisted minimally invasive cardiac surgery. Int. J. Med. Robotics Comput. Assist. Surg. 3, 355–364 (2007)
18. Jayender, J., Patel, R.V., Michaud, G., Hata, N.: Optimal Transseptal Puncture Location for Robot-Assisted Left Atrial Catheter Ablation. In: Yang, G.-Z., Hawkes, D., Rueckert, D., Noble, A., Taylor, C. (eds.) MICCAI 2009. LNCS, vol. 5761, pp. 1–8. Springer, Heidelberg (2009)
19. Sciavicco, L., Siciliano, B.: A solution algorithm to the inverse kinematic problem for redundant manipulators. IEEE Transactions on Robotics and Automation 4, 403–410 (1988)
20. Merlet, J.P.: Jacobian, manipulability, condition number, and accuracy of parallel robots. Journal of Mechanical Design 128, 199–206 (2006)

GPU-Accelerated Robotic Intra-operative Laparoscopic 3D Reconstruction

Markus Moll[1], Hsiao-Wei Tang[2], and Luc Van Gool[1,3]

[1] Katholieke Universiteit Leuven, ESAT-PSI/IBBT, Department of Electrical Engineering, Heverlee, Belgium
{Markus.Moll,Luc.VanGool}@esat.kuleuven.be
[2] Katholieke Universiteit Leuven, PMA, Department of Mechanical Engineering, Heverlee, Belgium
[3] Swiss Federal Institute of Technology (ETH), D-ITET/Computer Vision Laboratory, Zürich, Switzerland
VanGool@vision.ee.ethz.ch

Abstract. In this paper we present a real-time intra-operative reconstruction system for laparoscopic surgery. The system builds upon a surgical robot for laparoscopy that has previously been developed by us. Such a system is valuable for surgeons, who can get a three dimensional visualization of the scene online, without having to postprocess data. We gain a significant speed increase over existing such systems by carefully parallelizing tasks and using the GPU for computationally expensive subtasks, making real-time reconstruction and visualization possible. Our implementation is also robust with respect to outliers and can potentially be extended to be used with non-robotic surgery. We demonstrate the performance of our system on ex-vivo samples and compare it to alternative implementations.

1 Introduction

Minimally invasive surgery (MIS) has become an important tool in surgery, as it greatly reduces the risks for the patient and leads to faster over-all recovery. In MIS, the surgeon operates through small incisions only, where a view into the body is provided through an endoscope. We are specifically dealing with laparoscopy, which is MIS in the abdominal. Nowadays, such images are usually taken by a video camera mounted on the endoscope and are then displayed on a separate screen. Robot assisted surgery (RAS) has also become more and more popular in this field, where today Intuitive Surgery is dominating the market with their Da Vinci system.

The downside of MIS is that it requires a lot of training from the surgeon. This is mainly caused by the indirect interaction and feedback, with the surgical instruments and the video camera being the surgeons hands and eyes. A great part of the problem is caused by the unusual vision that an endoscope provides. Firstly, the perception of three dimensional structure is greatly reduced because the image is displayed on a screen. Secondly, the surgeon usually only sees a small part of the body cavity, which makes it harder to navigate.

N. Navab and P. Jannin (Eds.): IPCAI 2010, LNCS 6135, pp. 91–101, 2010.

For the former problem, stereo endoscopes have been introduced but have not become widely accepted. The reason for that is that the only reasonable way to display stereoscopic video is by using goggles, which isolate the surgeon from his surroundings.

The computer vision community has actively worked on solutions for these problems, notably by Koppel et al. [6,7] and Wengert [13]. The early work of Koppel et al. concentrates on estimating camera pose to correct the image orientation. To achieve this, only a small number (around 20) of features are tracked using a window search tracker. Full window search is relatively slow, so they use FFT to speed it up. They also describe how to create novel views by fitting a low order polynomial to these points. Wengert's work consists of an intra-operative system for 3D reconstruction relying on camera pose estimates from an external optical tracker. His system works at 2–8 frames per second for a resolution of 384x288 pixels, depending on the number of features[1]. The near real-time speed is achieved by using SURF features[2] and the efficient selection of candidate matches in the feature matching stage. He already noted that off-loading work to a graphics processor could yield a great speed up.

In recent years, graphics processors (GPUs) have become more and more powerful and at the same time more and more versatile. Graphics processors feature a large number of processor cores running with shared memory. They have virtually no caches when compared to general purpose processors, and the memory latency is instead hidden by the strong parallelism. In earlier GPUs, some of these processors could only perform special tasks, but in modern *unified shader architectures*, all these processors can share the same workload.

We use the GPU to gain a significant performance increase over previous implementations. This allows us to process the image stream at video-rate, i.e. at 25 frames per second. To the best of our knowledge, our system is the only such system achieving real-time performance. We have implemented an affine feature drift prevention mechanism in Cg, Nvidia's shader language, as feature drift severly impacts the quality of the reconstruction. We use GPU and CPU in a multi-threaded fashion, so that GPU and CPU work can actually be done in parallel and very efficiently be pipelined (see Figure 1), allowing us to—whenever necessary—spend more computation time per frame at the expense of increased latency. We have also implemented a proper way to deal with outlying points in the bundle adjustment step, as outlying points tend to still occur even in the presence of drift prevention, e.g. through moving highlights on otherwise uniform surfaces.

2 Methods

We start by giving an overview of the individual units of our system. After an image from the video stream is captured with a frame grabber, we correct for lens distortion, which tends to be quite large in endoscopes. This simplifies the

[1] For example, a scene with on average 251 features resulted in a frame rate of 4.5 frames per second.

subsequent tracking and 3D reconstruction which assume that local image patch deformations are approximately affine. As this sampling step can be efficiently performed on the GPU, its cost is negligible. From the undistorted image, we extract image patches and subsequently track them. We have used our own surgical robot to move the endoscope. From this robot, we constantly obtain position estimates. With the information from the new image frame, we triangulate new points where this is possible and refine existing points non-linearly. In the end, we create a triangle mesh from these points for visualization. We project the current video frame onto that mesh to texture it, very much like a video beamer. In the following subsections we will give more detailed information on some of these steps.

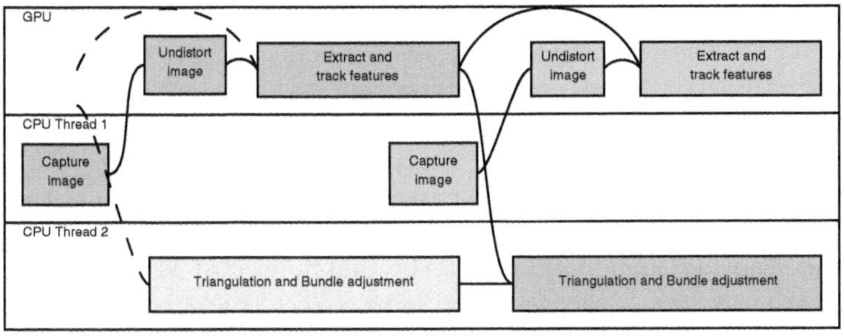

Fig. 1. Overview of the reconstruction part with data dependencies. GPU and CPU processing can be pipelined efficiently to increase throughput.

2.1 Image Undistortion

Typical endoscopic images show a fairly large amount of image distortion. Because this interferes with the remaining processing steps, the very first thing we do is to undistort these images on the GPU. Our distortion model consists of all three of radial distortion, tangential distortion and thin prism distortion. Let $\mathbf{x}_d = (x_d, y_d)^T$ be a point in the distorted input image and $\mathbf{x}_u = (x_u, y_u)^T$ be the corresponding point in the undistorted image, then the relation between these is commonly modeled as

$$\mathbf{x}_d = \mathbf{x}_u + \delta_{\text{radial}}(\mathbf{x}_u) + \delta_{\text{tangential}}(\mathbf{x}_u) + \delta_{\text{prism}}(\mathbf{x}_u) \quad (1)$$

$$\delta_{\text{radial}}(\mathbf{x}_u) = (k_1\|\mathbf{x}_u\|^2 + k_2\|\mathbf{x}_u\|^4 + k_3\|\mathbf{x}_u\|^6)\mathbf{x}_u \quad (2)$$

$$\delta_{\text{tangential}}(\mathbf{x}_u) = \begin{pmatrix} 2t_1 x_u y_u + t_2(3x_u^2 + y_u^2) \\ t_1(x_u^2 + 3 * y_u^2) + 2t_2 x_u y_u \end{pmatrix} \quad (3)$$

$$\delta_{\text{prism}}(\mathbf{x}_u) = \mathbf{p}\|\mathbf{x}_u\|^2 \quad (4)$$

Here, k_i, t_i and $\mathbf{p}$ are the distortion parameters which have to be estimated in advance.

2.2 Feature Extraction and Tracking

For feature tracking we use the classic Lucas-Kanade tracking method based on Shi and Tomasi's interest point detector (KLT)[12]. This has turned out to be robust with respect to the relatively high image noise, and can also be computed very efficiently. Shi and Tomasi define key points as points which are reliably trackable, i.e. in whose neighborhood there is considerable gradient variation. If $\Omega(\mathbf{x})$ denotes a small window around the point $\mathbf{x}$ in the image I, then key points are extracted at local minima of the smaller eigenvalue of

$$\sum_{\mathbf{z}\in\Omega(\mathbf{x})} (\nabla I|_{\mathbf{z}})^T \nabla I|_{\mathbf{z}}$$

In contrast to e.g. SURF[2] or SIFT[9] features which come with discriminative descriptors, KLT features cannot reliably be redetected once they are lost, as the Shi and Tomasi detector has relatively low repeatability and the descriptors (the local image patches) are not invariant to any geometric or photometric changes.

However, when camera poses are externally measured, a feature loss can be dealt with by simply starting with a new set of tracks, assuming that the external camera pose correctly aligns the two otherwise independent reconstructions. It is also worth noting that in that case the matching cost is typically quadratic and thus rather costly. If the only goal is to collect tracks to build a 3D model, KLT features promise to be faster and most robust, as has also been shown for example in [5].

We have chosen to perform both feature tracking and interest point detection on the GPU, as prior experiments with a CPU based implementation on top of OpenCV have shown that these steps are the most time consuming. Tracking naturally lends itself to parallelization because all points can be tracked independently. This fits modern GPUs perfectly, because they are designed for data parallelism, where the same task has to be performed on multiple data. As one of the most time consuming steps is the accumulation of gradients over a local window, a GPU implementation further benefits from the GPU's texture units, which are designed for image sampling tasks. We have implemented a GPU algorithm of the drift-resistant KLT tracker from Zinsser et al.[15], based on the GPU tracker by Zach[14]. We refer to the respective authors for a more detailed discussion of the GPU KLT implementation.

Feature drift not only occurs in very long sequences, but also during lighting changes, especially in the presence of specularities, which are quite common in endoscopic surgery. The tracking method of Zinsser et al. continuously estimates an affinely distorted registration of the feature's very first image patch and the patch in the current image, and discards tracks if the difference becomes too large, thus avoiding feature drift. To this end, they use an affine lighting model such that if $I(\mathbf{x})$ are the points in the first patch and $J(\mathbf{x})$ are those in the most recent patch an iterative update

$$\underset{\Delta A, \Delta\mathbf{b}, \alpha, \beta}{\arg\min} \sum_{\mathbf{x}} (\alpha I(\Delta A\,\mathbf{x} + \Delta\mathbf{b}) + \beta - J(\mathbf{x}))^2$$

is found. ΔA and $\Delta \mathbf{b}$ are small updates to an estimated affine distortion $A\mathbf{x}+\mathbf{b}$ of the patch and α and β are used to adjust for intensity changes. The resulting linear least squares problem is solved by a Gauss-Newton iteration. We have implemented the above algorithm in the Cg shader language, taking care of the data layout to benefit from the GPU SIMD instructions.

2.3 Bundle Adjustment

While the robot provides the vision system with pose estimates, it is not stiff enough for these estimates to be correct. The problem is magnified by the relatively large leverage from the endoscope, in that small angular errors in the robot readings can have a huge impact on the camera position. Furthermore, initially point positions are chosen so as to minimize errors in the views that contribute to their creation. If the point track continues, errors in additional views will not be taken into account. Therefore, it is usually advisable to optimize both structure and motion through bundle adjustment. We employ local bundle adjustment, which has proven to be useful in online problems [10,4]. In local bundle adjustment, only a small subset of the most recent views is optimized after every iteration. This reduces the problem size considerably and thus allows to find a solution in real-time.

If additive zero-mean Gaussian noise is assumed on the image position measurements, then the solution that minimizes the sum of squared image errors is the maximum likelihood estimate. However, in real settings this assumption is usually violated, as features can drift or jump even when using drift-resistant trackers, and single outlying measurement can have arbitrary influence on the estimate. We found it necessary to deal with outliers, as ignoring them resulted in substantial pose estimation errors and inferior structure estimates. A commonly chosen approach is to remove outliers prior to running the bundle adjustment. However, besides being inherently arbitrary because of thresholding, this also suffers from outlier masking problems if the initial estimate is too far from the optimum. Similar to [4], we chose to re-weight the individual image errors such that their squared norm follows a more robust error measure, i.e. for a set of 3D points $\mathbf{X}_i$ with corresponding image measurements $\mathbf{x}_{i,j}$ we solve the least squares problem

$$\min \sum_{i,j} \left\| \sqrt{\rho\left(\|\mathbf{x}_{i,j} - \Pi_j(\mathbf{X}_i)\|^2\right)} \frac{\mathbf{x}_{i,j} - \Pi_j(\mathbf{X}_i)}{\|\mathbf{x}_{i,j} - \Pi_j(\mathbf{X}_i)\|} \right\|^2 \tag{5}$$

which is equivalent to minimizing

$$\sum_{i,j} \rho\left(\|\mathbf{x}_{i,j} - \Pi_j(\mathbf{X}_i)\|^2\right) \tag{6}$$

Here, $\Pi_j(\mathbf{X}_i)$ denotes the projection of the i-th 3D point into the j-th image. We actually use two different functions ρ, the first is the Cauchy distribution likelihood, the second is Tukey's bi-weight function. The Cauchy distribution looks similar to the Gaussian distribution at first glance, but its tail is heavier, so that gross outliers do not have as large an influence. Tukey's bi-weight function features a so-called re-descending influence function, i.e. the influence of gross outliers is actually approaching zero. It is highly efficient at Gaussian distributions but, because it completely ignores outliers above a certain threshold, it actually does not lead to a unique solution and its performance heavily depends on the initial estimate. Therefore we first use the Cauchy likelihood to converge to a better guess and only then use the bi-weight function. The remaining problem is that of finding a good scale of the data, i.e. a good outlier threshold. We use the *median absolute deviation*, which is a highly robust scale estimator.

We have added the robustness functionality and some speed improvements to the SBA package by Lourakis [8] which we use in our system.

2.4 Experiments

In order to evaluate how our system performs, we have done experiments with an apple for the sake of simplicity, and have furthermore conducted experiments on both an ex-vivo uterus and a skull.

We have used a Storz laser laparoscope on the Storz telecam SL pal system for the apple sequences, and the same endoscope in conjunction with Storz HD equipment for the other two sequences. However, in all cases only half frame PAL resolution of 384×288 pixels was recorded with a generic PAL video grabber from S-Video inputs in order to avoid interlacing.

The apple experiments were run in our lab on an Intel Q9300 2.5GHz equipped with a GeForce 8800 GTS graphics board. For the other experiments, we used an Intel core i7 2.8GHz with a GeForce 8800 GTX card.

In order to compare the performance of alternative tracking methods, we have recorded video data together with pose estimates. These were replayed afterwards so that all algorithms ran on the exact same data.

3 Results

Figure 4 shows reconstructions of a skull as well as an ex-vivo uterus. The skull has also been scanned in a structured light scanner to obtain high quality 3D reconstructions that our results can be compared to. To this end, we created a point cloud model from the points that were reconstructed during the course of the whole sequence. We then manually aligned the unstructured point cloud obtained from our system to the structured light scan and found the best similarity transform of the point cloud model by the iterative closest point method (ICP). We have recorded the root mean square residual errors as a measure of goodness of these fits and thereby of the reconstructions that our system created. The results can be found in Figure 6(b).

For evaluation, we have replaced the GPU tracker in our system by a number of other tracking methods. We have used the same GPU tracker, but without the drift detection and correction as well as the OpenCV KLT implementation with and without drift correction.

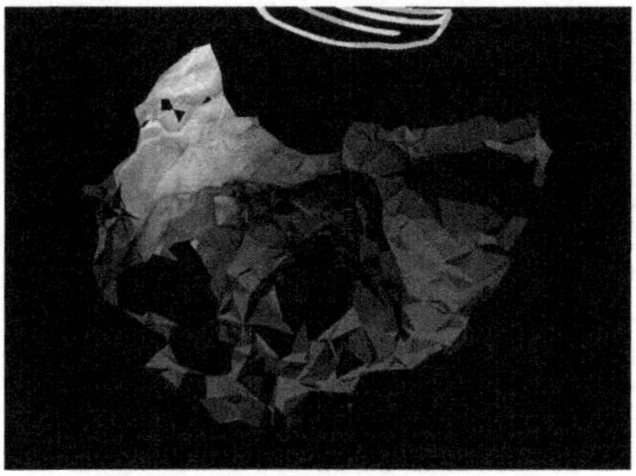

(a) skull reconstruction

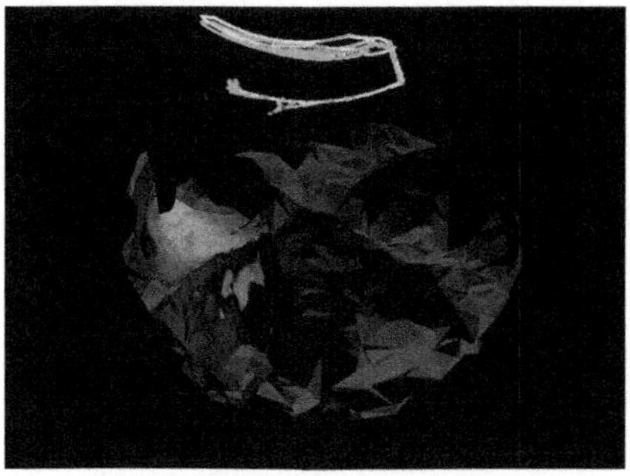

(b) skull reconstruction

Fig. 2. Results of our system on a sequence of the base of a skull. The pyramids indicate camera position, green pyramids signify refined poses.

We attempted to compare the tracker with SIFT or SURF by mimicking a "tracker" that would only match the strongest keypoints from image to image. However, the resulting tracker failed to produce any reasonable results in our test setup. Timing and accuracy results of these alternative implementations are given in Figure 6. It is also interesting to look at the number of inlying reconstructed points at the end of the sequences in Figure 3. The affine drift correction increases the number of inliers for both GPU and CPU implementations. The relatively high number of inliers in the OpenCV implementation is due to our not restricting the proximity of newly detected features to existing ones in the OpenCV implementation. The GPU tracker prevents clustered feature points.

Algorithm	Uterus Sequence	Skull Sequence
GPU	7865	4945
GPU drift corr.	8658	5138
OpenCV	17542	7309
OpenCV drift corr.	21894	16217

Fig. 3. Number of inliers after reconstruction of the complete sequence

We have also artificially increased the image size to 768x576 by upsampling the image. The system still only dropped 120 of 1770 frames, achieving a framerate of on average 23–24 frames per second at full PAL resolution. However, we performed the upsampling on the graphics card so this number does not account for the larger data transfer that would normally occur.

4 Discussion

The timing results presented in the previous section show that while the GPU implementations are indeed faster, with multi-core processors the gap has become relatively small. The question might arise whether a GPU implementation

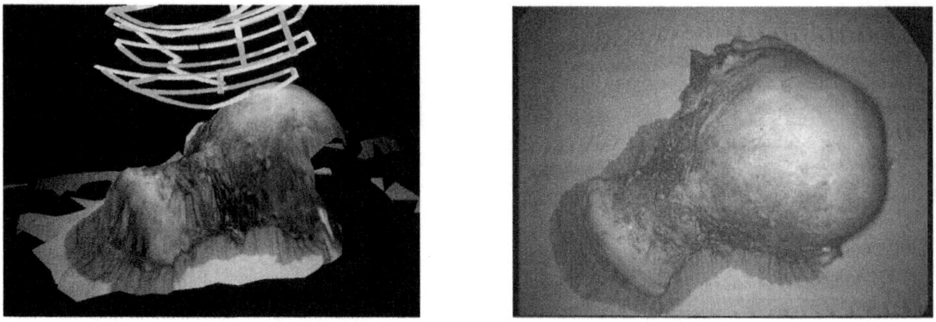

(a) uterus reconstruction (b) uterus video frame

Fig. 4. Results of our system on a sequence of an ex-vivo uterus. The pyramids indicate camera position, green pyramids signify refined poses. Meshing artifacts can be seen near the ground in the uterus.

is beneficial, given that the CPU implementations do not perform much worse. However, it is important to notice that the tracking algorithms in the CPU implementations are also parallelized and made use of all available processor cores, leaving no further computing power to other processes. To us, using the GPU for highly parallelizable tasks seems very attractive as it leaves the general purpose CPU free for other purposes. Also, we could not further investigate how the runtime increases with increasing image sizes or increasing feature count and whether or not there is a significant constant overhead.

The KLT tracking performance was generally good. As can be seen in the results section, adding the drift correction step increased the number of inliers and decreased the residual error at the same time, leading to larger reconstructions with smaller errors. There is of course a certain trade-off between this improvement and the additional run-time cost one has to pay, but that has to be considered in the actual case at hand individually. It needs to be noted that we have implemented the drift correction in OpenCV ourselves and have tried to support as many border cases as the original OpenCV tracking code. Because of that, our implementation sacrifices speed for generality, so timings for that method have to be interpreted with some care.

We have not tried to evaluate a full SIFT or SURF based reconstruction method, as this would necessarily have quite a different design. Matching only temporally close, strong features was unsuccessful, so a feature database comprising a large part of the system's history would have to be built. However, as the size of that database increases, the number of candidate matches becomes larger and matching therefore takes more time.

Wengert used SURF features, but basically degraded the matching to a simple tracking by imposing strong geometric constraints on the position of candidate matches. This is however not general enough and will only work for triangulated features whose 3D positions are already known. Wengert extends this to two and three-view cases using epipolar constraints and trifocal point transfer.

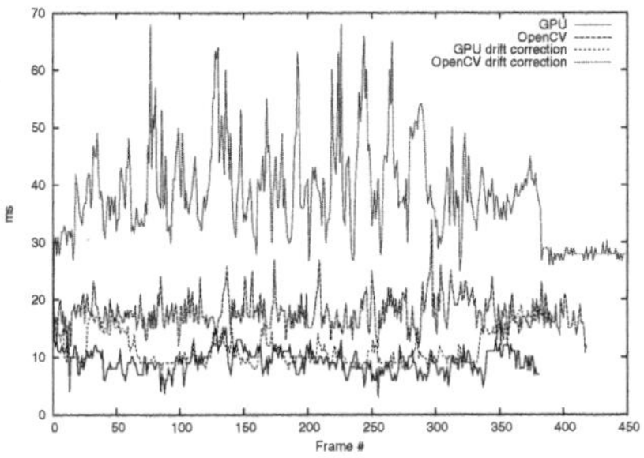

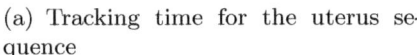

(a) Tracking time for the uterus sequence

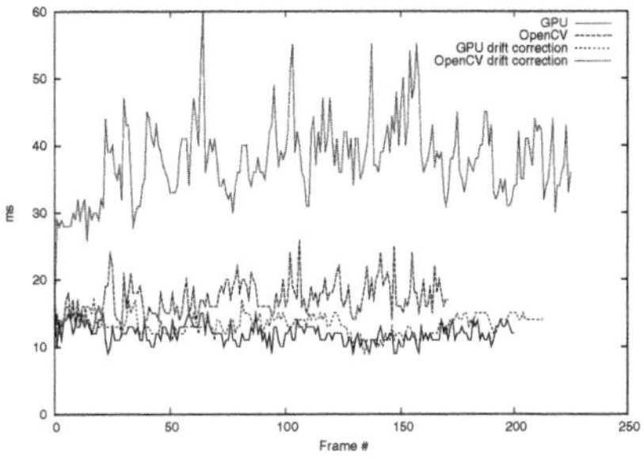

(b) Tracking time for the skull sequence

Fig. 5. Experimental timing results

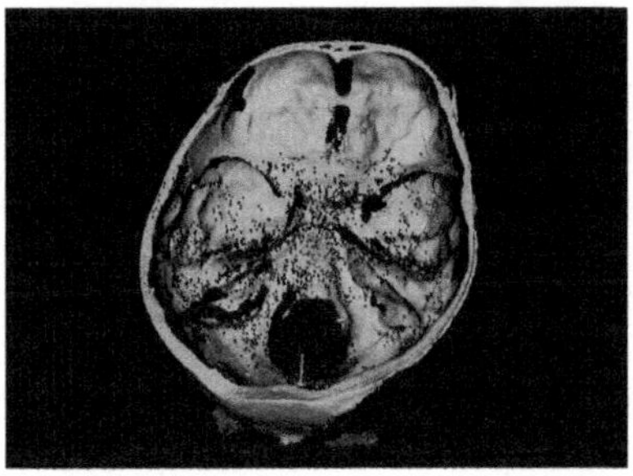

(a) The structured light scan of the skull with aligned point cloud

Algorithm	**ICP error**
GPU	4.790656
GPU drift corr.	2.204764
OpenCV	5.516799
OpenCV drift corr.	1.961356

(b) Residual RMS ICP errors in mm

Fig. 6. The high quality skull model used for evaluation and ICP registration errors

But the worst case number of fundamental matrices that need to be considered is quadratic in the number of views. Likewise, it is our understanding that trifocal point transfer amounts to a simple triangulation method that strongly underestimates errors in one of the two views.

Under these circumstances, KLT achieves a far higher match count. However, when it is necessary to do pose estimation as in hand-held laparoscopic surgery without any external tracking, SURF or similar features are needed for the case that all tracks are lost, for example due to blood or water in front of the lens. Wengert's system offers the advantage of the theoretical capability to be used for pose estimation, although the speed would suffer tremendously.

We feel that in these circumstances it is better to only add a few landmark SURF features that are sufficient to estimate the pose but use KLT tracking on many more features for structure estimation. This way, real-time performance can be maintained while the pose can be re-established after feature loss.

Also, currently we have to build the triangle mesh in a separate step, as the construction thereof takes too much time for integration into the system. We currently use the alpha shape reconstruction suggested by Wengert, and have taken the implementation from CGAL[1]. However, on its own the time required for meshing is negligible and can thus be done intra-operatively as well. All meshes were created in significantly less than one second. Although the triangle mesh creation needs time, mapping the current video image to it as a live texture is fast and is integrated into the processing loop. It seems interesting to experiment with point-based visualization methods (textured splatting) in order to achieve better live visualization than displaying the point cloud.

At the current stage, the 3D visualizations seem to be a promising addition to the information provided to the surgeon, while measurements based on it should be treated with care.

5 Conclusion and Future Work

We have demonstrated a real-time intra-operative 3D reconstruction system that can provide the surgeon with additional three-dimensional information for approximately rigid structures. We are convinced that the results concerning both timing and reconstruction quality are satisfactory for the target application. While we could not test our robotic system during real surgery, we have good reason to believe that performance will be similar.

We are planning to use the extracted 3D information for robot guidance, for example to keep a fixed distance to the surface for laser ablation, or to detect and avoid collisions. We hope to further improve the reconstruction quality significantly by using higher definition video, but because of hardware limitations in the grabber device, no such videos were taken for our tests. Earlier experiments on higher resolution material lead us to think that structure estimates will greatly benefit from that. Finally we would like to extend the work beyond rigid structures by using the presented method to create a model for tracking non-rigid deformations, similar to e.g. [11].

References

1. CGAL, Computational Geometry Algorithms Library, `http://www.cgal.org`
2. Bay, H., Tuytelaars, T., Gool, L.J.V.: Surf: Speeded up robust features. In: Leonardis, A., Bischof, H., Pinz, A. (eds.) ECCV 2006, Part I. LNCS, vol. 3951, pp. 404–417. Springer, Heidelberg (2006)
3. Bouguet, J.Y.: Pyramidal implementation of the lucas kanade feature tracker, description of the algorithm. Tech. rep., Intel Corporation Microprocessor Research Labs (2000) (from the OpenCV documentation)
4. Engels, C., Stewénius, H., Nistér, D.: Bundle adjustment rules. In: Proceedings of Photogrammetric Computer Vision. The International Archives of The Photogrammetry, Remote Sensing and Spatial Information Sciences (2006)
5. Klippenstein, J., Zhang, H.: Quantitative evaluation of feature extractors for visual slam. In: Proceedings of the Fourth Canadian Conference on Computer and Robot Vision (2007)
6. Koppel, D., Wang, Y.F., Lee, H.: Image-based rendering and modeling in videoendoscopy. In: Proceedings of the 2004 IEEE International Symposium on Biomedical Imaging: From Nano to Macro, April 2004, pp. 269–272. IEEE, Arlington (2004)

7. Koppel, D., Wang, Y.F., Lee, H.: Robust and real-time image stabilization and rectification. In: Proceedings of the Seventh IEEE Workshop on Applications of Computer Vision/IEEE Workshop on Motion and Video Computing, vol. 1, pp. 320–355. IEEE Computer Society, Los Alamitos (2005)
8. Lourakis, M.I.A., Argyros, A.A.: The design and implementation of a generic sparse bundle adjustment software package based on the levenberg-marquardt algorithm. Tech. Rep. 340, Institute of Computer Science - FORTH, Heraklion, Crete, Greece (August 2004), http://www.ics.forth.gr/~lourakis/sba
9. Lowe, D.G.: Distinctive image features from scale-invariant keypoints. International Journal of Computer Vision 60(2), 91–110 (2004)
10. Mouragnon, E., Lhuillier, M., Dhome, M., Dekeyser, F., Sayd, P.: 3d reconstruction of complex structures with bundle adjustment: an incremental approach. In: Proceedings of the 2006 IEEE International Conference on Robotics and Automation, May 2006, pp. 3055–3061. Orlando, Florida (2006)
11. Salzmann, M., Hartley, R., Fua, P.: Convex optimization for deformable surface 3-d tracking. In: Proceedings of the 2007 IEEE International Conference on Computer Vision (2007)
12. Shi, J., Tomasi, C.: Good features to track. In: IEEE Conference on Computer Vision and Pattern Recognition (CVPR 1994), June 1994, pp. 593–600 (1994)
13. Wengert, C.: Quantitative Endoscopy. Ph.D. thesis, ETH Zürich (2008)
14. Zach, C., Gallup, D., Frahm, J.M.: Fast gain-adaptive klt tracking on the gpu. In: Proceedings of Computer Vision and Pattern Recognition Workshops, pp. 1–7 (2008)
15. Zinßer, T., Gräßl, C., Niemann, H.: Efficient feature tracking for long video sequences. In: Rasmussen, C.E., Bülthoff, H.H., Schölkopf, B., Giese, M.A. (eds.) DAGM 2004. LNCS, vol. 3175, pp. 326–333. Springer, Heidelberg (2004)

A Minimally Invasive Multimodality Image-Guided (MIMIG) Molecular Imaging System for Peripheral Lung Cancer Intervention and Diagnosis

Tiancheng He[1,2], Zhong Xue[1], Kelvin K. Wong[1], Miguel Valdivia y Alvarado[1], Yong Zhang[1], Weixin Xie[2], and Stephen T.C. Wong[1]

[1] The Center for Bioengineering and Informatics, The Methodist Hospital Research Institute and Department of Radiology, The Methodist Hospital, Weil Cornell Medical College, Houston, Texas, USA

[2] Intelligent Information Institute, Shenzhen University, Shenzhen, China

zxue@tmhs.org

Abstract. The once-promising computed tomography (CT) lung cancer screening appears to result in high false positive rates. To tackle the common difficulties in diagnosing small lung cancer at an early stage, we developed a minimally invasive multimodality image-guided (MIMIG) interventional system for early detection and treatment of peripheral lung cancer. The system consists of new CT image segmentation for surgical planning, intervention guidance for targeting, and molecular imaging for diagnosis. Using advanced image segmentation technique the pulmonary vessels, airways, as well as nodules can be better visualized for surgical planning. These segmented results are then transformed onto the intra-procedural CT for interventional guidance using electromagnetic (EM) tracking. Diagnosis can be achieved at microscopic resolution using a fiber-optic microendoscopy. The system can also be used for fine needle aspiration biopsy to improve the accuracy and efficiency. Confirmed cancer could then be treated on-the-spot using radio-frequency ablation (RFA). The experiments on rabbits with VX2 lung cancer model show both accuracy and efficiency in localization and detecting lung cancer, as well as promising molecular imaging tumor detection.

Keywords: image-guided intervention, peripheral lung cancer, image computing, molecular imaging.

1 Introduction

Lung cancer is the most common cause of cancer-related death in men and women. The American Cancer Society estimated over 210,000 new lung cancers and about 160,000 deaths from lung cancer for the United States in 2007. Deaths from lung cancer in the nation outnumbered the cumulative deaths from colon, breast, and prostate cancers. Peripheral lung cancer constitutes more than half of all lung cancer cases. However, computed tomography (CT) diagnosis is known to result in high false positive rates to confirm malignancy [1] (most studies reported false positive

N. Navab and P. Jannin (Eds.): IPCAI 2010, LNCS 6135, pp. 102–112, 2010.

rates between 10% and 20% [2]). It is believed that the key to improving long term survival rate of patients with lung cancer is early detection, accurate localization and diagnosis, and novel therapies [1, 3]. The Mayo Clinic experience shows that when high risk individuals are screened for lung cancer with CT, the likelihood that they undergo a thoracic resection for lung cancer is increased by 10-fold [4]. To tackle the common difficulties in identifying small lung lesions (<1.5cm) at an early stage, an image-guided therapy approach is most promising.

In this paper, we introduce a minimally invasive multimodality image-guided (MIMIG) intervention system for early detection of peripheral lung cancer. The approach relies on initial pre-procedural CT imaging to locate small lesions. From the pre-procedural scan, pulmonary vessels, airways, as well as nodules can be segmented for better visualization during surgical planning, which can be transformed to intra-procedural scan using deformable registration for guiding the intervention. Electromagnetic (EM) tracking is embedded in the system to visualize the probe location in 3D CT, so physicians can efficiently perform the intervention by referring to the feedback from the visualization. After successfully targeting the lesion, fiber-optic molecular imaging is used for diagnosis through microendoscopy, and the confirmed malignant tumor can be treated immediately using radio-frequency ablation (RFA). MIMIG can also be used for fine needle aspiration biopsy to improve the accuracy and efficiency.

The proposed MIMIG system consists of the following components: 1) an electromagnetic (EM) tracking device for real-time tracking of the needle introducer; 2) coherent software for real-time localization and visualization of multiple devices being tracked on the intra-procedural CT images; 3) a fiber-optic microendoscope for fluorescence molecular imaging diagnosis and a radio-frequency ablation needle for localized therapy. New image computing modules are incorporated in the system for improved visualization and accuracy, and modular design of the functions in the Philips PMS Informatics Infrastructure (PII). PII is a commercial software development environment for the development, integration, deployment, monitoring and support of inter- and intra-enterprise healthcare solutions that deliver clinical functionality to the point of need, allowing us to implement these new functions conveniently through dynamic-link libraries. We hypothesize that MIMIG will allow us to accurately and efficiently detect small peripheral lung cancer and treat it at an earlier stage on-the-spot. In the experiments, the MIMIG system and the molecular imaging module have been validated using eight rabbit models, and the results show accuracy and efficiency in localization and detecting lung cancer.

2 The MIMIG System

2.1 System Overview

The MIMIG lung intervention system consists of one workstation for computing and visualization, an electromagnetic (EM) tracking system for localizing the position of the needle, a microendoscopy imaging system, and a needle-based treatment device such as radiofrequency ablation probe. The intervention and diagnosis is performed in the CT room. In this paper, we introduce and validate the MIMIG system using the lung intervention experiments for live rabbits. Although MIMIG has been embedded with a molecular imaging system, it can also be applied to other applications such as image-guided biopsy and ablation for improving the accuracy and efficiency.

A. System hardware

In addition to the MIMIG workstation developed based on the PII platform, we adopt the NDI Aurora EM tracking system and the Valleylab Cool-tip ablation system for tracking the interventional probe and performing lung cancer treatment if necessary. CellVizio 660 fiber-optic microendoscopy system is utilized to capture the molecular images, and for this purpose the IntegriSense 680 fluorescent contrast agent is used to label $\alpha_v\beta_3$ integrin expressed in malignant cancer cells. During the past two years, we setup all the hardware and developed the software modules to complete a functional prototype system, and tested it on live rabbits. In another parallel study [5], we confirmed that the subcutaneous A547 nude mice tumor highly expresses $\alpha_v\beta_3$ integrin and labeled well with IntegriSense 680. This further supports the feasibility of applying MIMIG for lung cancer diagnosis.

Fig. 1 shows some pictures of the MIMIG system. The portable MIMIG system (Fig. 1(a)) can be used in the CT room to help physicians accurately guide the probe to the target and to perform precise molecular imaging, fine-needle biopsy, as well as radiofrequency ablation. In our experiments, the MIMIG system and the molecular imaging module have been validated using rabbit models, and Fig. 1 (b) shows a rabbit experiment. The rabbit experiments not only validate the accuracy and efficiency for localization of lung cancer using MIMIG system but also show the feasibility for detecting lung cancer using molecular imaging.

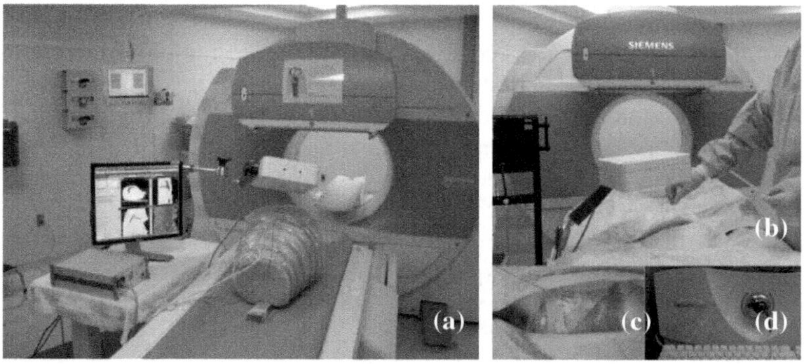

Fig. 1. System setting and interventional experiments. (a) The setting of the system; (b) rabbit intervention experiment; (c) picture of the probe; (d) the CellVizio system.

B. System workflow

The workflow paradigm of the image-guided diagnosis and therapy system is implemented by using a modular multimodality image guidance platform. In this system, peripheral lung cancer diagnosis is accomplished based on morphologic and molecular imaging information obtained from different imaging modalities. Fig. 2 illustrates the workflow of the MIMIG system. If the nodule size detected from CT is small, the MIMIG system will be used for further diagnosis or treatment. Traditional method will be used for larger nodules. The MIMIG system is used to confirm the initial diagnosis using real-time fiber-optic fluorescence molecular imaging and to guide the treatment for the small lesions. After injection of optical contrast agent (e.g., IntegriSense 680) the MIMIG system can guide accurately the interventional needle to the right location, and molecular imaging diagnosis can be accomplished by using CellVizio 660 system. Our rationale is that high sensitivity and specificity diagnosis can be achieved for small peripheral lung cancer through accurate intervention and molecular imaging. Compared to the previous systems which focus on precise targeting using EM tracking [6-10], MIMIG not only provides new image computing modules but also presents an on-the-spot treatment solution so that the confirmed malignant lesion can be treated onsite by using radiofrequency ablation. MIMIG significantly shortens the duration between diagnosis and treatment and reduces the healthcare cost involved in this procedure.

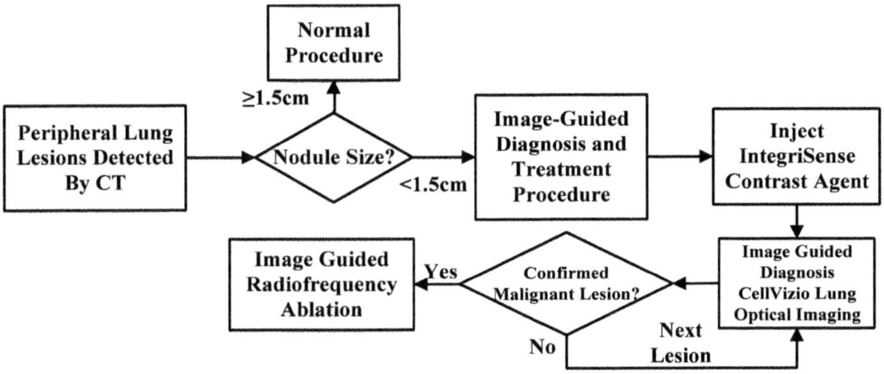

Fig. 2. The workflow of image-guided diagnosis and treatment for peripheral lung cancer

C. System software

The MIMIG software modules are constructed from the visual application builder of PII. PII enables one unified application development environment and provides implicit compatibility of shared components, which enables optimally tuned pre-clinical or clinical workflow. By using standardized interfaces, information models and API's, it provides the complete spectrum of applications between console and enterprise software, common schemas for configuration, preferences, and databases.

Standard informatics infrastructure and applications have been implemented in the PII system. The informatics infrastructure utilized in MIMIG includes workflow design, DICOM protocol, data input/output, and data repository. The standard applications that MIMIG used include 2D/3D visualization and interaction with the current workflow and imaging data, human interface functions, multi-modality image fusion, EM tracking and molecular imaging data stream interface.

Most importantly, PII allows extension of new components, thus our new image processing modules of the MIMIG system were implemented using based on this extendable feature. Fig. 3 illustrates how a new function is incorporated in the PII platform. For example, a new component in the new image segmentation can be first constructed in the PII visual application builder using XML and C# languages. C# codes define the classes of the services that the segmentation component will provide, including data input, output, and functions. XML provides the properties of this component used by the PII visual application builder. Then the detailed implementation of the image segmentation function can be written either in C or C++ language and compiled as an external dynamic-link library (DLL). Finally the segmentation function can be easily called by using a program wrapper. In this way, any new functions can be easily embedded in the PII system, and used in the visual application builder to provide the flexibility of reconfiguring the MIMIG system.

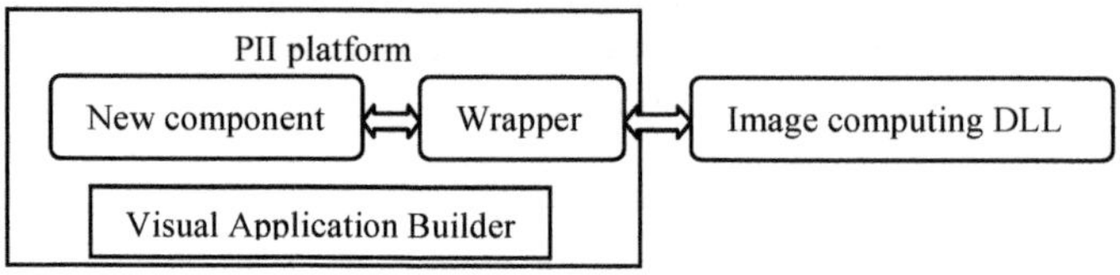

Fig. 3. Illustration of adding a new component/function to PII platform

Using PII platform we implement the real-time visualization and guidance functions for EM-based intervention tools. The major functions implemented include: 1) automatic lung field and vessel segmentation, as well as the visualization for path planning from pre-procedural images; 2) saving and loading the segmentation results and path planning data for intra-procedural use; 3) registering the pre-procedural image, segmentation results and the path planning data onto the intra-procedural images for better visualization; 4) visualization of the segmentation results of vessels and nodules in both volumetric and surface meshes; 5) image guidance based on the EM-tracking and CT images to determine the location of the needle in the CT image in different views; 6) enabling multiple devices (needles) tracking from the EM system and visualize them in the PII MIMIG system; and 7) performing data fusion between microendoscopy and the CT image-based guidance system.

2.2 Novel Software Modules and Features

We developed novel image computing tools including segmentation [11], registration [12], and microendoscopy image sequence processing for MIMIG. The pre-procedural images can be segmented for better visualization during surgical planning, and since fast segmentation is needed for intra-procedural images, the segmentation results will be transformed onto the intra-procedural images for visualization during the intervention. Using these tools fast and accurate image segmentation and registration algorithms are developed for better visualization during surgical planning and intervention, and alignment of pre-procedural and intra-procedural images; microendoscopy is used for lung cancer diagnosis, and cancerous lesions is treated on-the-spot using RFA. The software modules were implemented using C++ language as an external DLL and incorporated in to the PII platform. With properly designed software interface, they can also be embedded in other open-source platforms such as the Image-Guided Surgical Toolkit (IGSTK).

A. Lung field and blood vessel segmentation

A lung field and pulmonary vessel segmentation tool is developed for MIMIG. First, the background and the cavity areas are automatically detected using 3D region growing; then, 3D morphological operations are performed to filter out the noise and fill the holes in the segmentation results; finally, a novel Vascularity-Oriented LEvel Set (VOLES) algorithm [11] is proposed for pulmonary vessel segmentation. The results show it outperforms traditional level set method on pulmonary vessel segmentation. Using manual points in twenty patients the results show that that VOLES obtained sensitivity rate of 96% and specificity rate of 97% for our datasets.

B. Deformable registration of lung parenchyma

The alignment of the pre-procedural lung CT images as well as the intra-procedural images is an important step to accurately guide and monitor the interventional procedure. We devised a robust joint serial image registration and segmentation method [12], wherein serial images are segmented based on the current temporal deformations so that the temporally corresponding tissues tend to be segmented into the same tissue type. Note that the simultaneous registration and segmentation framework had been studied in [13-15] for MR images. The advantage of our new algorithm is that no temporal smoothness about the deformation field is enforced so that our algorithm can tolerate larger or discontinuous temporal changes that often appear during image-guided therapy. Moreover, physical procedure models could also be incorporated to our algorithm to better handle the temporal changes of the serial images during intervention. The proposed algorithm has been applied to both simulated and real serial lung CT images and compared it with the free-form deformation (FFD) [16]. The dataset used in the experiments consists of anonymized serial lung CT images of lung cancer patients. The results show that the proposed algorithm yields more robust registration results and more stable longitudinal measures: the mean registration error is $0.9mm$ for image resolution $0.7\times0.7\times1.5mm^3$, and is $4.1mm$ for images with resolution $0.81\times0.81\times5\ mm^3$.

C. Quantification of microendoscopy images

To reliably detect tumor tissue with molecular labeling, we perform temporal motion correction and scene change detection across the image sequences: a smooth temporal motion model is used to estimate the shifting and small rotation of the image sequence, and a scene change signal is generated if the degree of matching between two consequent frames is low. For motion correction a novel fluorescence microendoscopy motion correction (FMMC) algorithm using both of normalized mutual information (NMI) and augmented unscented Kalman filter (AUKF) is developed. Using this method, the similarity between consequent frames after serial image registration is defined by NMI, and the longitudinal transformation across the serial images is also subject to the regularization of AUKF. In this way, we can obtain relatively longitudinally stable transformations to correct the motion along the video. To optimize the combined objective function of NMI and AUKF, an iterative optimization algorithm is designed, and the parameters are adjusted to the microendoscopy image sequence alignment.

3 Experiments and Results

3.1 Materials

The protocol has been revised and approved by the Comparative Medicine Program at our institute, and all the procedures were carried in our facilities. The lung tumor models were created using females White New Zealand Rabbits, the animals had weights of 2.2kg±200g. The initial VX2 tumor cell line was provided by the department of comparative medicine at MD Anderson. In order to propagate this cell line in our facility a tumor cell suspension was first inoculated in the limb of one rabbit, a tumor with a diameter around 20*mm* was noticeable after two weeks. From this tumor two cell suspensions were prepared, one for limb inoculation and the other one for lung inoculation. For this procedure the rabbits were anesthetized with general anesthesia, and the hair of the thoracic was shaved completely. The lung inoculation was performed under fluoroscopy guidance. Once a region of the lung was selected an 18G Chiba needle was introduced in the rabbit chest. In order to simulate a peripheral lung tumor the needle was placed at the base of the right lung and the depth of the needle was continuously assessed with different fluoroscopy views of the C-arm at 0, 45 and 90 degrees. Once the needle was in the desire location and adequate depth the VX2 cell suspension was injected. Five minutes later new fluoroscopic images of the rabbit chest were taken for pneumothorax assessment. No animal developed pneumothorax in our experiments. The VX2 tumor size was assessed with weekly CT until a desired size of ~15*mm* was attained.

On the day of the image-guided diagnosis experiment the rabbit was anesthetized with general anesthesia and taken to the CT facility. A pre-procedural CT scan with breath holding was performed. The data was then transferred to the MIMIG system using the build in DCMTK tool. This CT scan was used for image segmentation, tumor identification and surgical planning. After placing five or six active fiducials near the chest of rabbit, the coordinates of the fiducials in the EM-tacking space and the CT image space were registered using affine transformation. During intervention real-time tracking data including the location and orientation of the intervention devices were precisely measured by the EM sensors and mapped onto the CT image space in real-time. For the guidance, the user-friendly visualization interface was used.

Fig. 4 (a) shows the interface for surgical planning where the target point is manually selected as the center of the tumor, and the entry point indicates the location for puncturing the needle. For the surgical planning the pre-procedural CT volume has been segmented using our advanced lung volume segmentation algorithm and the lung lesions were labeled and visualized in both volumetric and surface meshes. A surgical planning interface has been provided for the operator to interactively create a path for the needle insertion. The orthogonal viewer (simultaneous axial, sagittal, and coronal view) provided a clear perspective about the depth, and direction of the needle should be used for reaching the tumor. Before puncturing the needle, we confirmed the needle tracking accuracy and location at the point of entry and ensured the line traced between the point of entry (skin) and the target (tumor) was planned according to the orthogonal viewer. This must be consistent in all the views displayed on the screen. A small (3mm) incision was made at the skin level for the needle.

Before the puncture the animal was breath hold again, avoiding any movement from the chest. Fig. 4 (b) shows the interface indicating that the needle tip had reached the target. Once the tumor (target) was reached we proceed to needle fixation, preventing movement due to the CT gantry of respiratory movements that may displace the needle from the target location. A post-procedural scan with breath holding was performed to verify the needle location.

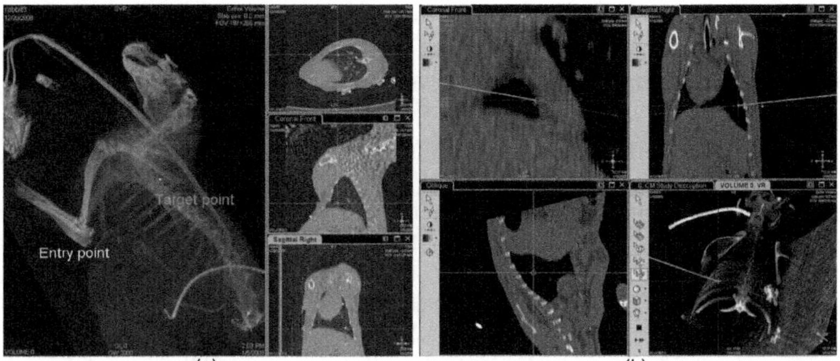

(a) (b)

Fig. 4. Visualization design. (a) Visualization of surgical planning; (b) screen shot of image guidance during the rabbit experiments.

3.2 Performance Evaluation

To evaluate the accuracy of the needle intervention, we calculated the distance between the manually selected needled tip from the confirmation CT and the target point obtained during surgical planning. Since the rabbit might move from the pre procedural to post-procedural scan, a global image registration was performed afterwards. Fig. 5 (a) shows a screen cut of the tumor and the arrow points to the target point in the pre-procedural CT. Fig. 5 (b) gives the corresponding slice, and the arrow points to the needle tip in the confirmation CT. Fig. 5 (c) shows the registered image. After these steps, the distance between these two points can be calculated. The result can be translated as the needle puncture accuracy.

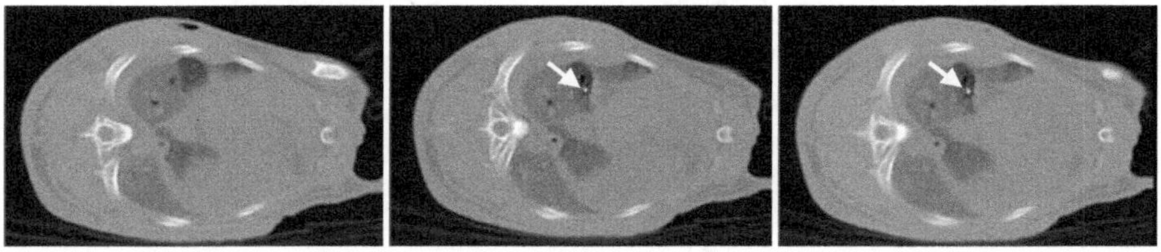

(a) (b) (c)

Fig. 5. An example of the intervention results. (a) The CT image with the tumor illustrated by the arrow before the puncture; (b) The confirmation CT after the puncture, and the arrow points indicates the needle tip; (c) The registered CT image of (b) to (a).

We did the experiments in eight rabbits, and they were numbered in the experiment time sequence. The first three experiments were performed without breath holding, while the later five were breath holding (by removing the ventilator) cases. We used distance between the target point in the pre-CT and the needle tip location in the confirmation CT (after global image registration using the FSL FLIRT program [17]) as the accuracy. Table 1 lists all the results. Overall the average distance without breath holding was 11*mm*, and the average error for the later five experiments with breath holding was 3.5*mm*, which means the lung movement caused by the breathing would impact the accuracy of intervention. After using the breath holding procedure, the accuracy of puncturing could be improved up to 70%.

Table 1. Accuracy of intervention experiments

Rabbit	Resolution (mm)	Accuracy (mm)
1	(0.27,0.27,1.20)	12.45
2	(0.26,0.26,1.20)	10.68
3	(0.29,0.29,1.20)	10.32
4	(0.28,0.28,1.20)	2.93
5	(0.23,0.23,1.20)	4.90
6	(0.28,0.28,1.20)	4.84
7	(0.28,0.28,1.20)	1.25
8	(0.25,0.25,1.20)	3.67

3.3 Quantitative Molecular Imaging Analysis

For validating the effectiveness of the microendoscopic procedure, we collected thirty microendoscopy video clips from the six rabbits' lung tumor to test the precision of our system. Fig. 6 shows the fluorescence microendoscopy images captured during our preliminary studies in the rabbit experiments. The motion of the image sequences

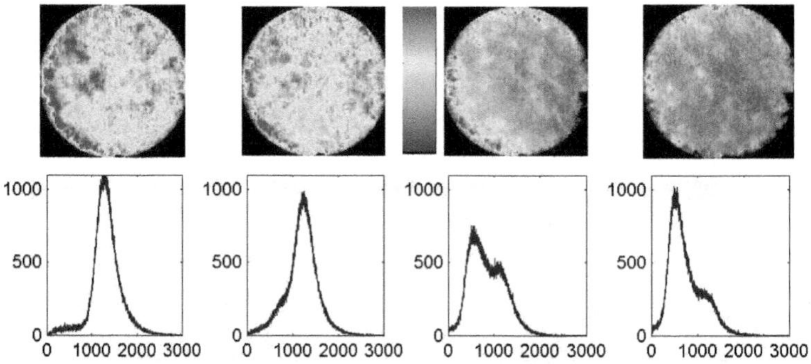

Fig. 6. Examples of the optical imaging of the rabbit experiments. Top: Four frames from the video. Bottom: histogram of images within a sliding time window (1 sec).

has been corrected, and the intensities are color-coded for better visualization. The histogram of the images within a one-second sliding window at each timepoint is shown in the second row. The first two frames show the molecular imaging results within the tumor and the next two gives the picture at the boundary of the tumor. From the histograms we can see that the intensity distributions of the images within a temporal sliding window are different within and outside the tumor, and there is a significant different contrast or distribution difference between images with non-labeled tissue and $\alpha_v\beta_3$-labeled tissue, where the histograms' peak value of non-labeled tissue images is around 500, and that of $\alpha_v\beta_3$-labeled tissue images is around 1500. Hence these histograms could be classified into two different groups with threshold value 1000 in order to determine whether the molecular imaging generates a positive response. We plan to establish the diagnostic criteria and extensively validate them in the lung cancer patient experiments.

3.4 Discussion

The advantage of MIMIG is that it could provide a convenient, efficient and accurate interventional tool for possible on-the-spot diagnosis and treatment, and it will gain more diagnostic power if a contrast agent is approved by FDA for human use in the future. Currently, the fine needle aspiration biopsy guided by MIMIG can be used to diagnose cancer for human, where the radiofrequency ablation can also be applied for confirmed cancerous cases. We plan to validate the MIMIG system in biopsy and RFA of peripheral lung cancer patients and to evaluate the clinical outcomes by comparing the group using MIMIG and the traditional repetitive CT-guided procedures.

Respiratory motion is always important especially for lung applications. In this system we use breath holding strategy to minimize the motion or image changes during intervention. We are currently working on an improved deformable image registration tool that not only models the temporal respiratory motion but also estimate the image according to the movement of the fiducials and respiratory belt. This motion also affects the stability of the microendoscopy imaging. In addition to the motion correction functions reported in this paper, the future work also focuses on modeling the intensity variations in molecular imaging caused by such motion.

4 Conclusion

In this paper, a MIMIG intervention system is designed for lung tumor intervention and molecular imaging diagnosis. After successfully targeting the tumor, molecular imaging can be used for onsite diagnosis, which could be followed by radio-frequency ablation treatment. The benefit of a 3D image-guided platform system relies in the design and planning of the needle trajectory for puncture using an orthogonal viewer (simultaneous axial, sagittal, and coronal view), which provides a clear perspective about the depth and the direction of the needle for reaching the tumor. The pilot study on eight rabbits showed the feasibility of on-the-spot intervention and tumor diagnosis. In the future work, we will evaluate the MIMIG system using lung cancer patient intervention experiments.

References

1. McWilliams, A., MacAulay, C., Gazdar, A.F., Lam, S.: Innovative Molecular and Imaging Approaches for the Detection of Lung Cancer and Its Precursor Lesions. Oncogene. 21(45), 6949–6959 (2002)
2. Wardwell, N.R., Massion, P.P.: Novel Strategies for the Early Detection and Prevention of Lung Cancer. Seminars in oncology 32(3), 259–268 (2005)
3. Hicks, R.J., Lau, E., Alam, N.Z., Chen, R.Y.: Imaging in the Diagnosis and Treatment of Non-Small Cell Lung Cancer. Respirology (Carlton, Vic.) 12(2), 165–172 (2007)
4. Bach, P.B., Jett, J.R., Pastorino, U., Tockman, M.S., Swensen, S.J., Begg, C.B.: Computed Tomography Screening and Lung Cancer Outcomes. Jama 297(9), 953–961 (2007)
5. Wong, K., Liu, J., Tung, C.H., Wong, S.T.: In Vivo Molecular Microendoscopy in Human Lung Cancer Mouse Model. In: World Molecular Imaging Congress, Montreal, Canada (2009)
6. Krucker, J., Xu, S., Glossop, N., Viswanathan, A., Borgert, J., Schulz, H., Wood, B.J.: Electromagnetic Tracking for Thermal Ablation and Biopsy Guidance: Clinical Evaluation of Spatial Accuracy. J. Vasc. Interv. Radiol. 18(9), 1141–1150 (2007)
7. Frantz, D.D., Wiles, A.D., Leis, S.E., Kirsch, S.R.: Accuracy Assessment Protocols for Electromagnetic Tracking Systems. Physics in medicine and biology 48(14), 2241–2251 (2003)
8. Barratt, D.C., Davies, A.H., Hughes, A.D., Thom, S.A., Humphries, K.N.: Optimisation and Evaluation of an Electromagnetic Tracking Device for High-Accuracy Three-Dimensional Ultrasound Imaging of the Carotid Arteries. Ultrasound in medicine & biology 27(7), 957–968 (2001)
9. Milne, A.D., Chess, D.G., Johnson, J.A., King, G.J.: Accuracy of an Electromagnetic Tracking Device: A Study of the Optimal Range and Metal Interference. Journal of biomechanics 29(6), 791–793 (1996)
10. Banovac, F., Tang, J., Xu, S., Lindisch, D., Chung, H.Y., Levy, E.B., Chang, T., McCullough, M.F., Yaniv, Z., Wood, B.J., Cleary, K.: Precision Targeting of Liver Lesions Using a Novel Electromagnetic Navigation Device in Physiologic Phantom and Swine. Medical physics 32(8), 2698–2705 (2005)
11. Zhu, X., Xue, Z., Gao, X., Zhu, Y., Wong, S.T.C.: Voles: Vascularity-Oriented Level Set Algorithm for Pulmonary Vessel Segmentation in Image Guided Intervention Therapy. In: IEEE International Symposium on Biomedical Imaging: From Nano to Macro, ISBI 2009, Boston, pp. 1247–1250 (2009)
12. Xue, Z., Wong, K., Wong, S.T.: Joint Registration and Segmentation of Serial Lung Ct Images for Image-Guided Lung Cancer Diagnosis and Therapy. Comput. Med. Imaging Graph. 34(1), 55–60 (2010)
13. Ayvaci, A., Freedman, D.: Joint Segmentation-Registration of Organs Using Geometric Models. In: IEEE Eng. Med. Biol. Soc., pp. 5251–5254. IEEE Press, New York (2007)
14. Droske, M., Rumpf, M.: Multiscale Joint Segmentation and Registration of Image Morphology. IEEE transactions on pattern analysis and machine intelligence 29(12), 2181–2194 (2007)
15. Pohl, K.M., Fisher, J., Grimson, W.E., Kikinis, R., Wells, W.M.: A Bayesian Model for Joint Segmentation and Registration. NeuroImage 31(1), 228–239 (2006)
16. Rueckert, D., Sonoda, L.I., Hayes, C., Hill, D.L., Leach, M.O., Hawkes, D.J.: Nonrigid Registration Using Free-Form Deformations: Application to Breast Mr Images. IEEE transactions on medical imaging 18(8), 712–721 (1999)
17. Denton, E.R., Sonoda, L.I., Rueckert, D., Rankin, S.C., Hayes, C., Leach, M.O., Hill, D.L., Hawkes, D.J.: Comparison and Evaluation of Rigid, Affine, and Nonrigid Registration of Breast Mr Images. Journal of computer assisted tomography 23(5), 800–805 (1999)

Simulating Dynamic Ultrasound Using MR-derived Motion Models to Assess Respiratory Synchronisation for Image-Guided Liver Interventions

Erik-Jan Rijkhorst, Daniel Heanes, Freddy Odille, David Hawkes, and Dean Barratt

Centre for Medical Image Computing, Department of Medical Physics and Bioengineering, University College London, London, United Kingdom
{e.rijkhorst,d.heanes,f.odille,d.hawkes,d.barratt}@ucl.ac.uk
http://cmic.cs.ucl.ac.uk

Abstract. Tracked intra-operative ultrasound can be registered to real-time synthetic ultrasound derived from a motion model to align pre-operative images with a patient's anatomy during an intervention. Furthermore, synchronisation of the motion model with the patient's breathing can be achieved by comparing diaphragm motion obtained from the tracked ultrasound, with that obtained from the synthetic ultrasound. The purpose of this study was to assess the effects of spatial misalignment between the tracked and synthetic ultrasound images on synchronisation accuracy. Deformable image registration of 4-D volunteer MR data was used to build realistic subject-specific liver motion models. Displacements predicted by the motion model were applied to acoustic parameter maps obtained from segmented breath-hold MR volumes, and dynamic B-mode ultrasound images were simulated using a fast ultrasound propagation method. To prevent synchronisation errors due to breathing variations between motion model acquisition and interventional ultrasound imaging from influencing the results, we simulated both the synthetic and the tracked ultrasound using a single motion model. Spatial misalignments of up to ± 2 cm between the tracked and synthetic ultrasound resulted in a maximum motion model breathing phase error of approx. 3 %, indicating that respiratory synchronisation of a motion model using tracked ultrasound is relatively insensitive to spatial misalignments.

Keywords: dynamic ultrasound, motion models, synchronisation, breathing, image guidance.

1 Introduction

Minimally- and non-invasive liver interventions, such as radio-frequency ablation and high-intensity focused ultrasound, rely on accurate image guidance to compensate for intra-operative respiratory motion. Over the past few years, several

N. Navab and P. Jannin (Eds.): IPCAI 2010, LNCS 6135, pp. 113–123, 2010.

methods for quantifying organ motion using 4-D CT or MR based motion models have been presented [1–4]. Such models can be used in combination with intra-operative imaging, such as B-mode ultrasound, to spatially align pre-operative images to the patient's anatomy during an intervention [5–8], allowing for a more accurate treatment of a target region.

Apart from spatial registration, accurate real-time temporal synchronisation of a motion model with the patient's breathing is equally important [4, 9]. To achieve this, a surrogate breathing signal needs to be available during intervention, for example by tracking skin markers [1] or using a navigator to track diaphragm motion [2, 4, 10].

The purpose of this study was to assess the effects on synchronisation accuracy of a pre-operative motion model with a subject's breathing due to spatial misalignment between tracked interventional ultrasound and real-time synthetic ultrasound derived from the motion model. Deformable image registration of free-breathing volunteer MR data was used to build a subject-specific liver motion model as a function of breathing phase. To obtain acoustic parameter maps, breath-hold MR volumes were segmented into liver, blood, lung, and ribs. The maps were deformed by applying the displacements predicted by the motion model, and a fast ultrasound propagation simulation was used to compute dynamic B-mode ultrasound images. One such simulated ultrasound sequence was used to represent the tracked ultrasound, while a second sequence, computed at a slightly different location to simulate spatial misalignment, represented the real-time synthetic ultrasound. A navigator window was positioned at the diaphragm in both simulated sequences, from which surrogate breathing signals and a motion model phase error were computed.

2 Materials and Methods

We propose the following scenario for synchronising a motion model to a subject's breathing during an intervention (Fig. 1). Prior to intervention, real-time

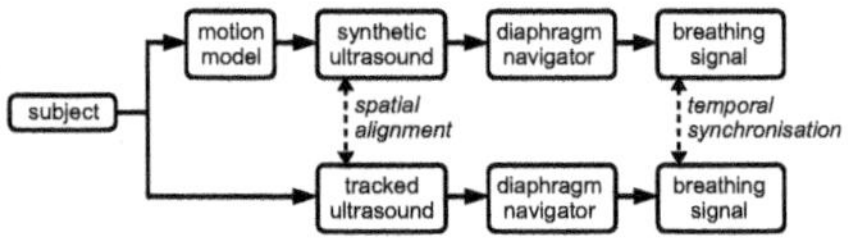

Fig. 1. Scenario for synchronising a motion model to a subject's breathing. Note that in this study both the tracked and synthetic ultrasound were simulated using a single motion model.

MR images are acquired and deformable image registration is used to obtain a motion model. High-resolution breath-hold MR images are segmented into different tissue types to allow the computation of simulated ultrasound images.

During intervention, tracked dynamic B-mode ultrasound images of the moving diaphragm are continuously acquired. Using the tracking information, these images can be aligned spatially with the motion model co-ordinate system. A fast ultrasound simulation technique produces a synthetic dynamic B-mode sequence at the tracked location of the real ultrasound. These can be registered to the tracked ultrasound to improve spatial alignment between the motion model and the subject [5, 8]. Furthermore, by placing navigator windows at the moving diaphragm in both the tracked and synthetic ultrasound sequences, two breathing signals can be obtained, which may be used to synchronise the motion model with the breathing.

In this paper, assuming this scenario, we computed a synchronisation error measure due to spatial misalignment between the tracked and synthetic ultrasound. Instead of using real tracked ultrasound, we simulated it using the motion model in the same way as was done for the synthetic ultrasound. This prevented introducing additional synchronisation errors due to variations in a subject's breathing which may occur between motion model acquisition and interventional ultrasound imaging, and which are of potentially larger magnitude than the synchronisation errors due to misalignment. Furthermore, the breathing signal obtained from the simulated tracked ultrasound acts as a "ground-truth", which would not be available if real tracked ultrasound would have been used. The following sections present the different parts of our computations in more detail.

2.1 MR Data Acquisition

Data were acquired for three healthy volunteers using a 1.5 T cylindrical bore Philips Achieva MR scanner at Guy's Hospital, London. A fast 3-D T1-weighted gradient echo sequence (THRIVE) was used to obtain high-resolution scans during breath-hold, and 4-D (3-D+time) real-time scans during free breathing. Parallel imaging with a 32-channel coil array using a SENSE acceleration factor of 8 resulted in scan times of approx. 16 seconds per breath-hold volume, and 1 second per real-time volume, respectively. A respiratory signal, obtained from a pneumatic bellow placed around the chest of each volunteer, was recorded during all scans.

The breath-hold scans were acquired at exhale with a voxel size of $1.4 \times 1.4 \times 1.7$ mm^3 and a field-of-view of $400 \times 400 \times 270$ mm^3 covering the whole abdomen. To reduce the time needed for a single real-time scan, the sequence parameters were modified to decrease the spatial resolution to $1.5 \times 1.5 \times 4$ mm^3, while keeping a similar FOV. A total of $N^{\mathrm{acq}} = 40$ volumes were acquired over approx. 10 breathing cycles.

2.2 Deformable Registration of Real-Time Free Breathing Scans

To obtain a measure of breathing induced displacements throughout the liver, the real-time MR scans were registered using a non-rigid fluid registration method [11]. This method solves the time-dependent Navier-Lamé equations for a compressible viscous fluid resulting in a diffeomorphic transformation between source and target images. The registration is driven by image-derived forces and employs a full multi-grid scheme [11].

First, the real-time volume with a breathing phase closest to exhale was manually selected and used as the source (i.e reference) volume. This scan was registered to all other target volumes, resulting in a set of N^{acq} displacement fields for each volunteer.

To assess the registration accuracy, corresponding anatomical landmarks, including vessel bifurcations and points on the diaphragm, were picked manually in each volume, resulting in a set of N^{acq} points for each location. Landmark points were identified for each volunteer at five different locations distributed throughout the liver. The mean target registration error (TRE), defined as the mean of the Euclidean distance between each landmark point in the reference volume and corresponding points in the other volumes, was computed before and after registration.

2.3 Motion Model Breathing Phase from Respiratory Bellow Signal

To fit a motion-model to the registration results, the tissue displacement at each voxel must be known as a function of the breathing cycle. Since we would like to represent an average breathing cycle by sorting the sparse real-time data, and the amplitude of the bellow signal may vary across breathing cycles (see Fig. 2), we used the breathing phase instead [1, 12].

To compute the breathing phase from the bellow signal, it was first convolved with a Gaussian to obtain a signal with clearly defined minima at times $t_i^{\min}$, and maxima at times $t_i^{\max}$, $i = 1, ..., N^{\max}$. The minima were assigned a breathing phase of zero, while the phase of each maximum was set to the average phase over all maxima, $\bar{\phi}^{\max}$, calculated using

$$\bar{\phi}^{\max} = \frac{1}{N^{\max}} \sum_{i=1}^{N^{\max}} \frac{t_i^{\max} - t_i^{\min}}{t_{i+1}^{\min} - t_i^{\min}} , \tag{1}$$

where $N^{\max}$ is the total number of maxima. The breathing phase corresponding to each real-time scan, ϕ_j, was linearly interpolated as a function of its acquisition time t_j, using

$$\phi_j = \begin{cases} \left(\frac{t_j - t_i^{\min}}{t_i^{\max} - t_i^{\min}}\right) \bar{\phi}^{\max} & \text{for } t_i^{\min} \le t_j < t_i^{\max} \\ \bar{\phi}^{\max} + \left(\frac{t_j - t_i^{\max}}{t_{i+1}^{\min} - t_i^{\max}}\right)(1 - \bar{\phi}^{\max}) & \text{for } t_i^{\max} \le t_j < t_{i+1}^{\min} \end{cases} , \tag{2}$$

with $i = 1, ..., N^{\max}$ and $j = 1, ..., N^{\text{acq}}$.

2.4 Motion Model

With the method outlined in the previous section, each real-time scan was assigned a respiratory phase ϕ_i, which, together with the deformable registration results, gave a set of tissue displacements at each voxel location $\boldsymbol{r}$, denoted by

$$\boldsymbol{u}_i(\boldsymbol{r}) \equiv \boldsymbol{u}(\boldsymbol{r}, \phi_i) , \quad \text{with } i = 1, \ldots, N^{\text{acq}} . \tag{3}$$

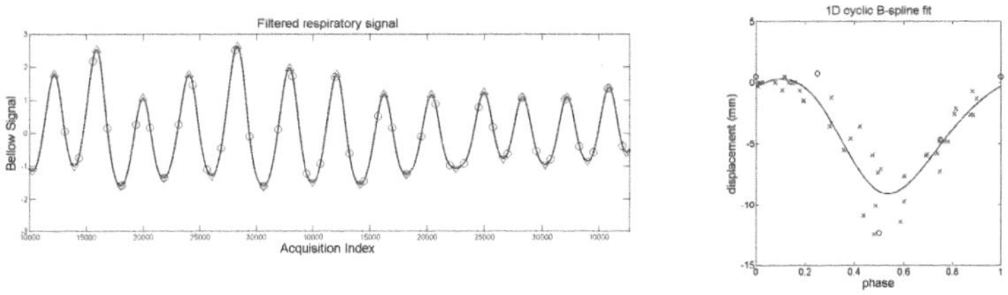

Fig. 2. Signal from a respiratory bellow (*left*) as a function of acquisition index illustrating variations in breathing amplitude. Open circles indicate the real-time MR acquisitions, whereas triangles indicate minima and maxima. B-spline fit to displacement data (*right*) as a function of phase at a single location in the liver. Open circles indicate the B-spline control points (i.e. the motion model coefficients).

To interpolate these displacement data, we used a 1-D cyclic homogeneous cubic B-spline with four control points as a fitting function, given by

$$\hat{\boldsymbol{u}}(\boldsymbol{r}, \phi) = \sum_{k=1}^{k=4} f_k(\phi)\boldsymbol{\beta}_k(\boldsymbol{r}) \ , \tag{4}$$

where $f_k(\phi)$ are the B-spline basis functions, and $\boldsymbol{\beta}_k(\boldsymbol{r})$ are the control point values (i.e. the motion model coefficients) at each location $\boldsymbol{r}$ and for each spatial direction x, y, and z. This particular fitting function was chosen because previous work had shown it to give the best approximation to the registration results [13].

By substituting equation (3) into (4), we obtain a set of N^{acq} equations for the known displacements $\boldsymbol{u}_i$, given by

$$\begin{bmatrix} \boldsymbol{u}_1(\boldsymbol{r}) \\ \boldsymbol{u}_2(\boldsymbol{r}) \\ \vdots \\ \boldsymbol{u}_{N^{\text{acq}}}(\boldsymbol{r}) \end{bmatrix} = \begin{bmatrix} f_1(\phi_1) & f_2(\phi_1) & f_3(\phi_1) & f_4(\phi_1) \\ f_1(\phi_2) & f_2(\phi_2) & f_3(\phi_2) & f_4(\phi_2) \\ \vdots & \vdots & \vdots & \vdots \\ f_1(\phi_{N^{\text{acq}}}) & f_2(\phi_{N^{\text{acq}}}) & f_3(\phi_{N^{\text{acq}}}) & f_4(\phi_{N^{\text{acq}}}) \end{bmatrix} \begin{bmatrix} \boldsymbol{\beta}_1(\boldsymbol{r}) \\ \boldsymbol{\beta}_2(\boldsymbol{r}) \\ \boldsymbol{\beta}_3(\boldsymbol{r}) \\ \boldsymbol{\beta}_4(\boldsymbol{r}) \end{bmatrix} . \tag{5}$$

From this over-determined system of linear equations, the unknown motion model coefficients $\boldsymbol{\beta}_k$ were found by computing the Moore-Penrose pseudo-inverse of the basis functions matrix $f_k(\phi_i)$ using singular value decomposition. Note that, since the basis functions are independent of $\boldsymbol{r}$, this inverse needs to be computed only once [3].

With the motion model coefficients known, equation (4) allows the computation of an approximate model displacement $\hat{\boldsymbol{u}}$ as a function of phase for every voxel location (Figure 2). Using the corresponding anatomical landmark points mentioned above, the mean target model error (TME), defined as the mean of the Euclidean distance between each landmark point in the reference volume and the corresponding locations predicted by the motion model for the other volumes, was computed for all volunteers.

2.5 Simulating Ultrasound Scan Lines

Synthetic ultrasound images were simulated using a fast propagation model similar to others described in the literature [5–8]. We assigned local impedance and absorption coefficients to different tissue types segmented from the breath-hold MR scan similar to [8], rather than using a conversion from CT Hounsfield units as in [5, 7].

Assuming a plane longitudinal acoustic wave propagating along a ray, and considering perpendicular reflection at a tissue interface i where the acoustic impedance changes from Z_{i-1} to Z_i, the ratio of reflected to incident intensity, $r_i^{\perp}$, is given by

$$r_i^{\perp} = \left(\frac{Z_i - Z_{i-1}}{Z_i + Z_{i-1}} \right)^2 , \tag{6}$$

with $i = 1, \ldots, N$, and boundary condition $r_1^{\perp} = 0$. Using a Lambertian reflection model, the intensity reflection ratio at an oblique interface can be written as

$$r_i = |\hat{\boldsymbol{x}} \cdot \hat{\boldsymbol{n}}_i| r_i^{\perp} = \frac{|\hat{\boldsymbol{x}} \cdot \nabla Z_i|}{\|\nabla Z_i\|} r_i^{\perp} , \tag{7}$$

with $\hat{\boldsymbol{x}}$ a unit vector along the ray direction, and $\hat{\boldsymbol{n}}_i$ the unit normal at the i-th interface. In practice, the inner product term is obtained by computing the gradient of the impedance, as indicated by the right-most term.

The ratio of transmitted to incident intensity up to the i-th interface is computed by tracing along each ray using

$$t_i = \prod_{j=1}^{j=i} \left(1 - r_j^{\perp}\right) , \tag{8}$$

whereas the ratio of absorbed to incident intensity can be written as

$$A_i = \prod_{j=1}^{j=i} \exp\left(-0.1 \ln(10) \alpha_j \Delta x\right) , \tag{9}$$

with Δx the distance between successive sampling points along the ray, and the local absorption coefficient α_i has the units of dB cm^{-1}. Combining equations (7), (8) and (9), the reflected intensity from the i-th interface, received at the transducer, is given by

$$I_i^{\mathrm{refl}} = I_0 \, t_i^2 \, A_i^2 \, r_i , \tag{10}$$

where the transmission and absorption terms are squared since the ultrasound wave is assumed to travel along the same path twice. The effects of finite beam width in the elevational direction were simulated by convolving I_r along the beam direction with a Gaussian, while the effects of multiple active transducer elements was taken into account by convolving I_r perpendicular to the beam direction with a 1-D triangular window function [6, 8, 14].

To obtain realistic speckle patterns representative of liver parenchyma, we applied a texture quilting technique using real ultrasound images as input [15, 16], as a computationally efficient alternative to performing extensive scattering simulations [6]. Inverse log-compression was applied to the texture map, resulting in a texture intensity I^{text}, which was blended with the reflected intensity (10) using

$$I^{\text{tot}} = w\, I^{\text{refl}} + (1 - w)\, t^2\, A^2\, I^{\text{text}}\ , \tag{11}$$

with blending weight w. The final log-compressed ultrasound scan line image was computed from

$$I^{\text{US}} = \log(1 + aI^{\text{tot}})/\log(1 + a)\ , \tag{12}$$

where a is the log-compression factor.

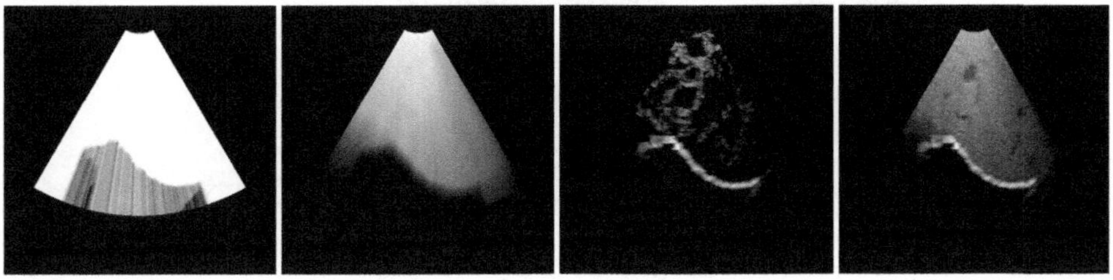

Fig. 3. Example of log-compressed simulated transmission, absorption, reflection, and final ultrasound B-mode image (*left-to-right*)

2.6 Simulating Dynamic B-Mode Ultrasound

To obtain 3-D impedance and absorption maps for the different tissues, we used semiautomatic methods to segment the breath-hold MR scan into liver, blood vessels, lung and ribs. The vessels were segmented using a Hessian-based multiscale filter [17]. Literature values for impedance and absorption coefficients were assigned to the segmented regions [18] (see Table 1), and Gaussian distributed noise was added to introduce small spatial inhomogeneities within regions of single tissue type.

Table 1. Acoustic impedance Z (in $10^6 \text{kg}\,\text{s}^{-1}\text{m}^{-2}$) and absorption coefficient α (in $\text{dB}\,\text{cm}^{-1}$) for tissue types considered in this study [18]

	liver	blood	lung	ribs
Z	1.65	1.61	0.50	7.8
α	0.94	0.18	12.0	20.0

To simulate a dynamic B-mode ultrasound sequence, we defined a sector-shaped region representing an ultrasound image at a location in the breath-hold MR volume (Fig. 4). The apical edge of this sector, representing the curvilinear ultrasound transducer face, was placed on the skin surface below the rib cage with the sector axis pointing upwards at an angle such that the liver, diaphragm, and part of the right lung were in view (Fig. 4). Please note that probe induced liver deformations were not taken into account.

Values for motion model B-spline control point coefficients $\boldsymbol{\beta}$ were obtained at regularly spaced points across the sector using linear interpolation. Displacements of these points were computed using equation (4) resulting in a warped sector point-set. The impedance and absorption coefficients were linearly interpolated across the warped sector, and equation (12) was used to simulate a B-mode sector scan (Fig. 3). By varying the breathing phase and repeating the simulation, a dynamic sequence of B-mode scans was obtained.

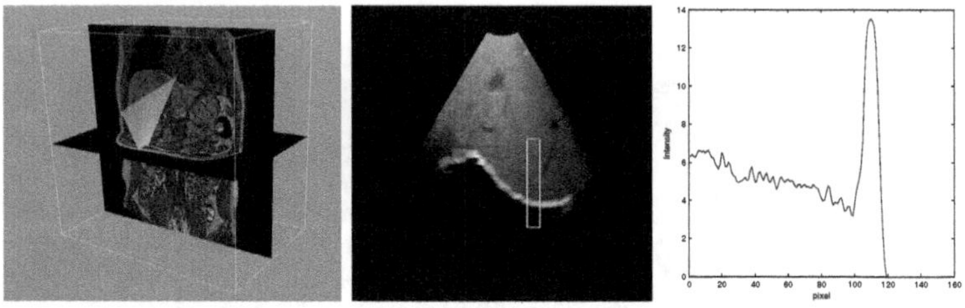

Fig. 4. Virtual ultrasound sector positioned inside the MR breath-hold volume (*left*), the resulting simulated B-mode image showing the diaphragm navigator window (*centre*), and the corresponding 1-D profile (*right*)

By combining a physics-based ultrasound propagation model with the texture maps our simulated ultrasound images contain sufficient characteristics of real ultrasound images, allowing acquisition of a breathing signal from the moving diaphragm, as explained in the next section.

2.7 Ultrasound Diaphragm Navigator Breathing Signal

Surrogate breathing signals were extracted from the simulated dynamic B-mode sequences by positioning a narrow navigator window at the diaphragm location [10] (see Fig. 4, centre image). By integrating across this navigator and computing the maximum of the resulting 1D profile (Fig. 4, right), a diaphragm navigator breathing signal s was obtained, which was normalised. This was done for both the tracked ultrasound and the synthetic ultrasound, resulting in the normalised signals s^{t} and s^{s}, respectively.

2.8 Synchronisation Accuracy: Motion Model Phase Error

The known relation $\phi(s^{\mathrm{s}})$ between the synthetic signal s^{s} and the motion model phase ϕ can be used to instantiate the motion model during an intervention using the signal s^{t} from the tracked ultrasound. In practice, spatial misalignments between the tracked and synthetic ultrasound result in differences between the signals s^{t} and s^{s}, leading to small errors in the phase ϕ at which the motion model is instantiated (Fig. 5). Since, in this study, we used a simulation to represent the tracked ultrasound, the "ground-truth" relation $\phi(s^{\mathrm{t}})$ is also known. This allows quantifying the synchronisation accuracy by the following phase error metric:

$$\Delta\phi = \phi(s^{\mathrm{t}}) - \phi(s^{\mathrm{s}}) . \tag{13}$$

3 Results and Discussion

Numerical results for the target registration and target model error are given in Table 2. The mean liver displacement of 4.6 ± 3.8 mm before correction was reduced to 2.5 ± 1.7 mm when applying the motion model, which is comparable to the real-time MR scan voxel size (1.5 mm in plane, 4 mm out of plane).

Table 2. Mean, standard deviation, and maximum displacement in mm of the corresponding anatomical landmarks (second column). For each volunteer five landmarks at different locations throughout the liver were used. Residual displacements after registration correction (TRE, third column), and after motion model correction (TME), are given in the third and fourth columns, respectively.

	displacement			TRE			TME		
volunteer	mean	σ	max	mean	σ	max	mean	σ	max
1	4.7	3.3	16.3	2.2	1.1	6.0	2.4	1.3	7.7
2	4.6	4.3	17.4	2.3	1.6	7.2	2.6	1.9	10.2
3	4.4	3.7	20.9	2.1	1.4	12.4	2.4	1.7	14.6
all	4.6	3.8	20.9	2.2	1.4	12.4	2.5	1.7	14.6

Deformable registration of a single real-time scan took around 30 minutes on a standard PC. To speed up the non-rigid registrations we are preparing to use a GPU accelerated registration method [19], and initial tests showed a computation time of approx. 60 seconds per registration.

The time needed to calculate the motion model coefficients $\boldsymbol{\beta}(\boldsymbol{r})$ across the complete volume by inverting equation (5) was approx. 2 minutes. Reslicing and interpolating the coefficients and simulating a single ultrasound image took of the order of a few seconds. Since we would eventually like to use our technique in clinical applications, real-time simulation of the synthetic ultrasound will be required, which can potentially be achieved using GPU techniques [6, 7].

Fig. 5 shows plots of the navigator signals and resulting phase error (13) due to translations along the superior-inferior axis of ± 2 cm of the tracked ultrasound with respect to the synthetic ultrasound, which represents an estimate of the upper limit of misalignment one may expect at the start of a treatment. The resulting maximum phase error was approx. 3 %, which indicates that the phase error is rather insensitive to alignment inaccuracies. This could potentially also be of importance for applications where the location of a diaphragm navigator used during pre-operative imaging is different from the location used during intervention [4].

Finally, comparing the tracked ultrasound signal directly to the bellow signal could be an alternative and more direct way for synchronising the motion

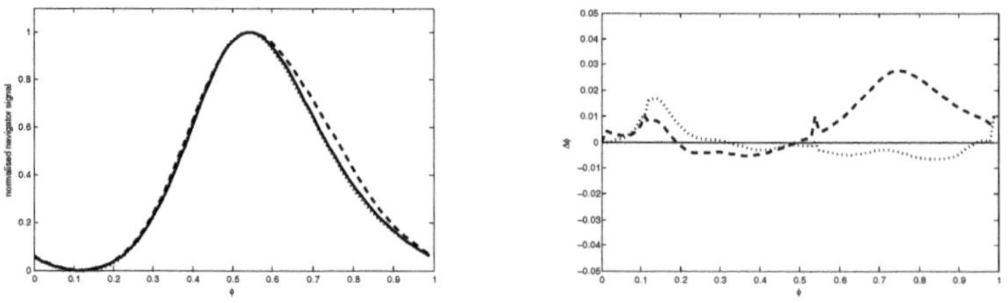

Fig. 5. Navigator signals (*left panel*) for the tracked (*solid line*) and synthetic ultrasound for misalignments in the superior-inferior direction of +2 cm (*dashed line*) and −2 cm (*dotted line*). Corresponding phase error $\Delta\phi$ (*right panel*) as a function of motion model input phase ϕ.

model to a subject's breathing. However, since these signals would potentially capture different breathing modes, like chest and abdominal breathing, a larger synchronisation error may result.

4 Conclusion

We presented a method for building a realistic liver motion model from MR scans obtained during breath-hold and real-time breathing. Applying the motion model to the segmented breath-hold volume, and using a fast ultrasound propagation model, dynamic B-mode sequences were simulated. A surrogate breathing signal was then computed by positioning a navigator window across the diaphragm, from which a motion model phase error, due to spatial misalignment between tracked ultrasound and synthetic ultrasound, was obtained. We found that for spatial misalignments of ±2 cm, the maximum phase error was approx. 3 %, indicating that synchronising a motion model to a subject's breathing is rather insensitive to inaccuracies in tracked ultrasound localisation.

Acknowledgments. We would like to thank Tobias Schaeffter for his help in acquiring the MR data, and Jamie McClelland for advice on motion models. This work was funded by EPSRC grant EP/F025750/1, and a UCL/UCLH Comprehensive Biomedical Research Centre (CBRC) grant (No. 96). Dean Barratt is funded by the Royal Academy of Engineering Research Fellowship scheme.

References

1. McClelland, J.R., Blackall, J.M., Tarte, S., et al.: A continuous 4D motion model from multiple respiratory cycles for use in lung radiotherapy. Medical Physics 33(9), 3348–3358 (2006)
2. Nguyen, T.N., Moseley, J.L., Dawson, L.A., et al.: Adapting liver motion models using a navigator channel technique. Medical Physics 36(4), 1061–1073 (2009)
3. White, M.J., Hawkes, D.J., Melbourne, A., et al.: Motion artifact correction in free-breathing abdominal MRI using overlapping partial samples to recover image deformations. Magnetic Resonance in Medicine 62(2), 440–449 (2009)

4. King, A.P., Boubertakh, R., Rhode, K.S., et al.: A subject-specific technique for respiratory motion correction in image-guided cardiac catheterisation procedures. Medical Image Analysis 13(3), 419–431 (2009)
5. Wein, W., Brunke, S., Khamene, A., et al.: Automatic CT-ultrasound registration for diagnostic imaging and image-guided intervention. Medical Image Analysis 12(5), 577–585 (2008)
6. Shams, R., Hartley, R., Navab, N.: Real-time simulation of medical ultrasound from CT images. In: Metaxas, D., Axel, L., Fichtinger, G., Székely, G. (eds.) MICCAI 2008, Part II. LNCS, vol. 5242, pp. 734–741. Springer, Heidelberg (2008)
7. Reichl, T., Passenger, J., Acosta, O., Salvado, O.: Ultrasound goes GPU: real-time simulation using CUDA. In: SPIE, vol. 7261 (2009)
8. King, A.P., Ma, Y.-L., Yao, C., Jansen, C., Razavi, R., Rhode, K.S., Penney, G.P.: Image-to-physical registration for image-guided interventions using 3-D ultrasound and an ultrasound imaging model. In: Prince, J.L., Pham, D.L., Myers, K.J. (eds.) IPMI 2009. LNCS, vol. 5636, pp. 188–201. Springer, Heidelberg (2009)
9. Ruan, D., Fessler, J.A., Balter, J.M., Keall, P.J.: Real-time profiling of respiratory motion: baseline drift, frequency variation and fundamental pattern change. Physics in Medicine and Biology 54(15), 4777–4792 (2009)
10. Timinger, H., Krueger, S., Dietmayer, K., Borgert, J.: Motion compensated coronary interventional navigation by means of diaphragm tracking and elastic motion models. Physics in Medicine and Biology 50(3), 491–503 (2005)
11. Crum, W.R., Tanner, C., Hawkes, D.J.: Anisotropic multi-scale fluid registration: evaluation in magnetic resonance breast imaging. Physics in Medicine and Biology 50(21), 5153–5174 (2005)
12. von Siebenthal, M., Székely, G., Lomax, A.J., Cattin, P.C.: Systematic errors in respiratory gating due to intrafraction deformations of the liver. Medical Physics 34(9), 3620–3629 (2007)
13. McClelland, J.R., Chandler, A.G., Blackall, J.M., Ahmad, S., Landau, D.B., Hawkes, D.J.: 4D motion models over the respiratory cycle for use in lung cancer radiotherapy planning. In: SPIE, vol. 5744, pp. 173–183 (2005)
14. Goldstein, A., Madrazo, B.L.: Slice-thickness artifacts in gray-scale ultrasound. Journal of Clinical Ultrasound 9(7), 365–375 (1981)
15. Efros, A.A., Freeman, W.T.: Image quilting for texture synthesis and transfer. In: SIGGRAPH 2001, pp. 341–346. ACM, New York (2001)
16. Zhu, Y., Magee, D.R., Ratnalingam, R., Kessel, D.: A virtual ultrasound imaging system for the simulation of ultrasound-guided needle insertion procedures. In: Medical Image Understanding and Analysis (2006)
17. Frangi, A., Niessen, W., Vincken, K., Viergever, M.: Multiscale vessel enhancement filtering. In: Wells, W.M., Colchester, A.C.F., Delp, S.L. (eds.) MICCAI 1998. LNCS, vol. 1496, pp. 130–137. Springer, Heidelberg (1998)
18. Curry, T.S., Dowdey, J.E., Murry, R.C.: Christensen's Physics of Diagnostic Radiology, 4th edn. Lea & Febiger, Philadelphia (1990)
19. Modat, M., Ridgway, G., Taylor, Z., et al.: Fast free-form deformation using graphics processing units. In: Computer Methods and Programs in Biomedicine (2009)

Rapid Image Registration of Three-Dimensional Transesophageal Echocardiography and X-ray Fluoroscopy for the Guidance of Cardiac Interventions

Gang Gao[1], Graeme Penney[1], Nicolas Gogin[2], Pascal Cathier[2], Aruna Arujuna[1], Matt Wright[1], Dennis Caulfield[3], Aldo Rinaldi[3], Reza Razavi[1], and Kawal Rhode[1]

[1] Division of Imaging Sciences, King's College London, London, UK
[2] Medisys Group, Philips Research, Paris, France
[3] Department of Cardiology, Guy's and St.Thomas' Hospital, London, UK

Abstract. The recent availability of three-dimensional (3D) transesophageal echocardiography (TEE) provides cardiologists with real-time 3D imaging of cardiac anatomy. X-ray fluoroscopy is the conventional modalilty that is used for guiding many cardiac interventions. Increasingly this is now supported using intra-procedure 3D TEE imaging. We hypothesize that the real-time co-registration and visualization of 3D TEE and X-ray fluoroscopy data will provide a powerful guidance tool for cardiologists. In this paper, we propose a novel, robust and efficient method for performing this registration. Our method consists of an image-based TEE probe localization algorithm and a calibration procedure. While the calibration needs to be done only once, the registration takes approximately 9.5 seconds to complete. The accuracy of our method was assessed by using both a crosswire phantom and a more realistic heart phantom. The target registration error for the heart phantom was less than 2mm. In addition, the accuracy and the clinical feasiblity of our method was evaluated in two cardiac electrophysiology procedures. The registration results showed in-plane errors of 1.5 and 3mm.

Keywords: Image registration, Cardiac intervention, Transesophageal echocardiography, X-ray fluoroscopy.

1 Introduction

Minimally-invasive cardiac interventions are carried out for the diagnosis and treatment of a broad range of cardiovascular diseases. These types of procedures are increasingly popular when compared to their more invasive counterparts because there is less morbidity to the patient with similar clinical outcomes of success. Examples of these procedures include those carried out for the repair of structural heart disease and cardiac electrophysiology (EP) procedures. The interventional devices, for example, catheters, are designed to be X-ray visible and can be seen throughout the part of their length that lies in the X-ray field of view (FOV). Two-dimensional (2D) X-ray imaging has been a dominant imaging modality for cardiac interventions. Typically, imaging can be performed at high frame rates (up to 30

N. Navab and P. Jannin (Eds.): IPCAI 2010, LNCS 6135, pp. 124–134, 2010.

frames per second) and therefore the cardiac motion and the motion of interventional devices do not cause significant motion artifacts in the acquired images. However, the use of X-ray fluoroscopy alone is inadequate for the guidance of procedures that require soft-tissue information, for example, the treatment of structural heart disease [1]. In addition, exposing patients, especially pediatric patients with congenital defects, to ionizing radiation carries a significant risk. On-going research is actively seeking to reduce the use of, or even replace, X-ray fluoroscopy in cardiac interventional procedures, especially for pediatrics [2]. Pre-operatively acquired magnetic resonance imaging (MRI) and computer tomography (CT) have been used with X-ray fluoroscopy to improve the guidance of cardiac interventional procedures [3]. However, the use of pre-procedural MR and CT imaging will produce roadmap images that are static and do not update with the intra-procedural situation. Additional steps are required to compensate for intra-procedural deformations, for example, caused by respiratory motion of the heart [4]. In contrast to MRI and CT, three-dimensional (3D) echocardiography is a real-time imaging modality that can be readily used in the catheter laboratory environment. It allows visualizing the exact cardiac pathomorphology and also the interventional devices and their surrounding structures. With recently emerging technologies such as 3D transesophageal echocardiography (TEE), the image quality and resolution of echocardiography has improved considerably. Recently, the clinical feasibility of 3D TEE was evaluated for guiding a variety of cardiac interventional procedures including atrial septal defect closure, patent foramen ovale closure, mitral valve / aortic valve repair and interventional EP procedures [5, 6]. The use of 3D TEE for guiding interventional procedures is on a rapid rise and this will be augmented by the introduction of smaller and higher quality transducers in the future. The miniaturization process is likely to lead to the availability of 3D trans-nasal probes that will remove the requirement for the use of general anaesthesia for prolonged procedures.

The purpose of this study was to develop a technique to combine 3D TEE and X-ray fluoroscopy images for the guidance of cardiac interventional procedures. A key step of our technique is the fast and robust image registration of 3D TEE and X-ray fluoroscopy data. The image registration of 3D ultrasound and X-ray fluoroscopy is challenging because of the lack of common information. Previously reported methods [7] rely on the use of additional tracking devices. However, the use of tracking systems has several disadvantages including the requirement of additional hardware, the requirement of modifications to the ultrasound probe, and, in the case of magnetic tracking systems, the sensitivity of these systems to metallic interference. Our method was built upon an image-based 2D-3D registration algorithm. It does not rely on tracking devices or modification to the TEE probe. Therefore, this method can be deployed easily to any cardiac catheterization laboratory. In the following sections, we will describe our method and validate its accuracy and robustness by using two different types of phantom. Its accuracy and clinical feasibility will also be evaluated in two patient studies.

2 Method

For our experiments we used a Philips iE33 ultrasound system with an X7-2t 3D TEE probe. X-ray imaging was performed using a Philips Allura Xper FD10 system.

2.1 Image Registration of 3D TEE and X-ray Fluoroscopy

The objective of 3D TEE and X-ray fluoroscopy registration is to find a transformation matrix $T_{us\_img \rightarrow X\text{-}ray}$ which transforms the TEE volume I_{us} from its own coordinate system to the X-ray coordinate system.

The transformation matrix $T_{us\_img \rightarrow X\text{-}ray\_img}$ consists of two rigid body transformation matrices T_{probe}, $T_{us\_img \rightarrow probe}$ and a projection matrix T_{proj}:

$$T_{us\_img \rightarrow X\text{-}ray\_img} = T_{proj} T_{probe} T_{us\_img \rightarrow probe} \tag{1}$$

While T_{probe} defines the 3D position of the ultrasound probe in X-ray space, $T_{us\_img \rightarrow probe}$ transforms the 3D ultrasound volume to the ultrasound probe space. Many of previously reported ultrasound image registration algorithms consisted of two steps: 1). Detect the 3D position of the ultrasound probe using optical or electromagnetic (EM) tracking devices; 2). Calibrate the ultrasound probe in the coordinate of the tracking device to calculate matrix $T_{us\_img \rightarrow probe}$. In this paper, we propose a method which does not use any additional tracking devices. Instead, an image-based localization algorithm was developed to estimate the 3D position of the TEE probe in X-ray space. A TEE calibration procedure was designed based on the probe localization algorithm.

2.2 Localization of the TEE Probe

Although the TEE probe is designed to be flexible (Fig.1a), its transducer is encapsulated in a rigid head. For simplicity, the rigid head of the TEE probe is referred to as "the TEE probe" in the following text. A Nano-CT scanner (http://www.skyscan.de) was used to reconstruct an ultra high resolution (0.2×0.2×0.2mm^3) 3D volume of the TEE probe, which reveals its contours and the internal structures (Fig.1b). To determine the 3D position of the TEE probe in X-ray space, the Nano-CT volume was registered with one or more X-ray images using a 2D-3D image registration algorithm.

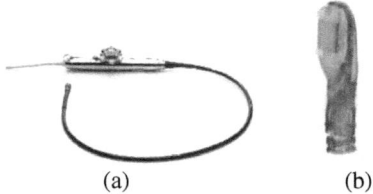

(a) (b)

Fig. 1. (a) Philips X7-2t 3D TEE probe was used in the experiments; (b) The ultra high resolution Nano-CT volume reveals the contours and the internal structures of the TEE probe

2D-3D image registration has been intensively studied in the past years [8, 9]. Clinically it was used to register pre-operative CT or MR volume of bones, blood vessels and medical devices to intra-operative X-ray images. During a 2D-3D image registration process, the algorithm repeatedly repositions the 3D volume in space and compares its projection, called the *digitally reconstructed radiograph* (DRR), with the X-ray image(s). At each iteration, an image comparison metric is used to calculate the similarity between the X-ray image(s) and the DRR. The three translation and three rotation parameters are changed according to the similarity measurement. The registration process continues until the similarity between the X-Ray image(s) and the DRR is maximized.

In this study, we implemented an intensity based 2D-3D registration algorithm similar to the one described in [8]. In our implementation, gradient difference was used as the similarity measurement while the standard Powell algorithm was used as the optimizer. The speed of the original algorithm was relatively slow because the reconstruction of DRR is computationally expensive. It could take minutes to complete a registration. Our implementation overcomes this issue by taking the advantage of the latest GPU technology. The DRR reconstruction time was reduced to less than 10 milliseconds for each estimated position. By using a standard computer workstation equipped with an Intel Quad-Core CPU (2.66GHz), 4GB RAM and an NVIDIA GeForce GTX 280 graphic card, the overall registration time between the Nano-CT volume and two X-ray images (1024×1024 with 0.17×0.17 pixel resolution) is around 9.5 seconds..

2.3 TEE Probe Calibration

The purpose of the calibration is to find the transformation matrix $T_{us\_img \rightarrow probe}$, which transforms the TEE volume to the coordinate system of the TEE probe which is defined by the Nano-CT. A calibration phantom which consists of a 9-litre water tank and two thin metal strings was used to help the calculation of $T_{us\_img \rightarrow probe}$. Nine metal landmarks which were visible in both X-ray and ultrasound were placed on the strings. The TEE probe was rigidly fixed beneath the strings during data acquisition. X-ray images were acquired from left anterior oblique (LAO) 45°, right anterior oblique (RAO) 45° and posterior-anterior (PA) projections. Simultaneously an ultrasound volume was acquired in full volume mode, giving the maximal volume coverage possible with the TEE probe. The following steps were adopted to determine the 3D position of the TEE probe: 1) The Nano-CT volume was registered with X-ray images acquired from PA; 2) the registration result from step 1) was used to initialize the registration between the Nano-CT volume and the X-ray acquired from LAO 45°. In the second step, the optimization of the 2D-3D registration was constrained to the projection direction of the X-ray system. The 3D positions of the landmarks, $P_{phantom, X\text{-}ray}$ can be reconstructed in X-ray space using a back projection algorithm from biplane X-ray images [10]. The third X-ray image was used to confirm the accuracy of the TEE probe localization and the landmark reconstruction.

The 3D positions of the landmarks, $P_{phantom, us}$ can also be identified manually from the ultrasound volume. $T_{us \rightarrow X\text{-}ray}$, the transformation from $P_{phantom, us}$ to $P_{phantom, X\text{-}ray}$ was calculated by using a landmark registration algorithm. By fitting the TEE probe position and $T_{us\_img \rightarrow X\text{-}ray}$ into equation (1), the calibration matrix $T_{us\_img \rightarrow probe}$ can be calculated. However, to minimize the calibration error, the error caused by the manual definition of the landmarks must be taken into account. Realistically, equation (1) should be rewritten as:

$$\varepsilon = T_{us\_img \rightarrow probe} P_{phantom,us} - T_{probe}{}^{T} T_{us \rightarrow X\text{-}ray} P_{phantom,us} \quad (2)$$

To solve equation (2), the calibration procedures described above were repeated three times with different probe positions. A hill-climbing optimization algorithm was employed to find $T_{us\_img \rightarrow probe}$ by minimizing error ε.

2.4 Accuracy Assessment

2.4.1 2D-3D Registration

In this study, we examined how the error in the 2D-3D registration could affect the accuracy of the overall TEE and X-ray registration. For our evaluation, we introduced a gold standard registration matrix which was found by manually registering the Nano-CT volume of the TEE probe to two X-ray images acquired from different angles. The Nano-CT volume was then perturbed from the registration position by $\pm\Delta\delta$ mm / degree in all six degrees of freedom (DOF) to generate new starting positions. The 2D-3D registration algorithm was used to correct the misalignment. To examine the accuracy of the registration, the 8 corners of the Nano-CT volume were used as the landmarks to calculate the mean target registration error (mTRE) in comparison to the gold standard (equation 3). A number of landmarks were also selected within the ultrasound FOV with from 1cm to 10cm depth to calculate the registration error, $mTRE^{depth}$. In this experiment, we examined different aspects of the registration algorithm, including the capture range, the robustness, the speed and the potential error for the target objects at different depths.

$$mTRE = \frac{1}{n}\sum_{i=1}^{n}\left\| \mathrm{T}_{registratin} P_{landmark}^{i} - \mathrm{T}_{gold} P_{landmark}^{i} \right\| \qquad (3)$$

2.4.2 Phantom Data

The calibration phantom was also used to validate the accuracy of our registration technique. Two TEE volumes that were not used in the calibration procedure were registered with the X-ray images. The TRE was the mean distance between the X-ray reconstructed landmarks and those defined on the TEE volumes.

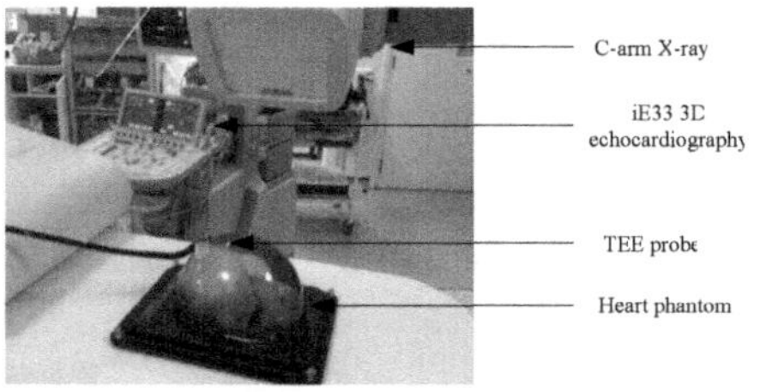

Fig. 2. The heart phantom experiment was performed in the catheter laboratory. The picture shows the experimental setup.

The accuracy of our method was further evaluated using a realistic heart phantom (`http://www.cirsinc.com`, Fig.2). The heart phantom is compatible with MRI and ultrasound but its visibility in X-ray is poor. A two-step strategy was used to evaluate the accuracy of the TEE and X-ray registration using this phantom. In the first step, a high resolution MR volume was acquired of the phantom and accurately transformed to the X-ray space using a landmark registration. More details about the landmark registration will be described below. In the second step, six TEE volumes were acquired from the heart phantom and transformed to X-ray space by using the proposed method. The MR volume which was transformed to X-ray space could therefore be used as a gold standard to evaluate the accuracy of the proposed method.

To achieve an accurate MRI and X-ray registration, 9 X-ray and MRI visible markers (`http://www.izimed.com/mri.shtml`) were placed on the surface of the phantom. A high resolution MR volume (1.0x1.0x1.0mm^3) of the heart phantom was acquired a day before the TEE and X-ray scans in the catheter laboratory. Between the MRI scan and the TEE scan, the heart phantom was carefully stored in order to avoid displacement of the markers. The 3D positions of the landmarks in MRI space and X-ray space were reconstructed from the MR volume and bi-plane X-ray images. The transformation between MRI space and X-ray space can be easily found by using the landmark registration. By transforming all the TEE volumes acquired from different probe positions and the MR volume to X-ray space, the TEE and X-ray registration error were assessed indirectly by calculating the mean distance between a set of landmarks identified from the TEE volume and the MRI surface.

2.4.3 Clinical Cases

We collected data from two cardiac EP procedures. Both of the patients had left atrial flutter and were under general anesthesia during the procedures. For the first patient, TEE and X-ray data were acquired after two deca-polar catheters were inserted into right atrium (RA), one forming a loop along the endocardial surface of RA and the other inserted in to the coronary sinus (CS). Both catheters were visible in the TEE volume. For the second patient, a transseptal puncture was performed to gain access to the left atrium (LA). TEE volumes were acquired after a lasso catheter and an ablation catheter were inserted into LA. The movement of the C-arm was limited by other equipment such as the life support system and the ultrasound scanner. X-ray images were acquired from PA and either RAO 30° or LAO 30° projections.

For both cases, the TEE volumes were acquired at the default depth setting (12cm) in full volume mode (volume size: 224×208×201, voxel size: 0.66×0.67×0.60mm^3). They were projected onto the X-ray images using the registration matrices. The accuracy of the TEE and X-ray registration were examined using the in-plane distance between the points defined on the catheter in the X-ray image and the center line of the same catheter in the TEE volume. This point-to-line distance (PTL) represents the in-plane registration error in our method.

3 Experimental Results

3.1 2D-3D Registration

5099 starting positions were generated using the procedures described in *2.4.1*. The Nano-CT volume was registered with two 1024×1024 X-ray images acquired from different C-arm positions during one of the clinical cases. The starting positions were distributed evenly in all six DOFs in a range of from 0 to 12mm in terms of mTRE. Fig.3 shows the registration results.

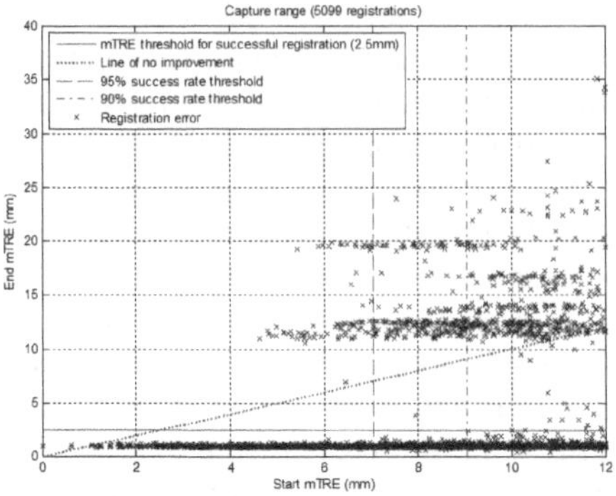

Fig. 3. 5099 new starting positions with mTRE range from 0-12mm were generated. The Y axis shows the end mTRE for each registration. Given that the mTRE threshold for successful registration is 2.5mm, the capture range for 95% success rate is 7.04mm and 9.05mm for 90% success rate.

The two vertical lines indicated the capture range were 7.04mm and 9.05mm with success rate of 95% and 90% respectively given that the mTRE threshold for success registration was set to 2.5mm. For all the other experiments carried out in this study, the 2D-3D registration algorithm was initialized by a manual registration which aligned the Nano-CT volume to within the capture range of the registration algorithm.

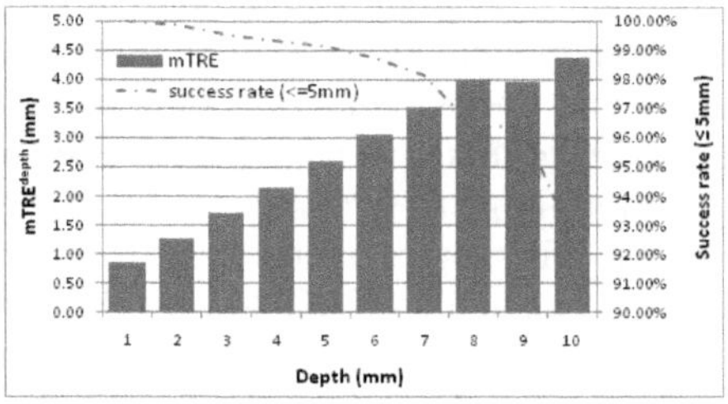

Fig. 4. Given a 2.5mm 2D-3D registration error, the columns showed the mean errors within the ultrasound FOV at different depths in terms of mTRE. While the maximum error could be up to 20mm, the dashed line shows the success rate ($\leq$ 5mm) for the targets at different depths.

The computational time of the 2D-3D registration depended on the starting position. For the 5099 registrations we did in this experiment, the mean computational time is 9.52 ± 4.23 seconds.

For all the successful registrations, $mTRE^{depth}$ was calculated using the landmarks defined within the ultrasound FOV. The results are shown in Fig. 4. Potentially, a small 2D-3D registration error ($mTRE \leq 2.5mm$) can create an error of 5mm at 10cm depth and 2.6mm at 5cm depth. In reality, it is unlikely that the target object (TO) is located at the far end of the ultrasound FOV. Clinicians often position the TO at the center (5-6 cm depth) of the FOV for best visualization.

For many cardiac interventional procedures, such as the treatment of atrial fibrillation, a sub-5mm clinical accuracy is sufficient for guidance. This is related to the size of the smallest target structures, for example the pulmonary veins. Fig.4 shows the success (($\leq$ 5mm) rate of the registration for targets at different depth given that less than 2.5mm mTRE was introduced by the 2D-3D registration.

3.2 Calibration

By using the calibration matrix, the last two volumes that were not involved in the calibration were transformed to the X-ray space and overlaid on the X-ray images (Fig.5). The mTREs were 4.6±1.1mm and 5.0±0.8mm respectively. The determination of the landmark positions from the TEE volume was difficult due to the noise and the shadowing effect of ultrasound. The mTREs show not only the registration error but also the subjective error in the determination of the landmark positions.

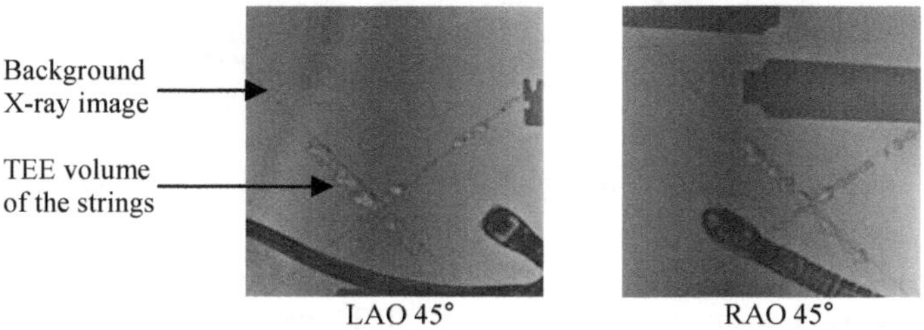

Fig. 5. The same TEE volumes acquired from the calibration phantom were overlaid onto the X-ray images acquired from LAO 45° and RAO 45°. The ultrasound volumes were clipped and thresholded to remove noise and other irrelevant structures for a better visualization.

3.3 Heart Phantom

Fig.6 shows the three image planes (X-Y, X-Z and Y-Z) of two TEE volumes which were transformed to the X-ray space. This mis-alignment between the two TEE volumes indicates the error produced by the TEE and X-ray registration. Fig.7 shows the composite TEE volume registered with the MR volume in X-ray space.

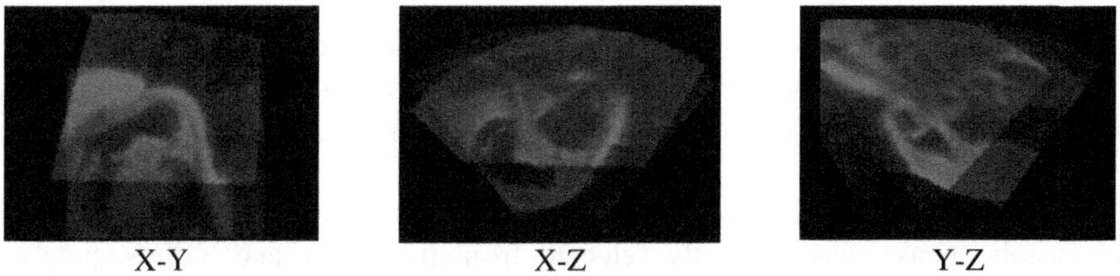

Fig. 6. By transforming the TEE volumes acquired from different probe position to the X-ray space, an ultrasound to ultrasound registration was effectively achieved. The three images show the three different image planes of two TEE volumes in X-ray space. The green image volume was acquired from probe position 1 while the red volume was acquired from probe position 2.

The endocardial surfaces of the heart phantom including left ventricle (LV), right ventricle (RV), left atrium (LA) and right atrium (RA) were reconstructed from the MR volume by using a manual segmentation tool. A total of 16 to 66 points were defined manually along the endocardial border from the TEE volumes. Both the MR surfaces and the TEE points were transformed to X-ray space. The point to surface distance which represents the registration error between TEE and MRI data is summarized in table 1.

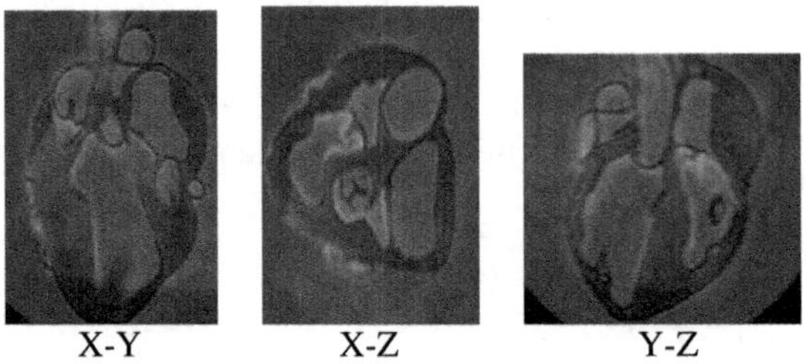

Fig. 7. The result of the registration between TEE (green) and MRI

Table 1. The point-to-surface error represents the error in the registration of TEE and MRI. For LV and RV, the points were defined on all the six TEE volumes, 10 for each volume. For LA and RA, points were defined on the volumes where the LA and RA borders were clearly visible.

	Num. of Points	Mean Error (mm)	STD (mm)	Max. Error
LV	66	2.0	1.5	4.7
RV	60	1.9	1.2	4.9
LA	22	1.5	0.8	2.8
RA	16	2.0	1.4	4.4
Overall	164	1.8	1.2	4.9

3.4 Clinical Studies

Fig. 8 shows the registration results of the patient data. To examine the accuracy of the registration, we choose the deca-polar catheter position in RV for the first patient and the lasso catheter for the second patient. The mean PTLs ($n = 5$) were 3.1±2.6 and 1.5±1.6mm, respectively.

At this stage, the data acquisition of TEE and X-ray were not synchronized. The end systolic phase was manually selected from the X-ray and TEE sequences to calculate the PTL. However, the catheter motion (caused by the cardiac motion) shown in the X-ray images was more considerable than that shown in the TEE volume. This is because the catheter motion shown in TEE was partly canceled by the motion of the TEE probe. At present, our 2D-3D registration algorithm is not fast enough to compensate the TEE probe motion in real-time. This error will be additive in the registration results.

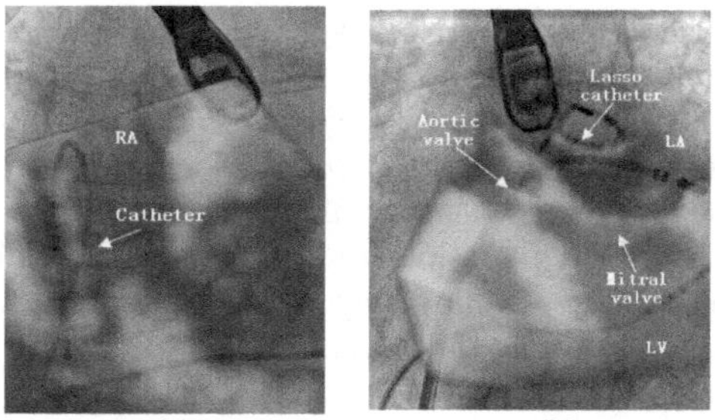

(a) (b)

Fig. 8. TEE volumes were registered with and overlaid onto the X-ray images. (a) For the first patient, the TEE volume shows a deca-polar catheter positioned in the right atrium. (b) For the second patient, a lasso catheter was inserted into the left atrium. For both patient data, the registration was successful as the catheters in the TEE volumes showed a good alignment with the background X-ray images.

4 Discussion

The results of both the phantom and clinical studies are encouraging in terms of the target registration accuracy achieved. The values of approximately 2mm achieved for the heart phantom and 1.5 and 3mm achieved for the clinical cases are well within the clinical accuracy requirement for most cardiac interventional procedures. The results for the calibration phantom study are less accurate at approximately 5mm. It is likely that is due to the errors associated with the manual localization of the markers in this phantom. Potentially the subjective errors can also reduce the accuracy of the calibration. However, those errors did not make a considerable impact in the registration result because they were partly compensated by the optimization algorithm adopted in our calibration procedure.

At present, our 2D-3D registration algorithm takes around 9.5 second to localize the position of the TEE probe using two 1024×1024 X-ray image. Potentially, the registration time could be further reduced by incorporating more sophisticated implementations such as the multiple-resolution technique. By using an EM tracking system, it is possible to track the TEE probe in real-time. However our method has three advantages when compared with the method of EM tracking. Firstly, for our method, there is no need to modify the TEE probe. For EM tracking, a sensor coil must be added.. Secondly, the accuracy of the EM tracking system relies on a metal-free environment. With the presence of the moving X-ray C-arm and other medical devices, the reliability of the EM tracking system is questionable. Thirdly, the methodology presented for the co-registration of 3D TEE and X-ray fluoroscopy data is better suited for the routine clinical workflow. Finally, the calibration matrix created in our method is very stable. The validity of the calibration depends on the stability of the position of the tracking devices. In clinical environment, the EM field generator can be moved either intentionally or accidentally, invalidating the calibration matrix. Our calibration matrix is directly associated with the X-ray coordinate system. It will be valid and accurate unless a different TEE probe or X-ray system is introduced.

The novelty of our method is that we employed an image-based 2D-3D registration algorithm to localize the TEE probe. The performance of the 2D-3D registration algorithm is usually data dependent. However, our task is more straightforward than previously reported studies. Firstly, the source object in our study is always the same. Secondly, the visibility and contrast of the TEE probe in the X-ray images is relatively constant and is unlikely to be affected by other objects because the density of the TEE probe is considerably higher than the soft tissues and the spine. The performance of our 2D-3D registration algorithm was carefully examined using a clinical data set. The authors acknowledged that the evaluation of a registration algorithm should involve multiple data sets. A more thorough study will be carried out when more clinical data become available. The other limitation of our study is that all processing is done off-line. However, the transition to real-time or near-real-time capability is relatively straightforward in this case, with all the required components already presents, including live data streaming from both X-ray and ultrasound systems. Our future work will focus on the implementation of the live functionality and also improvements in the visualization of the co-registered data.

5 Conclusion

In this study, we described a novel, efficient and fast TEE to X-ray fluoroscopy registration technique. The method was successfully evaluated in two phantom studies and two clinical cases. It is likely that such a co-registration and visualization technology is going to have a significant impact in the field of image-guided cardiac interventions.

References

1. Silverstry, F.E., et al.: Echocardiography-Guided Interventions. Journal of the American Society of Echocardiography 22, 213–231 (2009)
2. Razavi, R., et al.: Cardiac catheterization guided by MRI in children and adults with congenital heart disease. The Lancet 362, 1877–1882 (2003)
3. Rhode, K.S., et al.: A system for real-time XMR guided cardiovascular intervention. IEEE Trans. Med. Imaging 24, 500–513 (2005)
4. King, A.P., et al.: A subject-specific technique for respiratory motion correction in image-guided cardiac catheterization procedures. Medical Image Analysis 13, 419–431 (2009)
5. Barker, G.H., et al.: Usefulness of Live Three-Dimensional Transesophageal Echocardiography in a Congenital Heart Disease Center. The American Journal of Cardiology 103, 1025–1028 (2009)
6. Mackensen, G.B., et al.: Real-Time 3-Dimensional Transesophageal Echocardiography during Left Atrial Radiofrequency Catheter Ablation for Atrial Fibrillation. Circulation: Cardiovascular Imaging 1, 85–86 (2008)
7. Jain, A., et al.: 3D TEE Registration with X-Ray Fluoroscopy for Interventional Cardiac Applications. In: Ayache, N., Delingette, H., Sermesant, M. (eds.) FIMH 2009. LNCS, vol. 5528, pp. 321–329. Springer, Heidelberg (2009)
8. Penney, G.P., et al.: A Comparison of Similarity Measures for Use in 2D-3D Medical Image Registration. IEEE Trans. Med. Imaging 17, 586–595 (1998)
9. Hipwell, J.H., et al.: Intensity based 2D-3D registration of cerebral angiograms. IEEE Trans. Med. Imaging 22, 1417–1426 (2003)
10. Hawkes, D., et al.: The Accurate 3-D Reconstruction of the Geometric Configuration of Vascular Trees from X-Ray Recordings. Physics and Engineering on Medical Imaging, 250–275 (1987)

Patient-Specific Modeling and Analysis of the Mitral Valve Using 3D-TEE

Philippe Burlina[1,2], Chad Sprouse[1], Daniel DeMenthon[1], Anne Jorstad[1], Radford Juang[1], Francisco Contijoch[3], Theodore Abraham[4], David Yuh[5], and Elliot McVeigh[3]

[1] Johns Hopkins University Applied Physics Laboratory
[2] Dept. of Computer Science
[3] Dept. of Biomedical Engineering, School of Medicine
[4] Division of Cardiology
[5] Division of Cardiac Surgery, Baltimore, MD, USA

Abstract. We describe a system dedicated to the analysis of the complex three-dimensional anatomy and dynamics of an abnormal heart mitral valve using three-dimensional echocardiography to characterize the valve pathophysiology. This system is intended to aid cardiothoracic surgeons in conducting preoperative surgical planning and in understanding the outcome of "virtual" mitral valve repairs. This paper specifically addresses the analysis of three-dimensional transesophageal echocardiographic imagery to recover the valve structure and predict the competency of a surgically modified valve by computing its closed state from an assumed open configuration. We report on a 3D TEE structure recovery method and a mechanical modeling approach used for the valve modeling and simulation.

Keywords: Mitral valvuloplasty, patient specific modeling, 3D echocardiography, preoperative surgical planning.

1 Introduction

This paper addresses the problem of exploiting 3D Transesophageal Echocardiographic data (3D TEE) to recover the structure of the mitral valve and surrounding left heart anatomy, and to model the valve pathophysiology. The tools we are designing can be applied in cardiothoracic surgery (to develop systems aiding in preoperative valvuloplasty planning), in cardiology (for performing diagnostics), and for education and training of ultrasonographers and anesthesiologists (often responsible for intraoperative TEE acquisition). The mitral valve is an essential structure which ensures unidirectional blood flow from the left atrium to the left ventricle. One of the essential issues in characterizing valve pathologies and planning surgical valve reconstruction is the ability to predict the outcome of a given valvuloplasty surgical procedure. There are many options for valvuloplasty including the addition of a ring, the resection of part of the valve leaflets, or modifications to the chordae tendinae.

Valvuloplasty surgery involves cardiopulmonary bypass. A bypass procedure has associated risks which require that the surgeon make a decision within a relatively

N. Navab and P. Jannin (Eds.): IPCAI 2010, LNCS 6135, pp. 135–146, 2010.

bounded time frame, once he has gained access to the valve, regarding the course of the valvuloplasty. A preoperative planning process elucidating which valvuloplasty option is most likely to result in a successful outcome (i.e., a *competent* valve) would therefore be highly useful to the cardiothoracic surgeon.

We describe our work with regard to segmentation, structure recovery and modeling, to address the goal of predicting the ability of a modified valve to be competent: the ability of the valve leaflets to coapt and thereby prevent any blood regurgitation from the left ventricle back into the left atrium, a condition potentially resulting in congestive heart failure. We initiate our process with an open 3D valve structure at end diastole, which was derived by segmenting 3D TEE data and was edited by a physician to remove artifacts and reflect the planned surgical modifications. From the open valve structure, we then infer the configuration of the valve leaflets at or near the end of isovolumic contraction to characterize coaptation.

Early heart modeling efforts can be traced back to the pioneering work by Peskin [3][4] in the '70s and '80s, that introduced the "immersed boundary" (IB) approach [5], which is still being refined and extended [6]. Yoganathan [1][7] reported Fluid Structure Interaction methods (FSI) extending IB to solve for the left-ventricle motion using 3D incompressible Navier-Stokes equations. [8] uses FSI for heart valve modeling. Watton [6] extended IB to simulate a polyurethane replacement valve placed in a cylindrical tube, subject to physiologic periodic fluid flow. Einstein [9] reported a coupled FSI mitral model immersed in a domain of Newtonian blood. This model had anterior and posterior leaflets but did not include other structures such as the left ventricle. Espino's 2D modeling work [10] simulated the left ventricle-generated blood flow by adding a non-anatomical inlet at the left ventricular apex. Other notable recent efforts and related projects include [13][14][15][16][17] and [18]. Most prior modeling work does not exploit patient specific anatomical data, with some recent exceptions that are focused on higher resolution medical imaging modalities such as MRI and CT [11][12]. Our approach differs from prior work, in that it incorporates patient-specific anatomical and dynamic information derived from 3D TEE. 3D echocardiography has several shortcomings when compared to MRI and

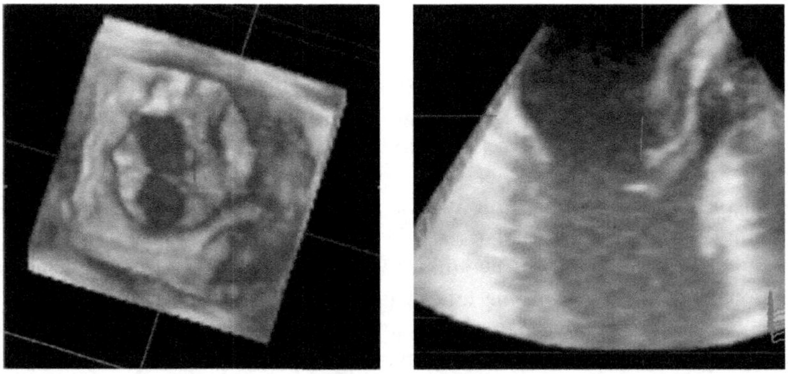

Fig. 1. A 3D TEE view of the mitral valve in the open position during diastole as seen from the atrium (left image) and a side view of the valve showing the anterior leaflet in front of the aortic valve (right image)

CT, including lower spatial resolution, and imaging artifacts including noise and obscuration. However, it has a number of advantages: it is non-ionizing, real-time, lower cost, it can be used pre- and intraoperatively, and allows interactive exploration.

Our valve mechanical modeling is also novel and takes its inspiration from methods characterizing cloth and sail behavior [21][22][23][24]. Sections 2 and 3 describe our approaches for structure recovery and modeling, while Sections 4 and 5 report experimental results and conclude.

2 Valve Segmentation

TEE segmentation is employed to recover the valve's static 3D structure that is then used in our mechanical modeling. We utilize an interactive user-in-the-loop approach that leverages two main automated methods to detect the valve leaflets and to find the boundaries of the heart's atrial and ventricular cavities.

A dynamic contour method is used to find the inner heart wall boundaries of the atrial and intraventricular cavities. This is complemented by a thin tissue detector that specifically finds the valve leaflets. The two methods are complementary, as the leaflets may not always be accurately segmented out by the dynamic contour approach, and the heart walls and valve annulus are generally not found by the thin tissue detector. The thin tissue detector models the local TEE intensity as Gaussian and then performs an analysis of the disparities of the eigenvalues associated with the intensity Hessian [25]. If one these eigenvalues is small when compared to the other two, this suggests the presence of a sheet or thin tissue structure. Another method we have used successfully to find thin tissues relies on morphological outlining.

The dynamic contour method used to find the heart inner walls exploits a level set approach and is summarized as follows: At time t=0, a dynamic contour is manually initialized in the atrial and/or intraventricular cavities. This dynamic contour is then obtained at any subsequent time t by considering an evolving function $\psi(x, y, z, t)$. The dynamic contour is found as $S(t)$, the zero level set of $\psi(.)$, i.e. $S(t) = \{(x, y, z) \mid \psi(x, y, z, t) = 0\}$. In our application, $\psi(.)$ evolves under a driving force which is designed to expand the contour until it reaches the intensity boundaries marking the inner walls of the atrial and ventricular cavities. An inhibition function $g(.)$, detailed later, stops the dynamic curve when it meets these walls boundaries.

Our specification of the evolution equation of $\psi(.)$ is inspired by the recent variational approach introduced by Li [19] that includes a penalty term $P(\psi)$ to evolve ψ so that, at all times, it closely approximates a signed distance function, a desirable feature for the determination of the zero level set $S(t)$. This penalty is expressed as

$$P(\psi) = \int_{\Omega} \frac{1}{2}\left(|\nabla \psi| - 1\right)^2 dxdydz \tag{1}$$

where $\Omega \subset \mathbb{R}^3$ is the domain of ψ. The time evolution equation is then expressed as

$$\frac{\partial \psi}{\partial t} = -\frac{\delta \varepsilon}{\delta \psi} \tag{2}$$

where the r.h.s. denotes the Gâteaux derivative. The energy $\varepsilon(\psi)$ is defined as

$$\varepsilon(\psi) = \mu P(\psi) + \varepsilon_m(\psi) \tag{3}$$

and includes a model energy term $\varepsilon_m(\psi)$ that drives the contour's evolution to the desired goals, with a balancing weight $\mu > 0$. The primary goal of $\varepsilon_m(\psi)$ is to expand or contract the contour by expanding or contracting its enclosed volume $V_g(\psi)$, while keeping this contour simple, which is done by constraining the boundary area $A_g(\psi)$. The term $\varepsilon_m(\psi)$ is therefore specified as

$$\varepsilon_m(\psi) = \lambda A_g(\psi) + \nu V_g(\psi) \tag{4}$$

where λ and ν are weights balancing the boundary area and volume terms. These terms are respectively expressed as

$$A_g(\psi) = \int_\Omega g\delta(\psi)\left|\nabla \psi\right| dxdydz \tag{5}$$

$$V_g(\psi) = \int_\Omega gH(-\psi)\; dxdydz \tag{6}$$

where $\delta(\psi)$ denotes the Dirac delta function, and $H(\psi)$ is the Heaviside function. The weight ν is chosen here to be negative so that the contour expands. We note that these terms contain the inhibition function $g(\cdot)$ mentioned earlier, that is designed to abate the motion of the dynamic boundary in places corresponding to the heart wall location. This location can be indicated by a change in intensity and the presence of an edge in the 3D TEE. If considering the presence of an edge, the function g can be designed as

$$g(x, y, z) = \frac{1}{1 + a\,|\nabla G * I(x, y, z)|^2} \tag{7}$$

where $\nabla G * I$ is the gradient of the Gaussian-smoothed TEE intensity. This function represents a 'negative' of the gradient magnitude map, taking small values for high gradient magnitudes, and values close to 1 for small gradient magnitudes.

This gradient-based definition of $g(.)$ might be unsuitable for echocardiography images with limited contrast. However, we have found that transesophageal echocardiography imaging, which allows a direct 'view' into the left heart complex and specifically the mitral valve, often exhibits good contrast when compared to other ultrasound imaging or heart echocardiography approaches such as transthoracic echocardiography. Alternatively, a term emphasizing image intensity can be used for echocardiographic imagery with lesser contrast. In this case the inhibition function

$g(.)$ is designed to measure the departure in intensity from the intensity of the heart wall cavity, expressed as

$$g(x,y,z) = 1 - \frac{M(I(x,y,z),m,\sigma)}{M_{\max}} \tag{8}$$

where $M(I(x,y,z),m,\sigma) = \left(I(x,y,z)-m\right)^2 / \sigma^2$, $M_{\max} = \max(M(.))$ over the entire TEE cube, and (m,σ^2) are the mean and variance computed over the initial inner patch specified by the dynamic contour at time zero within the heart inner cavity.

In sum, regrouping all terms together in Eq. (2), and using the Gâteaux derivative it can be shown that the evolution of ψ is finally expressed as

$$\frac{\partial\psi}{\partial t} = \mu\left[\Delta\psi - \mathrm{div}\left(\frac{\nabla\psi}{|\nabla\psi|}\right)\right] + \lambda\delta(\psi)\,\mathrm{div}\left(g\frac{\nabla\psi}{|\nabla\psi|}\right) + \nu g\delta(\psi) \tag{9}$$

where div denotes the divergence and Δ the Laplacian operators. This equation specifies a time-update evolution equation $\partial\psi/\partial t$ which corresponds to a form of steepest descent. This equation is discretized to evolve the function ψ so as to minimize the objective functional $\varepsilon(\psi)$.

3 Computation of the Closed Valve Configuration

In contrast to other work concerned with computation of the valve dynamics or the left heart hemodynamics [2], this paper reports on work aiming to design a mechanical model of the valve specifically developed to infer the closed position of the valve (at or near the end of isovolumic contraction during systole) from open position (at end diastole) or vice versa. This is of particular interest in cases where one desires to answer the following question: given a hypothetical, patient specific, valve geometry modified to reflect the planned valvuloplasty, or given a surmised configuration of the chordae tendinae, or given the placement of a ring, does the novel valve geometry have the potential to come to a closed position where the leaflets may coapt? As argued earlier, this capability is useful for surgical planning. This capability is also of interest for diagnostics or as a way of generating additional data for image simulation and rendering for education and training purposes.

The method we use for stationary modeling of the closed valve is inspired by shape-finding finite element approaches applied to fabric ([21] through [24]). We have chosen this approach because the valve leaflets are very thin structures made up of connective tissue with elastic properties (tensile, compressive and bending modulus) similar to some types of thin cloth and fabric. A related method was recently applied to model the shape of spinnaker sails for the Swiss team that won the 2007 America's Cup.

The valve modeling is performed as follows. A mesh is defined on the leaflets based on the segmentation results. At each node of the mesh we prescribe either displacements or forces. Forces modeled include those due to fluid pressure, gravity, linear elastic stress, collision with other portions of the mesh, and tethering of the valve to the chordae tendinae themselves attached to papillary muscles.

The specified initial configuration of the open mesh is used to specify the zero energy point for external (fluid, gravity, etc.), elastic, and tethering forces. The zero energy point for the collision force is the configuration in which all facets of the mesh are not contacting (more specifically, further apart than a distance δ). Our goal is to find the configuration of the valve system at closed position where all forces are at equilibrium. This steady state is found by solving an energy minimization problem where we seek a stationary point that corresponds to a minimum for the energy.

For any given displacement of the nodes from the initial open configuration, and for each node *i*, we define the total energy ϕ of the displaced system as

$$\phi = \sum_i \phi_i \tag{10}$$

along with the forces $\mathbf{F}_i = -\nabla \phi_i$. We consider the following additive components for the energy

$$\phi_i = \phi_i^X + \phi_i^E + \phi_i^T + \phi_i^C + \phi_i^K \tag{11}$$

including: ϕ_i^X , the external energy, ϕ_i^E , the elastic energy, ϕ_i^T , the tethering energy, ϕ_i^C the collision energy, and ϕ_i^K , the kinetic energy. The kinetic energy is neglected here since we are interested in directly solving for the system state in closed position where the velocity is negligible. The other significant energy terms are specified next.

External energy

The external energy results from external forces exerted on the leaflets such as the intraventricular blood pressure forces and gravity. This energy is assumed to be due to a set of fields of constant force $\{\mathbf{f}^k\}$ such that

$$\phi_i^X = -\sum_k \mathbf{f}^k \bullet \mathbf{d}_i \tag{12}$$

where $\mathbf{d}_i$ is the displacement of node *i*, and the index *k* ranges over the external force fields to which the leaflets are subject, including gravity and blood intraventricular force field. Gravity is not considered here since this term is negligible when compared to the energy due to intraventricular pressure. Our external force direction is specified so as to be oriented toward a 3D line that goes through the two commissure points of the valve (the points at which the two leaflets join).

Elastic energy

The elastic energy is given by

$$\phi_i^E = \sum_{\substack{\text{facets } j \\ \text{containing} \\ \text{node } i}} \frac{1}{2} \boldsymbol{\sigma}_j \bullet \boldsymbol{\varepsilon}_j \tag{13}$$

where $\boldsymbol{\varepsilon}_j = \left(\varepsilon_{xx}, \varepsilon_{yy}, \varepsilon_{xy}\right)^T$ is the strain vector determined from the fractional displacements of the nodes of the facet j [24] and $\boldsymbol{\sigma}_j = \left(\sigma_{xx}, \sigma_{yy}, \sigma_{xy}\right)^T = \mathbf{H}\boldsymbol{\varepsilon}_j$ is the stress vector of the facet j. Here,

$$\mathbf{H} = \frac{E}{1-\nu^2}\begin{pmatrix} 1 & \nu & 0 \\ \nu & 1 & 0 \\ 0 & 0 & 1-\nu \end{pmatrix} \tag{14}$$

is the elasticity matrix of the mesh, written in terms of Young's modulus of elasticity, E, and Poisson's ratio, ν. Note that while, in general, a hyperelastic assumption is used and may more accurately model certain biological tissue properties, we feel that this is unnecessary in the case of the valve modeling due to the leaflets' specific nature, i.e., very thin and flexible but highly inelastic. The small amount of leaflet stretching can be accurately modeled using a linear stress-strain relationship, while the primary mode of deformation is deflection of the leaflet. We assume that energy associated with folding along the edges of the finite elements is small compared to energy due to external forces and hence elastic resistance to leaflet deflection can be neglected.

Tethering energy

The tethering energy is used to include the effects of the chordae tendinae whose function is to restrict the range of motion of the leaflets thereby preventing prolapse in healthy valves. Since these chords are quasi-inextensible, this energy is specified as

$$\phi_i^T = \begin{cases} \Phi^t \dfrac{\left(\left|\mathbf{p}_i - \mathbf{q}_i\right| - r_i\right)^3}{\rho^3} & if \left|\mathbf{p}_i - \mathbf{q}_i\right| > r_i \\ 0 & otherwise \end{cases} \tag{15}$$

Where Φ^t is the strength of the tethering force, $\mathbf{p}_i$ is the position of the displaced node i, $\mathbf{q}_i$ is the position of the point to which node i is tethered, r_i is the chord length, and ρ is the scale of the range dependence of the force. Some of the nodes located at the leaflets' rims are selected and subject to tethering forces to simulate attachment to the primary mitral chordae tendinae. Secondary and tertiary chordae effects can be neglected for this application although their configuration does impact the overall systolic pressure distribution and they should be considered for dynamic simulation.

Collision energy

The collision energy ϕ_i^C is given by considering a repulsive force between all nodes

$$\phi_i^C = \sum_{\substack{facets\ T_j \\ containing \\ node\ i}} \ \sum_{\substack{facets\ T_k \\ not\ adjacent \\ to\ facet\ T_j}} \int_{T_j} d\mathbf{r}_j \int_{T_k} d\mathbf{r}_k e\left(\left|\mathbf{r}_j - \mathbf{r}_k\right|\right) \tag{16}$$

where the facet point $\mathbf{r}_j$ (resp. $\mathbf{r}_k$) spans the region of the facet T_j(resp. T_k) and $e(d)$ specifies a repulsive energy dependent on the distance d between the interacting facet points and is defined as

$$e(d)=\begin{cases}\Phi^C\left(1-\dfrac{d}{\delta}\right)^n & if\ d<\delta \\ 0 & otherwise\end{cases} \tag{17}$$

where Φ^C specifies the strength of the repulsive force. Defining the collision energy in such a fashion allows us to address self collision effects. The double summation is only considered between facets which are 'close' to each other, and we use an efficient tree-based range search to restrict the computational impact of this summation. This is an important consideration since the computation of the collision energy is a major factor contributing to total computational load. The range δ specifies the interacting node distance under which the collision force becomes active. Since the double integral term is evaluated by further discretizing points within the facet, this range should be set to a value that is of the order of the smallest distance between the mesh nodes. Therefore, at the final configuration, the remaining gap between colliding/coapting leaflets will be of the order of the mesh facet resolution. The mesh resolution can be tuned down to generate smaller gaps thereby trading slower convergence for finer precision. Since a planning tool is meant to allow the clinician to test various candidate solutions, a moderate mesh resolution that would still allow to answer the question of whether the leaflets have potential to coapt and the valve to be competent, should be sufficient.

The variation of total potential energy is a function of 3N displacement coordinates where N is the number of free nodes. We define a plane including the valve annulus and all 'top' nodes on the other side of this plane are kept static during the optimization process. To find the closed position of the leaflets given the distributed forces and imposed displacements, we find the configuration which minimizes the total energy by using the BFGS (Broyden Fletcher Goldfarb Shanno) quasi-Newton optimization process implemented in the Matlab Optimization Toolbox. Additional constraints may be used to augment this model: one such possibility is to add a constraint to model the addition of a ring around the valve annulus to simulate the surgical insertion of a ring to render the valve more competent.

4 Experiments

Intra-operative real-time 3D TEE full volume data of mitral valves were obtained from several patients using an iE33 Philips console fitted with a Philips X2-T Live 3D TEE probe (Philips Medical Systems, Bothell, WA). The data was semi-automatically segmented using the method described in Section 2. Examples of segmentation of 2D TEE planes and full 3D TEE cubes are shown in Figure 2. The automated segmentation was followed by visual inspection and user-in-the-loop correction to edit out artifacts due to ultrasonic imaging, and to complete some anatomical structures missing because of obscuration or limitations of the TEE field of view.

User intervention is also used to modify the valve in a way that reflects a plausible surgical valvuloplasty. Figure 2 shows segmentation results obtained using the level set inner heart cavities segmentation, and the thin tissue leaflet detection, prior to user intervention. The thin tissue methods give satisfactory results and, as expected, tend to omit sections of the annulus that can be reconstructed through the level set method. The level set method tends to do better with the intraventricular and atrial walls, which can then be combined with the thin tissue method for a complete segmentation. We found results to be generally acceptable although some challenges still remain: it is often difficult to completely discern where the valve ends and the chordae start. However this is to be expected since the chords' anatomy consists of an intricate extension of the valves' extremities, and both structures are made up of similar types of tissue that are rich in collagen and elastin fibers. The segmented valve was converted to a mesh and, as a final processing step, a nearest neighbor mesh smoothing filter was applied.

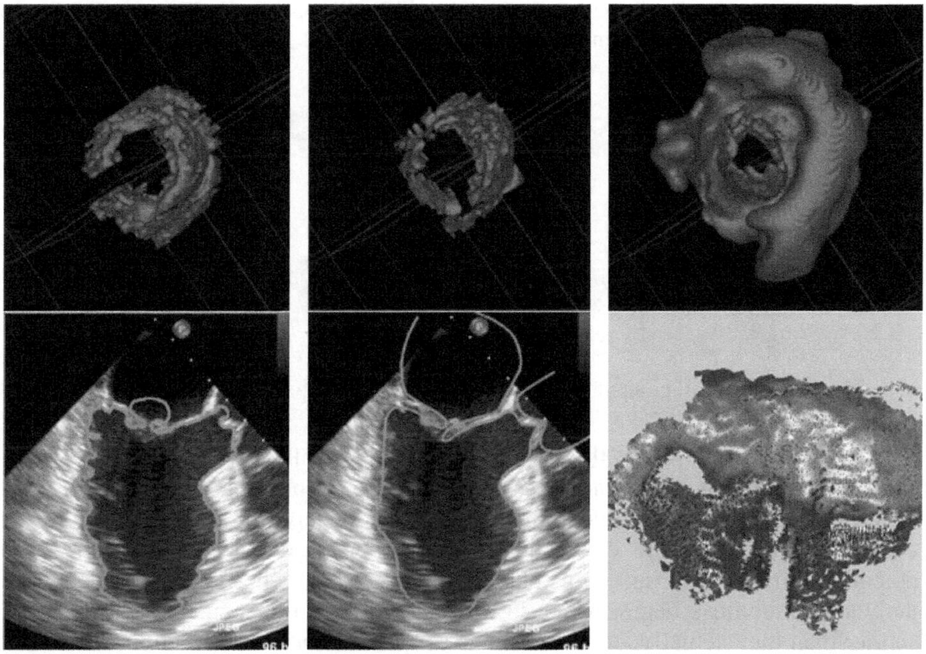

Fig. 2. 2D Examples of segmentation of the mitral valve and heart walls: using a morphology-based thin tissue detection (top left); using a Hessian-based thin tissue detection (top middle); using level sets (top right). 2D segmentation of a 3D TEE planar slice before and after user modifications (bottom left and middle); final 3D segmentation including valve and internal heart wall cavities with surface normals shown, after user modifications (bottom right).

The segmented 3D mesh obtained at a frame corresponding to the open valve position was used to model and predict the configuration at end systole (Figures 3 and above). Figure 3 shows the initial and final computed configurations. The color coded surfaces show in blue and orange the facets corresponding to the anterior and posterior

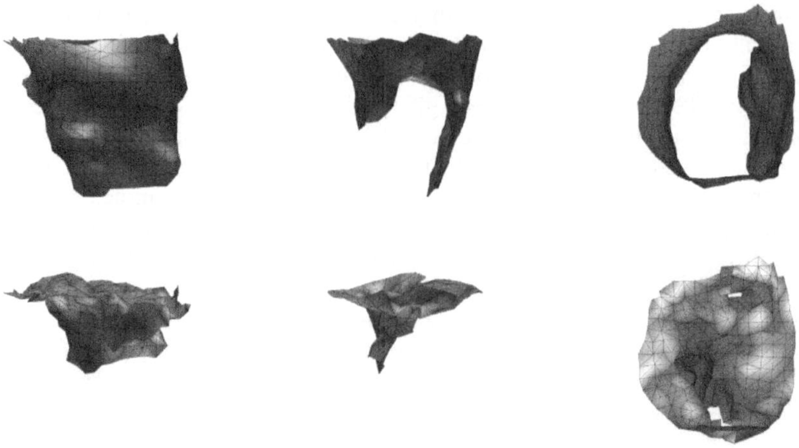

Fig. 3. Initial open valve configuration from TEE segmentation (top) and closed configuration computed by mechanical modeling at near end systole (bottom)

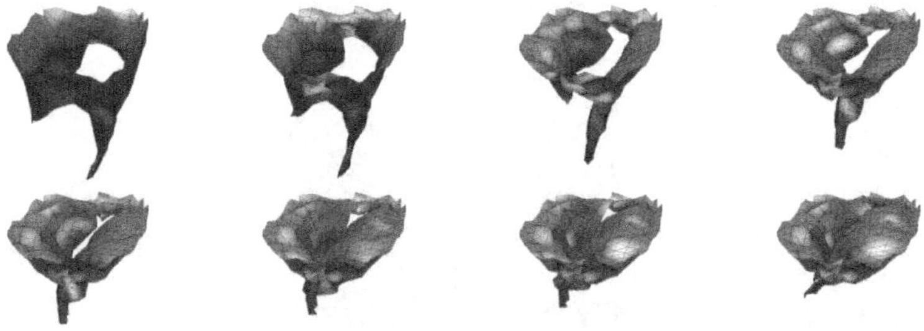

Fig. 4. Sequence of computed configurations taken at various intermediary iterations

leaflets. As is seen from the various views, the collision computation worked correctly as there is no surface crossing. In this example, the valve geometry was deemed to be capable of coapting everywhere except in an area close to the commissure points where the leaflets are too short to contact. This illustrates the potential difficulty during segmentation in discerning where the valve ends and the chordae tendinae begin, which in turn may lead to the segmented leaflets to be shorter than they actually are. A sequence of intermediary configurations in Figure 4 shows that although this model was developed to solve a stationary problem, the intermediary states give a plausible kinematic description of the leaflets' motion. This is because the kinetic energy of the valve leaflets is probably negligible when compared to the other energy terms during closure, in particular the external energy due to intraventricular pressure.

We performed experiments using several 3D TEE sequences taken from patients at JHU SOM. Validation was carried out by manual registration and comparison of (a) the closed valve configuration predicted at end systole from the segmented open valve captured at end diastole, with (b) the actual closed valve structure segmented at end systole (see Figure 5) and found an average difference of 4 to 5 mm. This is a

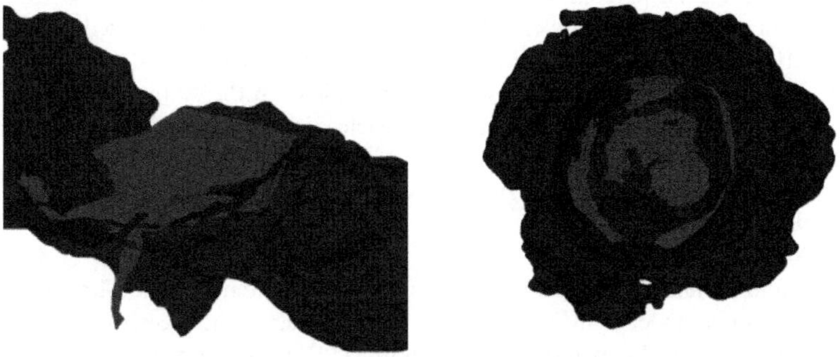

Fig. 5. Comparison of computed closed configuration (red) overlaid and registered with closed configuration segmented from 3D TEE (blue) acquired at end systole (side and top views). Close inspection reveals a good fit between the computed and actual configurations. We also inferred differences which are of the order of the errors made by the segmentation step, indicating good performance for the modeling step.

promising result considering that the TEE resolution is of the order of 1 mm and segmentation has an average error of about 1 to 2 mm depending on the method used.

5 Conclusions

We proposed a novel patient-specific mitral valve surgical planning method to help characterize the competency of a virtually modified valve. The novelty of our approach is twofold: (a) we exploit prior structural information derived from segmentation of 3D TEE, and (b) we propose a novel valve leaflet modeling approach based on the modeling of cloth. Preliminary results are presented and show the promise of the approach. Future goals are to address certain limitations of the segmentation and modeling methods, augment the model by incorporating physiological blood pressure forces, and carry out further clinical validation.

References

[1] Sacks, M.S., Yoganathan, A.P.: Heart valve function: a biomechanical perspective. Philos. Trans. R. Soc. Lond. B. Biol. Sci. 362, 1369–1391 (2007)

[2] Sprouse, C., Yuh, D., Abraham, T., Burlina, P.: Computational Hemodynamic Modeling based on Transesophageal Echocardiographic Imaging. In: Proc. IEEE Engineering in Medicine and Biology Conference, Minneapolis (September 2009)

[3] Peskin, C.S.: Flow patterns around heart valves. a digital computer method for solving the equations of motion. Albert Einstein College of Medicine, Ph.D (1972)

[4] Peskin, C.S.: Mathematical aspects of heart physiology: Courant Institute of Mathematical Sciences (1975)

[5] Peskin, C.S., McQueen, D.M.: A 3D computational method of blood flow in the heart: 1. immersed elastic fibers in a viscous incompressible fluid. Journal Computational Physics 81, 372–405 (1989)

[6] Watton, P.N., Luo, X.Y., Singleton, R., Wang, X., Bernacca, G.M., Molloy, P., Wheatley, D.J.: Dynamic modeling of prostetic chorded mitral valves using the immersed boundary method. In: IEEE Conf. Engineering in Medicine and Biology Society (2004)
[7] Vesier, C.C., Lemmon, J.J.D., Levine, R.A., Yoganathan, A.P.: A three-dimensional computational model of a thin-walled left ventricle. In: Proceedings of the 1992 ACM/IEEE conference on Supercomputing (1992)
[8] Loon, R.v., Anderson, P.D., van de Vosse, F.N.: A fluid-structure interaction method with solid-rigid contact for heart valve dynamics. Jounal of Computational Physics 217, 806–823 (2006)
[9] Einstein, D., Kunzelman, K., Reinhall, P., Nicosia, M., Cochran, R.: Non-linear fluid-coupled computational model of the mitral valve. J. Heart Valve Dis. 14, 376–385 (2005)
[10] Espino, D., Watkins, M.A., Shepherd, D.E.T., Hukins, D.W.L., Buchan, K.G.: Simulation of blood flow through the Mitral Valve of the heart: a fluid structure interaction model. In: Proc. COMSOL Users Conference (2006)
[11] Hu, Z., Metaxas, D., Axel, L.: Computational modeling and simulation of heart ventricular mechanics with tagged MRI. In: ACM symposium on Solid and physical modeling 2005 (2005)
[12] Hammer, P., Nido, P.d., Howe, R.: Image based mass spring model of mitral valve closure for surgical planning. In: SPIE Medical (2008)
[13] Bassingthwaighte, J.B.: Design and strategy for the Cardionome project. Adv. Exp. Med. Biology (1997)
[14] Delinghette, H.: Integrated cardiac modeling and visualization. In: Int. Conf. Medical Image Computing and Computer-Assisted Intervention (2008)
[15] INRIA-REO, The INRIA REO group (2008)
[16] Santos, N.D.D., Gerbeau, J.-F., Bourgat, J.F.: A partitioned fluid-structure algorithm for elastic thin valves with contact. Comp. Meth. Appl. Mech. Eng. 197 (2008)
[17] Astorino, M., Gerbeau, J.-F., Pantz, O., Traoré, K.-F.: Fluid-structure interaction and multi-body contact. Application to the aortic valves, INRIA RR 6583 (2008)
[18] EU, The virtual physiological human EU project (2008)
[19] Li, C., Xu, C., Gui, C., Fox, M.: Level Set Evolution without Re-Initialization: A New Variational Formulation, pp. 430–436 (2005)
[20] Corsi, C., Saracino, G., Sarti, A., Lamberti, C.: Left ventricular volume estimation for real-time three-dimensional echocardiography. IEEE Trans. Medical Imaging 21 (2002)
[21] Maître, O.L., Huberson, S., Souza de Cursi, E.: Unsteady Model of Sail and Flow Interaction. Journal of Fluids and Structures 13, 37–59 (1998)
[22] Charvet, T., Huberson, S.G.: Numerical Calculation of the flow around sails. European Journal of Mechanics 11, 599–610 (1992)
[23] Hauville, F., Mounoury, S., Roux, Y., Astolfi, J.E.: Equilibre dynamique d'une structure idealement flexible dans un ecoulement: application a la deformation des voiles. Journees AUM AFM. Brest (2004)
[24] Arcaro, V.F.: A Simple Procedure for Shape Finding and Analysis of Fabric Structures, `http://www.arcaro.org/tension`
[25] Huang, A., Nielson, G., Razdan, A., Farin, G., Baluch, D., Capco, D.: Thin structure segmentation and visualization in three-dimensional biomedical images: a shape-based approach. IEEE Transactions on Visualization and Computer Graphics 12, 93–102 (2006)

Evaluation of a 4D Cone-Beam CT Reconstruction Approach Using an Anthropomorphic Phantom

Ziv Yaniv[1], Jan Boese[2], Marily Sarmiento[3], and Kevin Cleary[1]

[1] Imaging Science and Information Systems Center, Department of Radiology, Georgetown University Medical Center, Washington, DC, USA
[2] Siemens AG Healthcare, Forchheim, Germany
[3] Siemens AG Healthcare, Malvern, PA, USA

Abstract. We have previously developed image-guided navigation systems for thoracic abdominal interventions utilizing a three dimensional (3D) Cone-Beam CT (CBCT) image acquired at breath-hold. These systems required the physician to perform the intervention in a gated manner, with actions performed at the same respiratory phase in which the CBCT image was acquired. This approach is not always applicable, as many patients find it hard to comply with the breath-hold requirement. In addition the physician's actions are limited to a specific respiratory phase. To mitigate these deficiencies we have developed and implemented a retrospectively gated acquisition protocol using a clinical C-arm based system. The resulting 4D (3D+time) image is then used as input for the navigation system. We evaluate our reconstruction approach using a computer controlled anthropomorphic respiring phantom. The phantom is respired using respiratory rates of 12, 15 and 20 breaths per minute, and three amplitudes corresponding to shallow, normal, and deep breathing patterns. We show that the gated images have a better contrast to noise ratio and sharper edges than the images reconstructed without gating. Thus we are able to acquire an intra-operative data set that potentially provides better navigation accuracy, using 3D images at arbitrary points in the respiratory cycle without requiring the patient to hold their breath during image acquisition.

1 Introduction

The use of image-guided navigation systems has grown in the past decades, as these systems enable minimally invasive interventions, reducing trauma to the patient. To date, these systems have primarily been applied in procedures dealing with rigid or semi-rigid anatomical structures such as those found in orthopedics and neurosurgery. More recently, developers of image-guidance systems have shifted their focus to thoracic-abdominal soft tissue interventions [1–3]. Commercial systems for soft tissue interventions have also started appearing on the market. Examples of such systems are the PercuNav system from Traxtal Inc., a Philips Heathcare Company, (Toronto Canada) and the iGuide CAPPA system from Siemens AG Healthcare (Erlangen, Germany).

N. Navab and P. Jannin (Eds.): IPCAI 2010, LNCS 6135, pp. 147–156, 2010.

These systems provide guidance based on a three dimensional (3D) image, usually, diagnostic quality CT or MR. This requires that patients hold their breath during image acquisition and that the intervention be carried out at the same respiratory phase in which the image was acquired. As a result, the intervention is performed in a gated manner, with actions limited to a specific respiratory phase. Most often the end expiration phase is used as this is the respiratory phase that has the best reproducibility [4].

Improvements in flat panel detector technology have led to the introduction of interventional C-arm based Cone Beam CT (CBCT) systems that provide reconstructions with sufficient soft tissue resolution for various interventional procedures [5]. By replacing the use of diagnostic CT with C-arm based CBCT the complexity of a procedure's workflow is potentially reduced. Instead of acquiring the CT images in a separate location and transferring the patient to the interventional suite, both imaging and intervention are carried out in the same location.

Based on our experience developing image-guidance systems that utilize either CT or CBCT [3], we conclude that the current guidance approach is sub-optimal for thoracic-abdominal interventions. In many cases, patients are not cooperative and cannot hold their breath during image acquisition. This is often due to sedation or their underlying medical condition. When this is not an issue, subsequent breath-holds after image acquisition do not always correspond to the same respiratory phase, reducing the guidance accuracy.

C-arm based CBCT systems can potentially be used to acquire 4D (3D+time) images. The acquisition and use of a 4D CBCT image for navigation guidance removes the requirement for breath-hold during image acquisition, and will potentially improve navigation accuracy. Instead of an image corresponding to a specific respiratory phase, the system uses images that reflect the position of underlying anatomical structures throughout the respiratory cycle. We are currently pursuing this research with the aim of using 4D CBCT to guide radiofrequency ablation of large (>3cm) tumors in the liver.

A straightforward approach to 4D CBCT acquisition is gated reconstruction. The acquired projection images are binned according to their respiratory phase or amplitude after which 3D reconstructions are performed separately for each bin [6]. This approach requires a dense spatio-temporal sampling. That is, each bin must contain enough spatial information such that it does not trade motion artifacts for reconstruction artifacts due to a sparse spatial sampling along the gantry's trajectory. When using clinical C-arm based systems, scan times are most often less than 30s. These systems are designed for fast rotations, as the intended image acquisition protocols assume patients hold their breath. This results in a sparse spatial sampling if projection images are binned according to a respiratory signal, leading to reconstruction artifacts. This is slightly less of an issue for CBCT systems used in radiation therapy. These on-board systems typically have rotation times longer than 1min.

A theoretical improvement over straightforward gating was presented in [7], using a 3D motion compensated reconstruction approach. This approach assumes the availability of a pre-operative 4D motion model that is consistent with the intra-operative respiratory motion. This approach was later successfully used in the radiation therapy setting, with 1min CBCT gantry rotation and motion models derived from 4D CT [8]. This approach is not applicable for most image-guided interventions as no pre-operative motion model is available.

We next describe our proposed 4D CBCT reconstruction method using a clinical C-arm system and its evaluation, using a computer controlled anthropomorphic respiring phantom.

2 Materials and Methods

In this work we use the Axiom Artis dFA (Siemens AG Healthcare, Erlangen, Germany) clinical C-arm based CBCT system. We have previously shown, in a simulation study, that a C-arm rotation of 80s using this system's calibration parameters would yield a 4D gated reconstruction of sufficient quality [9]. Unfortunately, the system design is such that it cannot be slowed down. It is optimized for fast rotations, with the longest possible rotation time being 25s. This is insufficient for a gated reconstruction approach as the spatial sampling associated with each respiratory phase is very sparse due to the limited number of respiratory cycles sampled in 25s.

Given the acquisition properties of our system we adopted the reconstruction approach proposed in [10] for reconstruction of gated cardiac images. In that approach the C-arm performs multiple back and forth sweeps. In our case, the C-arm performs five 25s sweeps. In each sweep 166 images are acquired uniformly covering an orbit of 200°. In total, 830 images are acquired in 125s. This specific choice of number of sweeps and number of images per sweep was based on the maximal size of the hardware's image buffer. It should be noted that the back and forth motions are only approximately identical. We ignore these minor differences during reconstruction and use the same C-arm parameters irrespective of the direction of rotation.

After acquiring the projective images, they are retrospectively labeled with a label in $[-1, 1]$ using the amplitude of a respiratory signal obtained from the motion of a fiducial marker placed on the patient's skin. The signal is estimated from the fiducial's location in the projection images and is thus implicitly synchronized with image acquisition [11]. Unlike the standard hard binning approach where each projection image is associated with one respiratory phase we use the soft binning approach as described in [10]. That is, for every bin, defined by the respiratory signal, we use all 166 C-arm poses. For each pose we select the projection image that is closest to the desired respiratory amplitude. This approach strikes a balance between reducing reconstruction and motion artifacts. Finally, each of the 3D images from the 4D CBCT image is obtained using the system's filtered backprojection reconstruction.

To evaluate our gated reconstruction approach we use a computer controlled anthropomorphic respiring phantom. The phantom anatomy is based on the visible human data. The thorax encloses two cavities that serve as artificial lungs

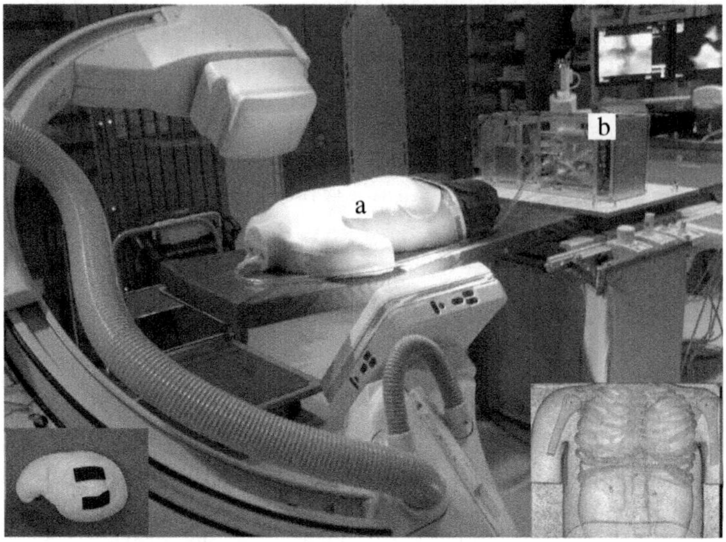

Fig. 1. Experimental setup (a) anthropomorphic respiring phantom and (b) computer controlled pump. Insets show volume rendering from a CT scan of the phantom and the foam liver placed inside the phantom's abdomen.

and artificial organs are placed inside the abdominal cavity [12]. Respiratory motion of the abdominal organs is induced by the motion of the diaphragm as air is pumped into and removed from the lung cavities. Respiration rate and volume are set using a computer controlled pump [13]. Given that our clinical application is navigated liver RFA, we place a foam liver model with a simulated tumor into the phantom's abdomen. This is our object of interest. It should be noted that the phantom only approximates respiratory motion and does not mimic the attenuation coefficients of human tissue.

For evaluation nine data sets were acquired. These correspond to three respiratory rates slow, medium, and fast, 12, 15 and 20 breaths per minute, and respiratory volumes representing shallow, normal and deep breathing. Figure 1 shows our experimental setup and a volume rendering of the phantom. In addition we acquired a CT scan (Siemens Somatom Sensation) and a CBCT scan with the phantom at rest. These serve as a gold standard, the best possible image quality obtained by these imaging systems.

The tumor was manually segmented in the 3D reconstructions. The segmentation is used as input for our evaluation. We use two image quality measures to evaluate reconstructions, Contrast to Noise Ratio (CNR) and the Gradient Magnitude in an Annulus (GM-A) defined by the segmentation boundary. The former assesses general image quality while the later reflects the influence of motion on the reconstruction. If the gating approach removes the blurring due to motion then the CNR is expected to change slightly as it is measured across the whole region of interest, tumor and surrounding tissue. The gradient magnitude

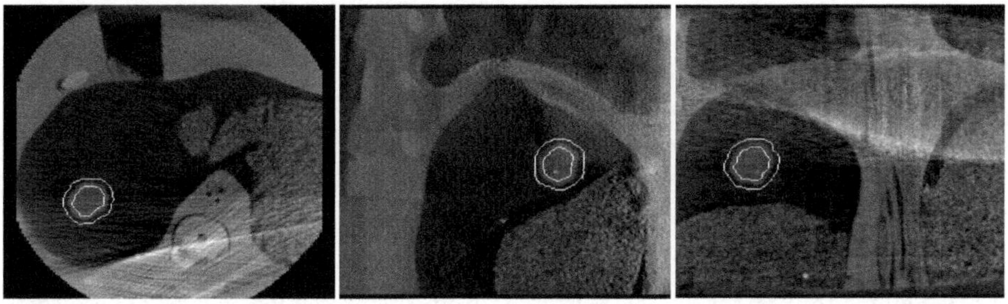

Fig. 2. Axial, Sagittal, and Coronal reformatted images of the anthropomorphic phantom with 3D annulus in which we compute the gradient magnitude

on the other hand is only evaluated at the border of the tumor and is expected to be more sensitive to the removal of motion blurring. On the other hand if the gating scheme introduces noise artifacts into the reconstruction then the CNR is expected to be lower and the gradient magnitude is expected to be higher. As a consequence these two quality values should be considered in conjunction, with the ideal results reflecting both higher CNR and gradient magnitude. Finally we also compare the estimated tumor size with and without gating to the size estimated by the segmentation of the stationary CT data.

The CNR formula we use is defined in [14]:

$$CNR = \frac{|\mu_{fg} - \mu_{bg}|}{\sqrt{(\sigma_{fg}^2 + \sigma_{bg}^2)/2}}$$

In our case the simulated tumor inside the foam liver serves as our foreground. The background is automatically defined by dilating the segmented tumor such that the volume of the surrounding background is approximately equal to the tumor volume.

Our second quality measure, GM-A, is defined by the segmentation boundary. This quality measure allows us to evaluate the effect of our gated reconstruction on motion artifacts, as these result in blurred object boundaries. To reduce the dependency on accurate tumor segmentation we evaluate the gradient magnitude in a 5mm annulus defined by the manual segmentation, as illustrated in Figure 2.

Finally, we compare the effect of our reconstruction approach on the estimated tumor volume, with the ground truth tumor volume obtained from a CT of the stationary phantom.

We compare the set of 3D images obtained from our 4D reconstruction approach to the standard 3D reconstruction. In our case we use the 166 projection images acquired in the first sweep of our multi-sweep acquisition as input to the standard 3D reconstruction approach. The input is thus similar to that acquired using the current clinical acquisition method and a freely breathing patient, without the need to perform a separate scan.

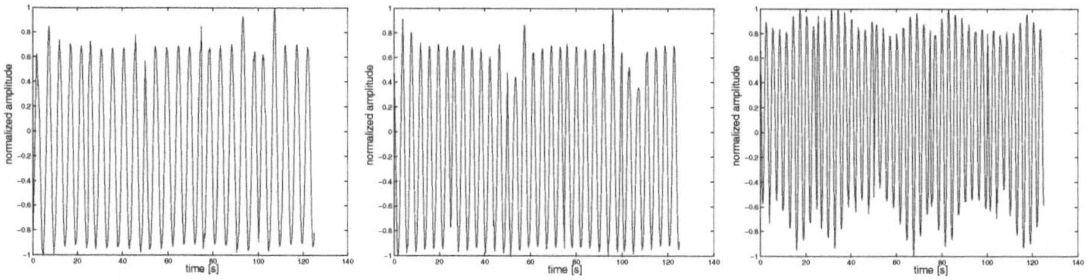

Fig. 3. Sample respiratory signals estimated from the projection images. These correspond, from left to right, to phantom respiration rates of 12, 15, and 20 breaths per minute.

3 Results

When working with our computer controlled respiring phantom we first confirmed that in all cases the respiratory signal obtained from the projection images was indeed consistent with the known respiratory pattern. This is illustrated in Figure 3.

We first visually evaluated our approach to generating a 4D CBCT data set by selecting coronal and sagittal reformatted images from the same spatial location of a 3D image created by our method and that created using the first C-arm sweep. Figure 4 illustrates this qualitative evaluation. In all cases our method was able to improve the visual quality of the data, primarily in the region of the diaphragm.

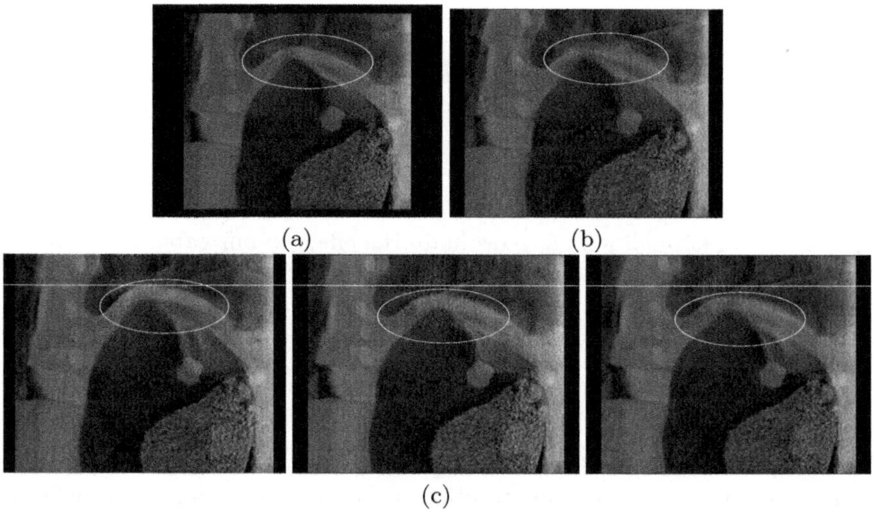

Fig. 4. Reformatted sagittal slices at the same spatial location (a) reconstruction from stationary phantom (b) reconstruction from free breathing data and (c) three respiratory phases reconstructed from gated data. Improved image quality is clearly evident next to the diaphragm (ellipse). The respiratory phases are visible with respect to the line placed at the top of the diaphragm location in the first image.

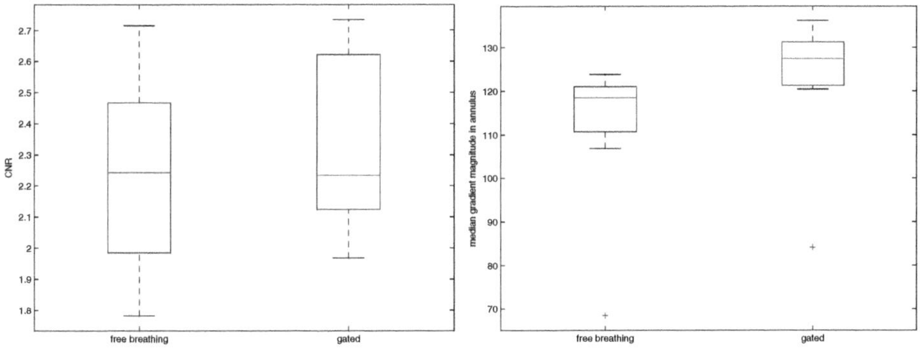

(a) (b)

Fig. 5. Comparison of (a) contrast to noise ratio and (b) median gradient magnitude in annulus, between reconstructions performed using the first sweep of the C-arm in our multi-sweep approach and a gated sweep. Standard values used in plot construction, box spans interquartile range, median marked inside box and maximal whisker length is set to 1.5 times inter quartile range.

We then quantitatively evaluated the 3D image quality obtained by our method and a 3D image obtained using the standard approach, ignoring the phantom's breathing. We start by assessing our ground truth data, a CBCT acquisition of the stationary phantom. The CNR for our ground truth is 2.85 and the GM-A is 117.43.

Figure 5 summarizes the evaluation for both our image quality measures, CNR and GM-A. The results show that the quality of the 3D images that comprise the 4D image is higher than that of the 3D image reconstructed from data that does not compensate for the respiratory motion. We also observed that for shallow breathing our approach does not improve the results irrespective of the respiratory rate but that for normal and deep breathing the results are improved for all respiratory rates, as summarized in Table 1.

Finally, we compared the estimated tumor volumes to the ground truth volume obtained from a CT of the stationary phantom. In our case the ground truth tumor volume is 10243.5mm^3. The median (std) error for the free breathing data was 262.10 (765.16)mm^3 and for the gated data it was 208.60(118.66)mm^3.

Table 1. Quantitative results from all nine data sets as a function of the respiratory rate and volume for corresponding gated(free breathing) data sets (a) CNR values and (b) median GM-A values

	shallow	normal	deep
slow	2.23(2.55)	2.72(2.32)	2.14(2.01)
medium	2.74(2.72)	2.29(2.24)	2.13(1.78)
fast	2.10(2.44)	2.59(2.21)	1.97(1.92)

(a)

	shallow	normal	deep
slow	134.33(119.60)	121.56(112.92)	84.14(68.47)
medium	123.27(123.83)	129.39(118.49)	120.45(106.88)
fast	127.44(123.53)	130.19(120.18)	136.15(111.96)

(b)

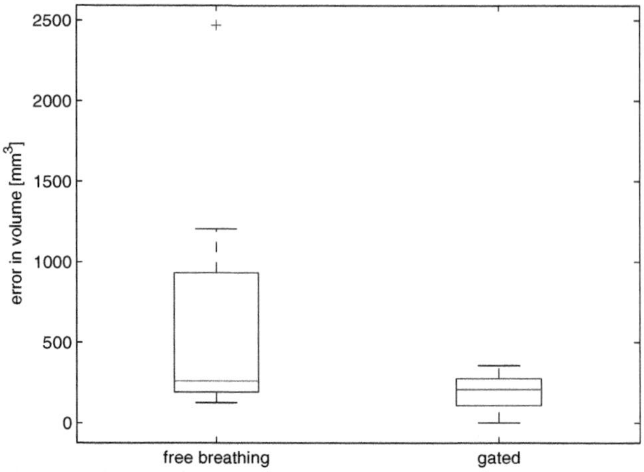

Fig. 6. Errors in tumor volume estimation as compared to a gold standard obtained from a CT of the stationary phantom. Standard values used in plot construction, box spans interquartile range, median marked inside box and maximal whisker length is set to 1.5 times inter quartile range.

Figure 6 summarizes this evaluation. Based on these results we conclude that our gating approach improves the volumetric estimation.

4 Discussion and Conclusion

We have presented a method for retrospective respiratory gating and 4D (3D+time) image reconstruction using an intra-operative C-arm based CBCT system. The proposed method was evaluated using a computer controlled anthropomorphic respiring phantom. We have shown that the proposed approach is able to compensate for the respiratory motion, producing a set of 3D images of improved quality over that available when performing reconstruction that ignores respiratory motion. This study has also shown that 4D CBCT can be readily acquired using currently deployed clinical systems without the need for any hardware modifications.

The use of such a 4D data set will enable data acquisition without requiring the patient to hold their breath during the process. In addition during the intervention breath-holds at arbitrary respiratory phases are accommodated, potentially improving targeting accuracy.

To date, the majority of phantom studies evaluating the effect of respiratory motion have utilized linear stages onto which objects with sharp edges were mounted (e.g. cubes, spheres). In this study we used an anthropomorphic respiring phantom that mimics abdominal respiratory motion. Abdominal motion is affected by the phantom's diaphragm, moving an anatomically correct model of the liver containing a tumor. This results in more realistic motion patterns.

While the end result is closer to human respiratory motion, our study was only conducted using uniform respiratory rates and amplitudes. As this study was an initial evaluation of our proposed reconstruction approach, we did not evaluate the effects of varying respiration rates and volumes during image acquisition. This further evaluation is planned for the near future. It should be noted that our phantom does not exhibit hysteresis and thus cannot fully mimic respiratory motion.

While in most cases our approach improved image quality, for shallow breathing it did reduce it, both for slow and fast respiratory rates. This is most likely due to the minimal motion, approximately 1mm, exhibited by our object of interest. It should be noted that in humans the motion magnitude is much larger, closer to that obtained by our normal, approximately 5mm, and deep breathing, approximately 10mm, motions.

Even with the improved image quality obtained by our method, it is still slightly lower than the image quality obtained when the phantom was stationary. Finally, when compared to diagnostic CT the quality of the images of the stationary phantom was considerably higher in CT with a CNR of 5.08 versus a CNR of 2.85 in the CBCT image. Thus, while the capability of C-arm based CBCT systems to differentiate between different materials has greatly improved it is still not at the level of diagnostic CT.

In thoracic-abdominal interventions, a pre-operative CT is most often available. We are currently investigating the use of this CT in conjunction with the intra-operative 4D CBCT. By registering the CT to each of the 3D images comprising the 4D CBCT image we will be able to provide 4D guidance with the high image quality of diagnostic CT.

Acknowledgement. This work was funded by NIH/NIBIB grant R01EB007195. The authors would like to thank Emmanuel Wilson for his help with the experiments.

References

1. Mundeleer, L., Wikler, D., Leloup, T., Warzée, N.: Development of a computer assisted system aimed at RFA liver surgery. Comput. Med. Imaging Graph. 32(7), 611–621 (2008)
2. Nicolau, S., Pennec, X., Soler, L., Buy, X., Gangi, A., Ayache, N., Marescaux, J.: An augmented reality system for liver thermal ablation: Design and evaluation on clinical cases. Medical Image Analysis 13(3), 494–506 (2009)
3. Yaniv, Z., Cheng, P., Wilson, E., Popa, T., Lindisch, D., Campos-Nanez, E., Abeledo, H., Watson, V., Cleary, K., Banovac, F.: Needle-based interventions with the image-guided surgery toolkit (IGSTK): From phantoms to clinical trials. IEEE Trans. Biomed. Eng. 57(4), 922–933 (2010)
4. Kimura, T., Hirokawa, Y., Murakami, Y., Tsujimura, M., Nakashima, T., Ohno, Y., Kenjo, M., Kaneyasu, Y., Wadasaki, K., Ito, K.: Reproducibility of organ position using voluntary breath hold method with spirometer during extracranial stereotactic radiotherapy. International Journal of Radiation Oncology, Biology, Physics 60(4), 1307–1313 (2004)

5. Wallace, M.J., Kuo, M.D., Glaiberman, C., Binkert, C.A., Orth, R.C., Soulez, G.: Three-dimensional C-arm cone-beam CT: Applications in the interventional suite. Journal of Vascular and Interventional Radiology 19(6), 799–813 (2008)
6. Li, T., Xing, L., Munro, P., McGuinness, C., Chao, M., Yang, Y., Loo, B., Koong, A.: Four-dimensional cone-beam computed tomography using an on-board imager. Med. Phys. 33(10), 3825–3833 (2006)
7. Li, T., Schreibmann, E., Yang, Y., Xing, L.: Motion correction for improved target localization with on-board cone-beam computed tomography. Phys. Med. Biol. 51(2), 253–267 (2006)
8. Rit, S., Wolthaus, J., van Herk, M., Sonke, J.J.: On-the-fly motion-compensated cone-beam CT using an a priori motion model. In: Medical Image Computing and Computer-Assisted Intervention, pp. 729–736 (2008)
9. Hartl, A., Yaniv, Z.: Evaluation of a 4D cone-beam CT reconstruction approach using a simulation framework. In: International Conference of the IEEE Engineering in Medicine and Biology Society (EMBC), pp. 5729–5732 (2009)
10. Lauritsch, G., Boese, J., Wigström, L., Kemeth, H., Fahrig, R.: Towards cardiac C-Arm computed tomography. IEEE Trans. Med. Imag. 25(7), 922–934 (2006)
11. Wiesner, S., Yaniv, Z.: Respiratory signal generation for retrospective gating of cone-beam CT images. In: SPIE Medical Imaging: Visualization, Image-Guided Procedures, and Display (2008)
12. Mazilu, D., et al.: Synthetic torso for training in and evaluation of urologic laparoscopic skills. J. Endourol. 20(5), 340–345 (2006)
13. Lin, R., Wilson, E., Tang, J., Stoianovici, D., Cleary, K.: A computer-controlled pump and realistic anthropomorphic respiratory phantom for validating image-guided systems. In: SPIE Medical Imaging: Visualization and Image-Guided Procedures, vol. 6509 (2007)
14. Perry, N., Broeders, M., de Wolf, C., Törnberg, S., Holland, R., von Karsa, L. (eds.): European guidelines for quality assurance in breast cancer screening and diagnosis (2006)

Determination of Pelvic Orientation from Ultrasound Images Using Patch-SSMs and a Hierarchical Speed of Sound Compensation Strategy

Steffen Schumann[1,⋆], Marc Puls[1], Timo Ecker[1], Tobias Schwaegli[2], Jan Stifter[2], Klaus-A. Siebenrock[1], and Guoyan Zheng[1]

[1] Inselspital, Orthopaedic Department, University of Bern, 3010 Bern, Switzerland
[2] Smith & Nephew Orthopaedics AG, Schachenallee 29, 5001 Aarau, Switzerland

Abstract. In the field of computer assisted orthopedic surgery (CAOS) the anterior pelvic plane (APP) is a common concept to determine the pelvic orientation by digitizing distinct pelvic landmarks. As percutaneous palpation is - especially for obese patients - known to be error-prone, B-mode ultrasound (US) imaging could provide an alternative means. Several concepts of using ultrasound imaging to determine the APP landmarks have been introduced. In this paper we present a novel technique, which uses local patch statistical shape models (SSMs) and a hierarchical speed of sound compensation strategy for an accurate determination of the APP. These patches are independently matched and instantiated with respect to associated point clouds derived from the acquired ultrasound images. Potential inaccuracies due to the assumption of a constant speed of sound are compensated by an extended reconstruction scheme. We validated our method with in-vitro studies using a plastic bone covered with a soft-tissue simulation phantom and with a preliminary cadaver trial.

1 Introduction

Accurate acetabular cup placement in total hip arthroplasty (THA) procedures is very important for the clinical outcome [1, 2]. Misaligned cup prostheses could lead to a reduced range of motion, impingement or dislocation [3–5]. Computer assistance therefore potentially provides a means to support this critical step [6]. In navigated THAs, the APP is typically used as a reference plane to measure the correct cup orientation [7]. This plane is constructed using two landmarks from the bilateral anterior superior iliac spines (ASISs) and a landmark from the pubis symphysis region. These landmarks are usually digitized intra-operatively using a tracked pointer. In order to reduce the invasiveness, these landmarks are acquired percutaneously. This may result - especially for obese patients - in a certain inaccuracy, subsequently increasing the probability of cup misalignment

⋆ The authors would like to thank CTI for funding this project.

N. Navab and P. Jannin (Eds.): IPCAI 2010, LNCS 6135, pp. 157–167, 2010.

[8, 9]. A minor failure in detecting these landmarks can lead to an increased error in placing the cup implant [10].

In contrast, ultrasound imaging provides a non-invasive way to visualize subcutaneous bony structures. The use of calibrated B-mode ultrasound has been proposed by several groups for detecting landmarks [8, 11, 12] or for reconstructing patient-specific 3D models of the pelvis using SSMs [13–15]. The main challenge of achieving an accurate 3D reconstruction is imposed by a proper alignment of the sparse US-derived point data with the mean pelvis model. Only a close alignment to the target points can guarantee the success of the instantiation. While in [13, 15] the pelvis model was manually aligned, Foroughi et al. [14] used rigid registration. Another source of error occurs due to the deviation of speed of sound in the human body from the one assumed in the calibration procedure. According to Barratt et al. [16], the correct depth estimation could be biased by up to 5% due to variations in speed of sound. However, none of the existing approaches accounts for this depth localization problem.

In this paper, we propose a new method for reconstruction of the pelvic orientation based on point clouds segmented from tracked ultrasound images. Instead of directly matching a SSM of the complete pelvis, we constructed local patch-SSMs, which are independently matched to corresponding US-derived points. Moreover, we developed a hierarchical optimization scheme, which compensates for the speed of sound difference. We evaluated our approach with in-vitro studies using a soft-tissue simulation phantom attached to a plastic bone and with a preliminary cadaver trial.

2 Materials and Methods

2.1 Patch-SSM Construction

Computed tomography datasets of 20 different patients (average age: 61.9 years, mixed gender) were semi-automatically segmented using the software tool Amira (Visage Imaging, Richmond, Australia). The extracted pelvis surface models were then rigidly aligned in a common coordinate system based on their oriented bounding box. In order to establish dense correspondences between these training models, a non-rigid registration scheme was applied. One instance, whose size was closest to the average training model size, was selected as the reference. The other (floating) surface instances were then rigidly registered in an affine sense to the reference instance. For the subsequent non-rigid registration step, all surface instances were converted to bit-volumes. The floating instance volumes were then deformed with respect to the reference volume using diffeomorphic demons algorithm [17]. This method computes the displacement field between a reference and a floating image to optimally align both images. Therefore, the displacement fields between the reference volume and each floating instance volume are computed, describing the non-rigid relation between the datasets. The overall correspondences between the available training instances could then be determined by deforming the reference instance based on the computed displacement fields.

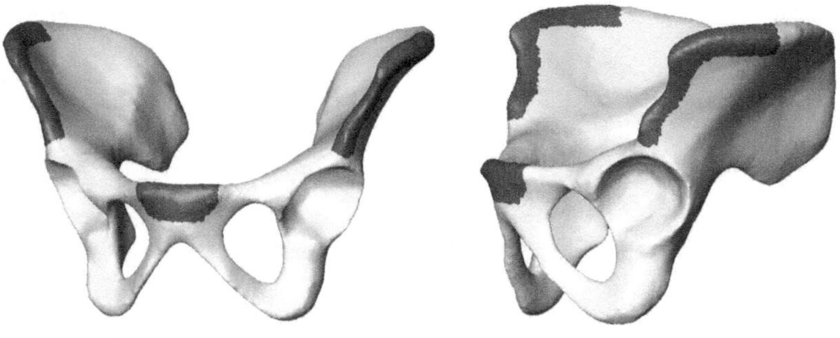

Fig. 1. Pelvic mean model with selected region patches

The patches were generated from the average pelvis model, computed from the aligned surface instances. The selection of the patches was performed by taking the prospective application into consideration. In this case we were mainly interested to reconstruct the APP. Therefore, following three regions were interactively defined, as shown in Fig. 1:

- o Iliac spine, left: Anterior superior iliac spine (ASIS) + Anterior inferior iliac spine (AIIS)
- o Pubis symphysis
- o Iliac spine, right: Anterior superior iliac spine + Anterior inferior iliac spine

As the correspondences between all the training instances have been established in the previous step, the patches could directly be extracted from each training model for each region. The inherent translational information due to different pelvis scales was eliminated by rigidly registering each single patch instance to the mean patch of the corresponding region. The variational shape information could then be analyzed using principal component analysis (PCA), resulting in modes of variation described by the eigenvalues and eigenvectors. The variations of the first eigenmode are depicted in Fig. 2.

2.2 Ultrasound Image Calibration and Segmentation

Ultrasound image datasets were acquired using the EchoBlaster US scanner (Telemed, Lithuania). In order to derive the spatial relationship of the acquired images, the pelvis and the ultrasound probe were equipped with reference bases, tracked by an infrared camera (NDI Polaris camera, Waterloo, Ontario, Canada). For this purpose, the ultrasound probe was calibrated using a special calibration phantom to a nominal speed of sound of 1540 m/s, resulting in the homogeneous calibration matrix $T_{calib} = {}^{im}_{US}T \cdot T_{scale}$. The matrix ${}^{im}_{US}T$ represents the constant transformation between the 3D global image coordinate-system (COS) and the COS of the reference base attached to the US probe (US-COS). T_{scale} is the scaling matrix, whereas s_x and s_y represent the scaling parameters (mm/pixel) in x- and y-direction, respectively (Eq. 1). These values are only valid for the type of

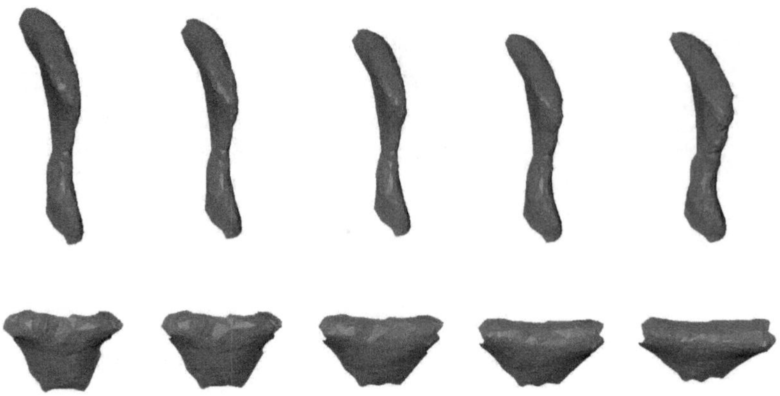

Fig. 2. First eigenmode variations of the left ASIS patch-SSM and the pubis symphysis patch-SSM

material, which is used for calibration. In order to account for different tissue parameters during intra-operative image acquisition, these parameters would need to be adjusted. As the scaling parameter s_y is directly related to the correct localization of structures in scanning direction, this factor needs to be optimized in order to compensate for the difference in speed of sound between the calibration and intra-operative use. The translation between the local image COS and the global 3D image coordinate system is described by s_{tx}. The respective coordinate-systems are illustrated in Fig. 3.

$$T_{scale} = \begin{bmatrix} s_x & 0 & 0 & s_{tx} \\ 0 & s_y & 0 & 0 \\ 0 & 0 & 1 & 0 \\ 0 & 0 & 0 & 1 \end{bmatrix} \quad (1)$$

The whole acquisition process was controlled by PiGalileo software application (Smith & Nephew Orthopaedics AG, Aarau, Switzerland). This application provides an online segmentation algorithm, automatically detecting the contour of bony structures. The segmentation of the US images is thereby restricted to a region of interest (ROI). This ROI and specific US imaging parameters (e.g. power, frequency, focus) have been assigned beforehand to a number of pelvic regions. During image acquisition, the surgeon has to select one of these predefined pelvic regions, whereof he is going to record the US images from. For each image column within the ROI, the algorithm collects the pixels with highest intensity. Within this collection, only pixels are extracted, which fit to a distinct segmentation pattern. For each pelvic region, a specific segmentation pattern was defined a priori. These patterns are based on empirical knowledge in terms of the potential appearance of the particular pelvic region on the US images. In order to assign the segmented point clouds to the corresponding regions, the surgeon is guided during acquisition to record ultrasound images from the following five anatomic regions:

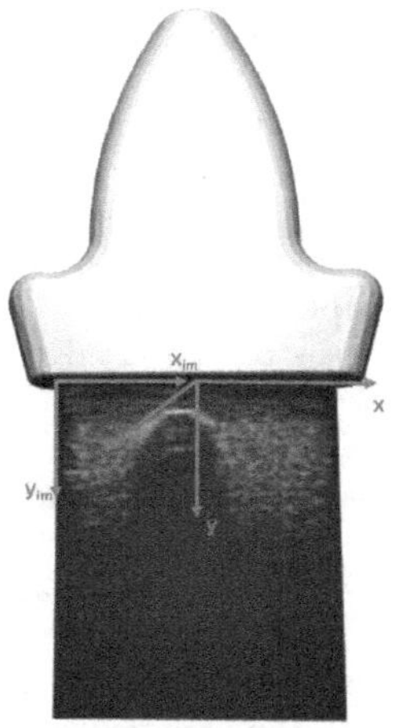

Fig. 3. Definition of local 2D and global 3D ultrasound image coordinate system

- o Anterior superior iliac spine, left patient side
- o Anterior inferior iliac spine, left patient side
- o Pubis symphysis
- o Anterior superior iliac spine, right patient side
- o Anterior inferior iliac spine, right patient side

After finishing the image acquisition, a post-processing step is performed to detect possible outliers. For each of the five extracted point clouds, hierarchical, single-linkage clustering based on euclidean distance metric is applied to remove outliers [18].

2.3 Reconstruction

The used reconstruction scheme is composed of three main steps, as illustrated in Fig. 4. Initially, the transformation between the intra-operative US and the SSM coordinate-system needs to be established. This step is realized by aligning the patch-SSMs with the US-derived point clouds. These patch-SSMs are then independently matched to the corresponding point cloud in the local reconstruction stage. In the last step, the complete pelvis-SSM is registered to the US points, revealing the final reconstructed APP. The local and global reconstruction methods are part of the hierarchical speed of sound optimization scheme.

Initial Alignment. At first, the mean patches are placed at the center of gravity of the corresponding point cloud. While the pubis symphysis patch is aligned based on the first two principal axes of the corresponding point cloud (Fig. 4, step 1.1), the iliac spine patches are aligned in two steps (Fig. 4, step 1.2). The ASIS and AIIS point clouds are derived from anatomical structures

Input: US points $_{im}p$ assigned to 5 different pelvic regions; 3 patch-SSMs; pelvis-SSM
Output: APP derived from pelvis-SSM, registered to optimized US points

1. **Initial Alignment of Patch-SSMs**
   1.1 Alignment of pubis symphysis patch
      1.1.1. Align pubis symphysis patch based on the 1st and the 2nd principal axes
   1.2 Alignment of iliac spine patches
      1.2.1. Align iliac spine patches to ASIS points based on the 1st principal axis
      1.2.2. Optimize rotation of the aligned iliac spine patches based on ASIS and AIIS points
   1.3 Rigidly register the bilateral iliac spine patches to ASIS points and the pubis symphysis patch to the assigned point cloud
2. **Local Patch-SSM Based Reconstruction**
   2.1 Optimize scaling factor of iliac spine patches based on AIIS points using method proposed by Barratt et al. [16]
   2.2 Update all US points based on optimized scaling factor (Eq. 2)
   2.3 Rigidly register the bilateral iliac spine patches to ASIS and AIIS points and the pubis symphysis patch to the assigned point cloud
   2.4 Instantiate patch-SSMs as described by Rajamani et al. [19]
   2.5 Establish dense correspondences by regularized deformation between instantiated patches and US points as presented by Zheng et al. [20]
3. **Global Pelvis-SSM Based Reconstruction**
   3.1 Align mean pelvis model with US points based on the correspondences, established in 2.5
   3.2 Register mean pelvis to US points using 3-stage registration method [20]
   3.3 Optimize scale based on all US points [16]
   3.4 Perform again non-rigid registration between mean pelvis and US points using the 3-stage registration [20]

Fig. 4. Algorithm description, consisting of three main steps

that are located at different depths within the human body. At the same time the ultrasound probe is calibrated for a constant speed of sound, which deviates from the actual speed of sound present in human soft-tissues. Therefore, the deeper the bony structure is located within the body (thus covered by a larger amount of soft-tissue), the increased is the error of localizing the bone surface. Due to this fact, we classified the ASIS region as most trustable and hence use only the ASIS points to align the iliac spine patch. In the first step, the first principal axis of each iliac spine patch is computed from the vertices assigned a priori to the ASIS region and aligned with the first principal axis of the corresponding ASIS point cloud. In the second step, the rotation around this newly determined axis is derived. This is done by computing a least squares fit, which minimizes the distance of the iliac spine patch to all US points (ASIS + AIIS). Fig. 5 shows the result after the automatic alignment. In case the automatic approach does not result in a proper alignment, it can be manually corrected. A manipulator handle is added to each patch, to interactively adapt its translation, rotation and scale. After the alignment is completed, the patches are rigidly registered to the associated cloud of points (Fig. 4, step 1.3). As the AIIS points are considered less trustable, these points are not involved for the registration of the iliac spine patches.

Local Reconstruction. In order to further integrate also the less trustable point clouds, the difference in speed of sound has to be compensated, which is related to the optimization of the scaling factor s_y (Fig. 4, step 2.1). This was done based on the approach proposed by Barratt et al. [16]. They introduced a self-calibration scheme for registration of US-derived points to surface data extracted from computed tomography (CT) images. As the US- and CT-images were acquired from the same patient, they only had to solve the speed of sound compensation problem. We employed this idea for the registration of point clouds to the corresponding mean patches. Unlike the situation in the work done by Barratt et al., we had to solve the shape instantiation and speed of sound compensation simultaneously. In order to optimize the scaling factor s_y for speed of sound compensation, a least squares fit is computed, minimizing the Euclidean distance between corresponding 3D points of the target patch (${}_{pat}P$) and 2D US-derived points (${}_{im}p$).

$$ {}_{pat}P = {}^{US}_{pat}T \cdot {}^{im}_{US}T \cdot T_{scale} \cdot {}_{im}p \qquad (2) $$

The matrices ${}^{im}_{US}T$ and T_{scale} were determined during the calibration process, as described in section 2.2. The transformation ${}^{US}_{pat}T$ describes the relation of the US-COS to the coordinate-system of the reference base attached to the patient. Eq. 2 is solved for s_y by finding corresponding point pairs ${}_{pat}P_i$ and ${}_{im}p_i$. At the beginning, the scaling factor is optimized taking only the AIIS points into account (Fig. 4, step 2.1). The optimized scaling parameter is then again plugged in Eq. 2, to update all US-derived points (Fig. 4, step 2.2). In the next step, the mean patches are rigidly registered to the updated point clouds. As the scaling-factor is now corrected for the AIIS-points, these points are also used to register the iliac spine patches (Fig. 4, step 2.3). To establish dense correspondences, the patch-SSMs are instantiated by computing the optimal shape parameters as described by Rajamani et al. [19] (Fig. 4, step 2.4). After the instantiation step, regularized deformation, as presented in [20], completes the non-rigid registration (Fig. 4, step 2.5). The final reconstructed patches are illustrated in Fig. 5.

Global Reconstruction. Within the global reconstruction scheme, the scaling parameter is further optimized using the complete pelvis model. This pelvis-SSM was constructed from the database of training surface models. As the correspondences between the training models were already established, the shape variation could directly be computed using PCA.

As dense correspondences between the intra-operative US- and the SSM-COS were already established in the local reconstruction scheme based on the patch-SSMs, the mean pelvis model could directly be aligned (Fig. 4, step 3.1). In

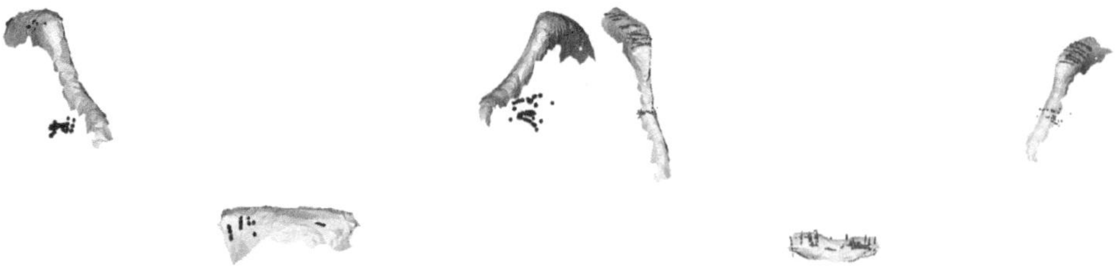

Fig. 5. Initial alignment of patches based on data obtained from phantom (left); instantiated patches after local reconstruction (right)

the next step, the pelvis-model is registered in an affine sense, instantiated and deformed involving all US-derived points (Fig. 4, step 3.2). Subsequently, another speed of sound optimization step is computed based on all five point clouds (Fig. 4, step 3.3). This step is required, as the pubis symphysis region is normally located at a greater depth within the human body. Another cycle of rigid and non-rigid registration is repeated to finally reconstruct the APP-landmarks (Fig. 4, step 3.4).

3 Experiments and Results

In order to evaluate the accuracy of our method, we conducted two experiments. In the first study, in-vitro tests using a pelvic plastic bone with a custom-made soft-tissue simulation phantom were performed. In the second study, ultrasound data acquired from one cadaveric specimen were used to validate our method. In both cases ultrasound images were acquired from the bilateral ASISs and AIISs and from the pubis symphysis. In order to simulate the acquisition in the operation theater, a sterile cover bag was pulled over the ultrasound probe. We then applied our method based on the acquired ultrasound datasets for reconstructing the APP. The respective landmarks were defined beforehand based on the mean pelvic model. The reconstructed APP landmarks positions were determined by transferring this information to the reconstructed pelvis model. The ground truth APP was established via direct pointer digitization. For the in-vitro study, the soft-tissue simulation phantom was detached from the pelvis model for landmark digitization. For the cadaver trial, three small regions of the pelvis were dissected to digitize the APP. The reconstruction error was then measured by comparing the reconstructed APP with the ground truth APP, expressing the error in terms of degrees for anteversion and inclination angle.

In the first study, three ultrasound datasets of the phantom were acquired and analyzed. In this study the plastic pelvis model was arranged in supine position. After fixing the reference base to the iliac crest, the soft tissue simulation phantom was attached to the model. This phantom, made from silicone, is specially designed to match to the plastic model. The experimental setup is shown in Fig. 6. For each dataset about 125 ultrasound images were acquired, resulting in approximately 2800 segmented points. While the reconstruction of the first dataset

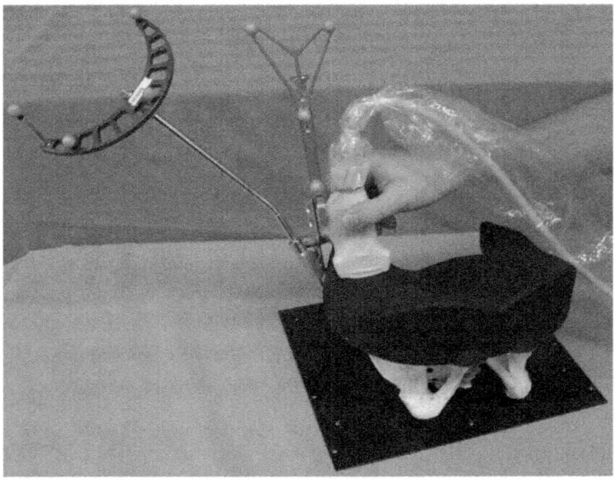

Fig. 6. Experimental setup of phantom study: Plastic pelvis with soft-tissue simulation phantom and reference base attached; ultrasound probe with sterile cover bag pulled over and reference base attached

was done fully automatic, an interactive step was required for the second and third dataset. As not all outliers were eliminated, remaining outliers were subsequently removed manually. Based on a manual inspection we omitted ultrasound images and associated point clouds, in order to avoid a bias on our results due to outliers. However, once all outliers were removed, the patches could be automatically aligned. Comparing the reconstructed APP with the ground truth APP resulted in an anteversion mean error of 0.99 ° and an inclination mean error of 0.95 ° . In the second study, 304 ultrasound images were acquired from the cadaveric specimen in supine position, providing 4884 US-derived points. Outlier points were automatically removed, whereas another interactive removal was required (see Fig. 7a). For the iliac spine patches, the automatic alignment had to be corrected manually. The final reconstructed pelvis model is visualized in Fig. 7b. In order to estimate the effect of the subjectiveness due to the user interaction, we evaluated the cadaver dataset three times. The results of the phantom and cadaver experiments are summarized in Table 1. The anteversion angle could be determined on average with an error of 0.89 ° , the inclination angle with an error of 1.13 ° . Also the effect of the user interaction was considerably low, which is represented by the standard deviation. In order to analyze the validity of the speed of sound optimization scheme, the updated 3D US-derived points were directly compared with some validation points, digitized on the pelvis surface of the cadaveric specimen. The successful speed of sound compensation is depicted in Fig. 7c.

Another approach to determine the pelvic coordinate system has been presented by Foroughi et al. [14]. This approach is also based on US images, acquired from only a few specific regions of the pelvis. The extracted US points were then rigidly registered to the mean model of a pelvis atlas, without taking a speed of sound difference into account. Several experiments were conducted, whereas the error was separated into translational and rotational components.

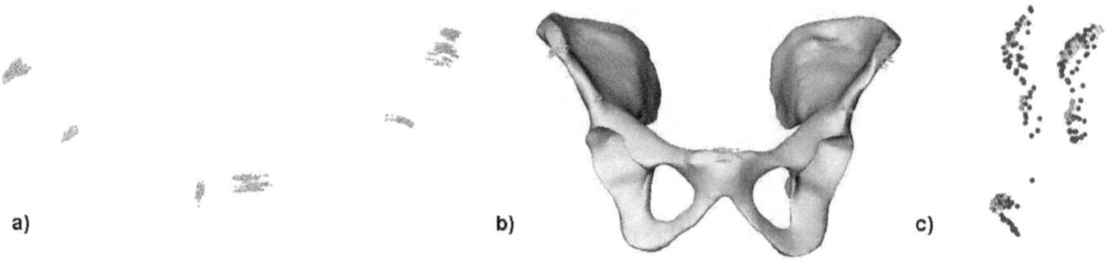

Fig. 7. (a) Point clouds derived from ultrasound images acquired from cadaveric specimen; (b) final reconstructed pelvis model; (c) validation points digitized on bone surface (blue) and US-derived points after speed of sound compensation

Table 1. Mean error of reconstructed angles (cadaver dataset was evaluated three times)

	phantom data 1	*phantom data 2*	*phantom data 3*	*cadaver data*
anteversion [°]	1.13	0.56	1.24	0.62±0.56
inclination [°]	0.93	0.38	1.55	1.67±0.03

The results of experiments with a dry bone and two cadaveric specimens were in the same range, as we have obtained with our method. However, the rotational error of the APP is expressed in different angles, which does not allow for a direct comparison.

4 Conclusion

B-mode ultrasound imaging has a great potential to replace currently used percutaneous pointer digitization for determining the APP. Several approaches have already been published, proposing the use of SSMs to reconstruct the pelvic shape and/or orientation. However, none of these methods presented a solution to compensate the difference in speed of sound between the calibration and the intra-operative use. We have developed a new method, which uses patch-SSMs to incrementally compensate for the speed of sound difference. After the initial alignment, these patches were independently fitted to the US-derived points based on a local reconstruction scheme. A complete pelvis model was then aligned based on the established correspondences, completing the hierarchical reconstruction strategy. Two experiments on phantom and cadaver data were conducted, showing promising results.

References

1. Murray, D.: The definition and measurement of acetabular orientation. J. Bone Joint Surg. Br. 75, 228–232 (1993)
2. McCollum, D., Gray, W.: Dislocation after total hip arthroplasty. Clin. Orthop. Relat. Res. 261, 159–170 (1990)

3. Lewinnek, G., Lewis, J., et al.: Dislocation after total hip replacement arthroplasties. J. Bone Joint Surg. Am. 60, 217–220 (1978)
4. Jaramaz, B., Nikou, C., et al.: Effect of cup orientation and neck length in range of motion simulation. Orthop. Res. Soc. 22 (1997)
5. D'Lima, D., Urquhardt, A., et al.: The effect of the orientation of the acetabular and femoral components on the range of motion of the hip at different head-neck ratios. J. Bone Joint Surg. Am. 82, 315–321 (2000)
6. Jolles, B., Genoud, P., et al.: Computer-assisted cup placement techniques in total hip arthroplasty improve accuracy of placement. Clin. Orthop. Relat. Res. 426, 174–179 (2004)
7. Tannast, M., Langlotz, U., et al.: Anatomic referencing of cup orientation in total hip arthroplasty. Clin. Orthop. Relat. Res. 436, 144–150 (2005)
8. Parratte, S., Kilian, P., et al.: The use of ultrasound in acquisition of the anterior pelvic plane in computer-assisted total hip replacement. J. Bone Joint Surg. Br. 90-B, 258–263 (2008)
9. Spencer, J., Day, R., et al.: Computer navigation of the acetabular component. J. Bone Joint Surg. Br. 88-B, 972–975 (2006)
10. Wolf, A., DiGioia, A., et al.: A kinematic model for calculating cup alignment error during total hip arthroplasty. J. Biomech. 38, 2257–2265 (2005)
11. Tonetti, J., Carrat, L., et al.: Clinical results of percutaneous pelvic surgery. computer-assisted surgery using ultrasound compared to standard fluoroscopy. Comput. Aided Surg. 6, 204–211 (2001)
12. Dardenne, G., Dusseau, S., et al.: Toward a dynamic approach of tha planning based on ultrasound. Clin. Orthop. Relat. Res. 467, 901–908 (2009)
13. Chan, C., Barratt, D., et al.: Cadaver validation of the use of ultrasound for 3d model instantiation of bony anatomy in image guided orthopaedic surgery. In: Barillot, C., Haynor, D.R., Hellier, P. (eds.) MICCAI 2004. LNCS, vol. 3217, pp. 397–494. Springer, Heidelberg (2004)
14. Foroughi, P., Song, D.: Localization of pelvic anatomical coordinate system using us/atlas registration for total hip replacement. In: Metaxas, D., Axel, L., Fichtinger, G., Székely, G. (eds.) MICCAI 2008, Part II. LNCS, vol. 5242, pp. 871–879. Springer, Heidelberg (2008)
15. Barratt, D., Chan, C., et al.: Instantiation and registration of statistical shape models of the femur and pelvis using 3d ultrasound imaging. Med. Image Anal. 12, 358–374 (2008)
16. Barratt, D., Penney, G., et al.: Self-calibrating 3d-ultrasound-based bone registration for minimally invasive orthopedic surgery. IEEE Trans. on Med. Imaging 25, 312–323 (2006)
17. Vercauteren, T., Pennec, X., et al.: Non-parametric diffeomorphic image registration with the demons algorithm. In: Ayache, N., Ourselin, S., Maeder, A. (eds.) MICCAI 2007, Part II. LNCS, vol. 4792, pp. 319–326. Springer, Heidelberg (2007)
18. Duda, R., Hart, P., Stork, D.: Pattern classification. John Wiley & Sons, Chichester (2000)
19. Rajamani, K., Styner, M., et al.: Statistical deformable bone models for robust 3d surface extrapolation from sparse data. Med. Image Anal. 11, 99–109 (2007)
20. Zheng, G., Rajamani, K., et al.: Use of a dense surface point distribution model in a three-stage anatomical shape reconstruction from sparse information for computer assisted orthopaedic surgery: A preliminary study. In: Narayanan, P.J., Nayar, S.K., Shum, H.-Y. (eds.) ACCV 2006. LNCS, vol. 3852, pp. 52–60. Springer, Heidelberg (2006)

Ultrasound Servoing of Catheters for Beating Heart Valve Repair

Samuel B. Kesner[1], Shelten G. Yuen[1], and Robert D. Howe[1,2]

[1] Harvard School of Engineering and Applied Sciences, Cambridge, MA
[2] Harvard-MIT Division of Health Sciences & Technology, Cambridge, MA

Abstract. Robotic cardiac catheters have the potential to revolutionize heart surgery by extending minimally invasive techniques to complex surgical repairs inside the heart. However, catheter technologies are currently unable to track fast tissue motion, which is required to perform delicate procedures inside a beating heart. This paper presents an actuated catheter tool that compensates for the motion of heart structures like the mitral valve apparatus by servoing a catheter guidewire inside a flexible sheath. We examine design and operation parameters and establish that friction and backlash limit the tracking performance of the catheter system. Based on the results of these experiments, we implement compensation methods to improve trajectory tracking. The catheter system is then integrated with an ultrasound-based visual servoing system to enable fast tissue tracking. In vivo tests show RMS tracking errors of 0.77 mm for following the porcine mitral valve annulus trajectory. The results demonstrate that an ultrasound-guided robotic catheter system can accurately track the fast motion of the mitral valve.

Keywords: Catheter, motion compensation, heart, ultrasound, visual servoing.

1 Introduction

Innovations in catheter technology have greatly expanded the range of procedures that interventional cardiologists can perform inside the heart using minimally invasive techniques. Procedures that are now performed using catheters include measuring cardiac physiological function, dilating vessels and valves, and implanting prosthetics and devices [1]. Nonetheless, catheters do not yet allow clinicians to interact with heart tissue with the same level of skill as in open heart surgery. A primary reason for this deficiency is that current catheters do not have the dexterity, speed, and force capabilities to perform complex or delicate tissue interactions.

Cardiac catheters are long and thin flexible tubes that are inserted into the vascular system and passed into the heart. Current robotic cardiac catheters, such as the commercially available Artisan Control Catheter (Hansen Medical, Mountain View CA, USA), permit a human operator to control the positioning of a catheter in the lateral direction and advance it through the vasculature [2]-[4]. However, these systems do not provide sufficient speeds to compensate for the motion of the heart. Fast motion compensation is required for many beating heart procedures to enable dexterous interaction and prevent the catheter from colliding with internal cardiac structures [5].

N. Navab and P. Jannin (Eds.): IPCAI 2010, LNCS 6135, pp. 168–178, 2010.

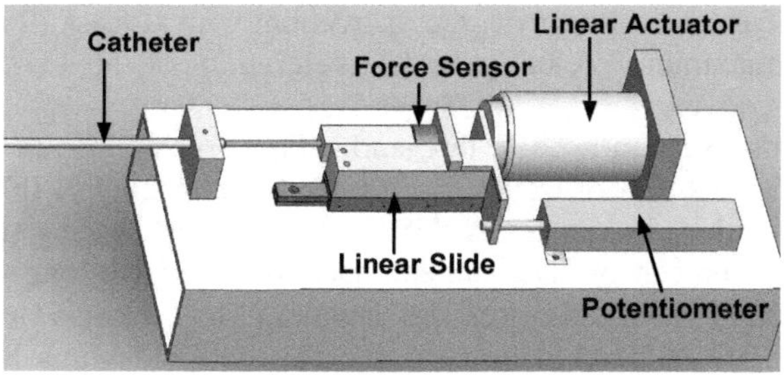

Fig. 1. Actuated catheter system prototype

Researchers have developed robotic approaches to compensating for the motion of the beating heart [6]-[8], but these techniques are directed at coronary artery bypass procedures that repair arteries on the external heart surface. In previous work, we developed robotic devices that compensate for the motion of internal heart structures with a handheld robotic instrument inserted through incisions in the heart wall [5], [9]-[11]. This work shows that single degree of freedom (DOF) servoing is sufficient to accurately track the motion of certain cardiac structures, including the human mitral valve annulus [9],[11]. This approach alleviates the risks associated with stopped heart techniques [12], but the necessity of creating incisions in the heart wall means that this approach is not minimally invasive.

This paper explores the viability of applying our successful robotic cardiac motion compensation techniques to catheters in order to minimize invasiveness. In the envisioned clinical system, an actuator at the base of the catheter system will drive a catheter guidewire inside a flexible sheath (Fig. 1). The sheath is manually advanced through the vasculature into the heart. A standard 3D ultrasound (3DUS) probe images the catheter tip and the tissue target, and real-time image processing algorithms track the catheter-tissue relationship. The guidewire tip is then translated in and out of the sheath to compensate for the cardiac motion and to perform repairs.

The paper begins with a description of the prototype actuated catheter system. Operation of this system reveals a number of challenges that result from quickly translating a guidewire inside a plastic sheath, particularly friction and backlash. This results in position hysteresis and significant tip trajectory errors. We characterize the relationship between catheter design parameters and performance. The insights from these experiments are then used to improve the catheter system tracking through mechanical design and compensation control. Finally, the catheter system is integrated with the ultrasound-based visual servoing system and evaluated with in vivo animal experiments. The results of these experiments demonstrate the feasibility of using catheters for beating-heart intracardiac repair.

2 System Design

The design parameters for the actuated catheter system were selected from the human mitral valve physiology values determined for our earlier handheld motion compensation instrument [5], [11]. The system's principal functional requirements are that it has a single actuated linear degree of freedom with at least 20 mm of travel that can provide a maximum velocity and acceleration of at least 210 mm/s and 3800 mm/s^2, respectively.

The experimental system used in this study (Fig. 1) is composed of a linear voice coil actuator with 50.8 mm of travel and a peak force of 26.7 N (NCC20-18-02-1X, H2W Technologies Inc, Valencia CA, USA), a linear ball bearing slide, and a linear potentiometer position sensor. The catheter sheaths are 85 cm long sections of PTFE (Teflon) tubing, and the guidewires are stainless steel close-wound springs. The geometry of the various combinations of sheaths and guidewires is detailed below. The catheter sheath and guidewire can be flexed as required by the vascular geometry (bent, twisted, etc.) while the guidewire is servoed by the base module.

A PID control system running at 1 kHz is used to control the position of the linear actuator at the base of the catheter. Commands to the linear actuator are amplified by a bipolar voltage-to-current power supply (BOP 36-12M, Kepco Inc., Flushing NY). The reaction forces between the guidewire and actuation mechanism generated by friction and forces applied to the tip of the guidewire are measured with a miniature force sensor (LCFD-1KG, Omega Engineering, Stamford CT, range: 10 N, accuracy: ±0.015 N). In the characterization tests that follow, the catheter tip position is measured with an ultra-low friction rotary potentiometer (CP-2UTX, Midori America Corp, Fullerton CA) connected to the catheter tip with a lightweight lever arm that converts the linear motion into rotation. For the subsequent in vivo studies, tip position is measured with an electromagnetic tracker and ultrasound imaging.

3 Performance Limitations

Operation of this prototype system reveals two principal performance limitations: the friction forces experienced by the guidewire, and the backlash behavior due to the guidewire-sheath interaction. These two issues degrade the trajectory tracking accuracy and response time of the actuated catheter end effector. Fig. 2 illustrates an example of the catheter tip failing to accurately track a desired trajectory. A large number of factors are involved in determining the friction and backlash properties of the catheter system. To understand how to best design and control this system, the experimental variables examined in this study include the gap size between the sheath and guidewire and the bending configuration of the catheter system, characterized by the bend radii and bend angles of the catheter sheath (Fig. 4).The catheter material properties and the external forces were held constant.

3.1 Friction

Experimental Methods. The first set of experiments examined the friction of the catheter system as a function of four different sheath-guidewire gap sizes (Table 1), three bending angles (90°, 180°, and 360°), and two bend radii (25 and 50 mm). The friction was calculated by commanding a series of constant velocities from the actuator in both the positive and negative directions. Force sensor readings during the constant velocity portion of the trajectory were averaged.

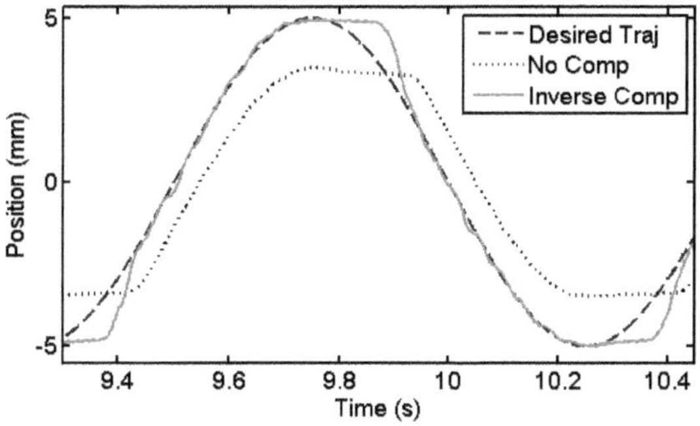

Fig. 2. A sinusoidal desired trajectory and the measured catheter tip trajectory with and without compensation

Friction Results. Fig. 4 presents a typical friction-velocity curve for this system. The observed behavior can be approximately described as constant dynamic Coulomb friction plus a component that varies linearly with velocity. For this case, the Coulomb term can be approximated as 1.0 N of friction and the velocity dependent term as 0.006 N/(mm/s).

The results of the friction experiments, summarized in Fig. 5, illustrate a number of trends. The data was analyzed with a three-way analysis of variance (ANOVA). The most significant trend is that the gap size has the strongest influence on guidewire friction ($p < 0.0001$). The gap size, i.e. the interior space between the guidewire and the inner wall of the sheath (Fig. 3), directly affects the normal forces applied to the guidewire by the sheath. The normal force is created by any sections of the sheath that might be pinched or kinked, locations where the catheter bending forces the guidewire

Table 1. Experimental catheter Dimensions

Symbol	Sheath Inner Diameter	Guidewire Diameter	Gap Size (G)
▽	1.6 mm	0.8 mm	0.8 mm
*	1.6 mm	1.5 mm	0.1 mm
○	2.4 mm	1.5 mm	0.9 mm
□	2.4 mm	2.2 mm	0.2 mm

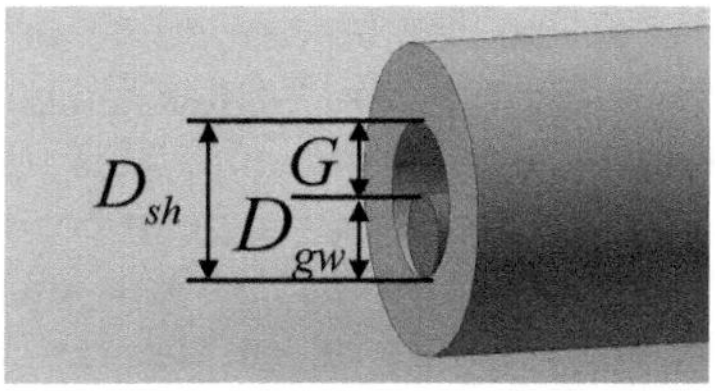

Fig. 3. Sheath and guidewire

to conform along the inner wall of the sheath, and discontinuities in either the guidewire or the sheath that cause the two components to come into contact. The small gap size amplifies these issues because smaller deformations in the catheter system cause the sheath and guidewire to interact. Therefore, increasing the gap size should decrease the friction forces experienced by the guidewire.

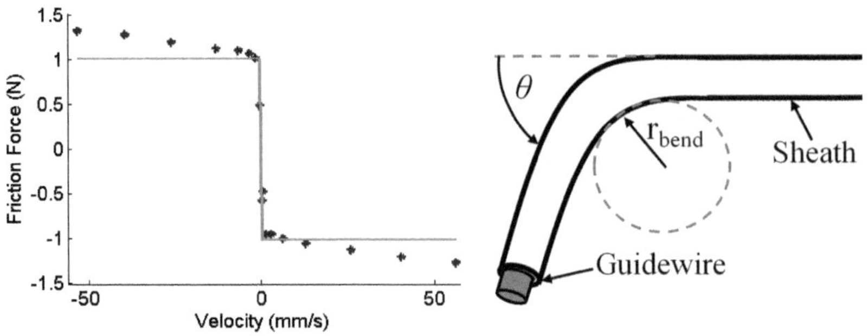

Fig. 4. Left: Friction force versus velocity for the catheter system. The points are experimental values and the line is a Coulombic model approximation of the data. Right: The bending configuration is specified by the bend angle (θ) and bend radius (r_{bend}).

The results also show that bend angle has an effect on the friction forces ($p = 0.004$). One reason for this trend is that bending causes the sheaths' cross sections to deform slightly. This deformation can pinch the guidewire, thus increasing the applied normal forces. Also, the bending of the sheath forces the inner guidewire to bend. The reaction forces generated by the conforming guidewire increase the normal force and therefore the friction on the guidewire.

The bending radius does not appear to have a significant impact on the friction measurements ($p = 0.64$), however only two radii (25 mm and 50 mm) were examined. These radii were selected because they are approximately the bend radii required to maneuver into the heart.

3.2 Backlash

Experimental Methods. The backlash properties of the sheath-guidewire system were investigated with the same experimental variables (gap size, bend angle, bend radius) as the friction experiments present above. The backlash was examined by commanding the base of the catheter system to follow a 1 Hz sinusoidal trajectory with an amplitude of 5 mm. This trajectory is a highly simplified version of a mitral valve annulus motion of a heart beating at 60 beats per minute (BPM).

The amount of backlash was quantified for each experiment as the width of the backlash hysteresis curve, determined by plotting the commanded trajectory versus the tip position trajectory. The width of the hysteresis is the amount of displacement commanded at the catheter base that does not result in movement at the tip. This backlash width is clearly seen when the commanded trajectory changes directions.

Backlash Results. The backlash data (Fig. 5) was analyzed with a three-way ANOVA. Bend angle has the clearest effect on backlash ($p < 0.0001$). The backlash width was proportional to the bend angle. The other parameter that was found to affect the backlash was the gap size ($p < 0.0001$). While the gap size value did not proportionally relate to backlash, the data does suggest that the larger the gap size, the larger the possible amount of backlash. Bend radius was not found to have a systematic effect on the backlash width ($p = 0.53$).

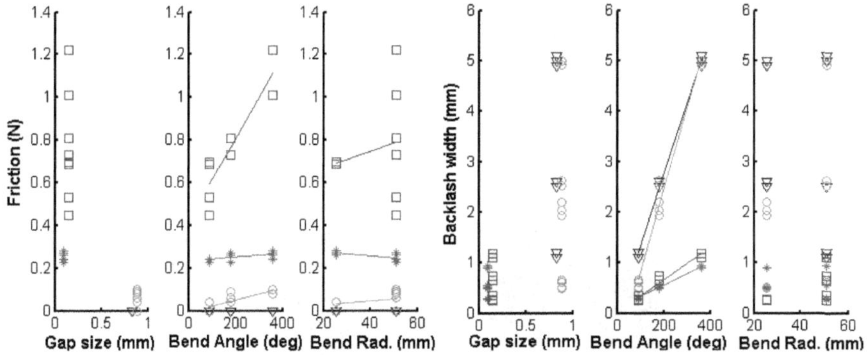

Fig. 5. Summary of the friction results (left) and backlash results (right) versus tested parameters. See Table 1 for symbols.

3.3 Compensation Techniques

The above results identify the major factors that affect catheter system trajectory tracking performance. This understanding can be used to improve performance through both mechanical design and control system modifications. Friction in the catheter system can be reduced through material selection, material coatings, and lubrication. Backlash can be decreased by reducing the gap between the guidewire and the sheath. However, reducing the gap will also increase the friction experienced by the guidewire.

Control compensation techniques can also reduce friction and backlash effects. For example, feedforward Coulomb friction compensation can be used to reduce the friction forces at the base module [18]. An enhanced control system can also reduce the backlash behavior by modifying the trajectory commanded at the base of the catheter. An example of a standard backlash deadzone compensating method is to solve for the inverse of the backlash [16]. This inverse compensation method is found by adding the system's trajectory tracking error to the original desired trajectory. The addition of the backlash position error term compensates for the deadzone behavior in the system and produces the originally desired trajectory at the output. This method, however, assumes the system can traverse the deadzone instantaneously and that the backlash width is constant and velocity-independent [16]. Fig. 2 presents an example of how inverse compensation can improve the catheter tip trajectory tracking. The use of inverse compensation improves the system tracking performance by reducing the mean absolute error (MAE) by 80%.

The results of the friction and backlash experiments, as well as further tests on more complex trajectories, show that backlash imposes more severe performance limitations than friction. In particular, each tip direction reversal requires that the base actuator traverses the entire deadzone in as short a time as possible (e.g. 9.8-9.9 sec in Fig. 2). Actuator force limitations mean this traverse takes long enough for significant errors to develop. Friction compensation, in contrast, can be accomplished to first order by feeding forward the estimated friction. While this changes sign at each direction reversal, the actuator bandwidth for rapid force changes is adequate to avoid

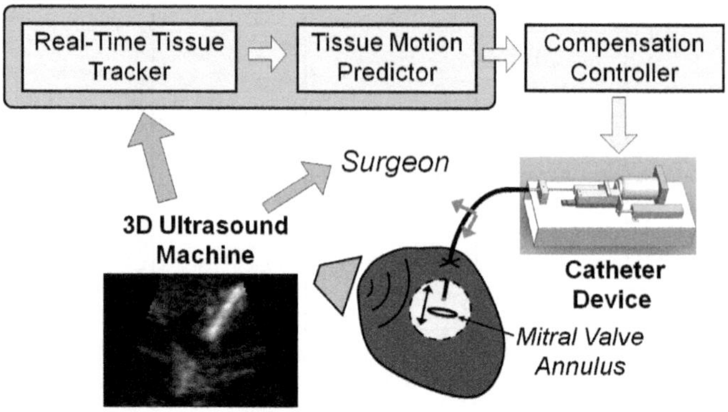

Fig. 6. Ultrasound image-based catheter servoing system

substantial errors. This design tradeoff leads us to select a small gap size for subsequent experiments to prevent significant backlash. A full investigation of compensation techniques will be explored in future research.

4 Image-Based Catheter Control

To investigate the feasibility of image-based catheter control, we integrated the catheter system described above with the ultrasound visual servoing system we developed in previous work [5], [9]-[11] and evaluated it in vivo. Controlling a catheter to follow the motion of internal cardiac structures requires real-time sensing of both the catheter tip and tissue target positions. 3D ultrasound must be used for guidance because it is currently the only real-time volumetric imaging technique that can image tissue through blood. In our original image guidance system, the tip of a hand-held instrument with a rigid shaft was introduced through a small incision in the heart wall. The instrument successfully tracked the tissue and in vivo experiments demonstrated its ability to lower interaction forces and place anchors in the mitral valve annulus. The ability to perform such tasks with a catheter would enable beating-heart intracardiac repairs to become minimally invasive.

In the ultrasound servoing system, 3D image volumes are streamed via ethernet to an image processing computer (Fig. 6). A GPU-based Radon transform algorithm finds the instrument axis in real-time [10]. The target tissue is then located by projecting the axis forward through the image volume until tissue is encountered; this allows the clinician to designate the target to be tracked by simply pointing at it with the catheter. To compensate for the 50-100 ms delay in image acquisition and processing, an extended Kalman filter estimates the current tissue location based on a Fourier decomposition of the cardiac cycle. Previous in vivo experiments showed that the rigid instrument system was capable of accurate tracking within the heart with an RMS error of 1.0 mm. See [9]-[11] for a detailed description of the system.

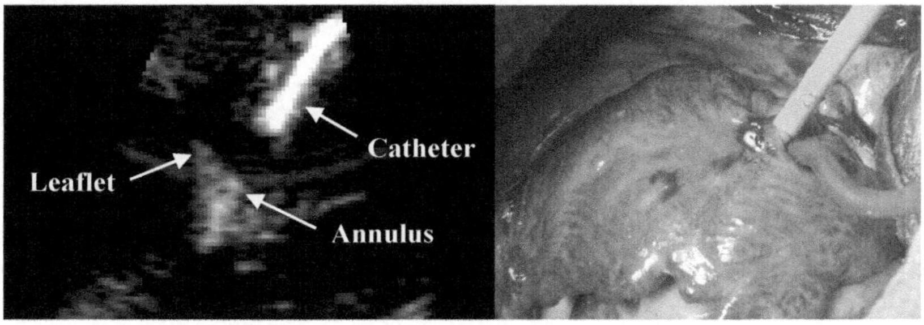

Fig. 7. Left: Ultrasound image showing catheter, mitral valve annulus, and mitral valve leaflets. Right: The catheter tool inserted into the left atrium.

4.1 In Vivo Evaluation

The image guidance system was evaluated in vivo on a 75 Kg porcine animal model. For this initial study, the actuated catheter was inserted into a beating heart via the top of the left atrium rather than the vasculature to give the surgeon easy access to the mitral valve. The 3D ultrasound machine probe was placed epicardially (SONOS 7500, Philips Healthcare, Andover, MA, USA). After the device was introduced into the beating heart, the surgeon used the ultrasound image to aim the catheter at the mitral valve annulus. The imaging system was then initialized and tracked the valve motion. See Fig. 7 for a 3DUS image of the catheter in vivo and an image of the catheter device being inserted into the porcine left atrium.

The catheter system used in this experiment was as described above, with a sheath with 1.6 mm inner diameter and a guidewire with a 1.5 mm outer diameter. An electromagnetic tracker (trakSTAR 1.5 mm sensor, Ascension Technology Corp., Burlington, VT, USA, measured RMS error of 0.3 mm) was affixed to the guidewire tip to assess control accuracy.

During the experimental trials, the catheter was fixed external to the heart in a shape with two 90° bends that roughly corresponds to the path from the femoral vein into the left atrium. The catheter was then positioned inside the left atrium so that the tip was 1-2 cm from mitral annulus. The catheter controller performs a simple calibration routine that estimates the magnitude of the friction force in the system. Next, the image processing routines locate the catheter using the Radon transform algorithm, and then project forward to find the target. The catheter is then servoed to maintain a constant distance between the catheter tip and the target.

4.2 Tracking Results

The catheter system was successful in tracking the mitral annulus tissue target. Fig. 7 shows a cross section through a typical ultrasound image volume, showing the catheter, mitral valve annulus, and edge of the valve leaflet. Friction compensation was used in this experiment, however deadzone compensation was not required because the mechanical design of the catheter system, including the selection of a guidewire and sheath with a small gap size, minimized the deadzone.

The catheter system was tested a number of times during this experiment. Fig. 8 shows a typical plot of the catheter tip trajectory and the position of the mitral valve

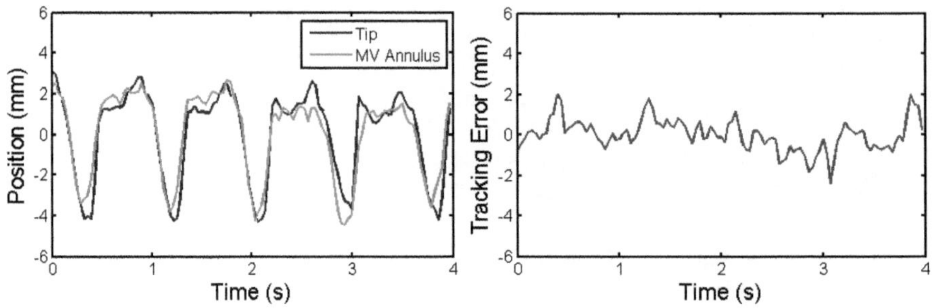

Fig. 5. Left: Trajectory of the catheter tip and the mitral valve annulus found by manual segmentation. Right: The catheter trajectory tracking error.

annulus. This plot was generated by manually segmenting the position of the catheter tip and valve structure from the 3DUS volumes three times and then averaging the values. The standard deviations of all of the segmented tip positions from the mean tip positions were less than 0.22 mm and the standard deviation of all of the segmented mitral valve annulus positions were less that 0.32 mm from the mean mitral valve annulus positions. Because of the seals required to prevent backflow of blood out of the heart, friction compensation values as high as 2 N were required for these experiments

The image guided catheter system tracked the valve motion with RMS errors less that 1.0 mm in all experimental trials. The RMS error for the trial presented in Fig. 8 was 0.77 mm. The tracking error, shown in Fig. 8, was caused by respiration motion not captured in the tissue tracking system, performance limitations of the actuated catheter caused by backlash and friction, and the small beat-to-beat variations in the valve motion not compensated for by the image tracking system.

5 Discussion

Robotic catheters have the potential to revolutionize intracardiac procedures by allowing clinicians to minimally invasively perform complicated surgical tasks inside the beating heart. One of the major technological challenges to realizing this concept is to compensate for the fast motion of cardiac tissue using a catheter. In this paper, we explored the mechanical challenges of servoing a guidewire inside a catheter sheath. Friction increased as a function of bending angle but decreased as a function of the gap size between the guidewire and the sheath. The size of the backlash deadzone was dependent on the gap size and the bending angle. Experiments showed that, compared to friction, backlash creates greater performance deficits and controller compensation is less successful. We therefore selected a small gap size that minimizes backlash at the expense of higher friction.

To investigate the feasibility of using image-based servoing to match catheter trajectories to the motion of cardiac structures, the catheter system was integrated with ultrasound imaging and an image processing system. Porcine in vivo studies showed that excellent tracking can be obtained, with RMS errors of less than one mm. These results are encouraging for the feasibility of this system performing more complicated surgical procedures in vivo.

The next step for this project will be to design adaptive controllers to improve the catheter tip tracking performance in vivo, as well as control the forces applied by the catheter to the cardiac tissue. Optimization of catheter materials and dimensions will be an important aspect of this effort. In addition, it will be essential to determine the durability of catheters under high guidewire velocities and repeated cycling. We note, however, that only a few thousand cycles are needed for a one-hour procedure, and we have operated catheters for this duration with negligible performance degradation.

To the authors' knowledge, the system described here is the first robotic catheter device that can compensate for the fast motion of structures inside the heart. It is interesting to note that this approach is complementary to current commercial catheter robot systems like the Artisan Control Catheter (Hansen Medical, Mountain View CA). That system achieves lateral deflection and sheath translation at roughly manual speeds and could be readily combined with the fast guidewire actuation system described here.

Future work will be required to extend this motion compensation technology to cardiac surgery applications that require additional DOF for end effector positioning and complex tissue trajectory tracking. In contrast to existing robotic catheter systems, fast motion in the lateral directions at approximately the same speeds as demonstrated in this study will be required for these applications.

6 Conclusion

This work demonstrates that single DOF robotic catheters can achieve the speed and tip position control required for specific intracardiac repair applications such as mitral valve annuloplasty. In addition, this study shows that catheter position can be accurately controlled using real-time image guidance in vivo. These results suggest that it is feasible to use catheters for beating heart procedures, which will enable intracardiac repairs that are both minimally invasive and avoid the risks of stopped-heart techniques.

Acknowledgments

The authors would like to thank Dr. Nikolay Vasilyev and Dr. Pedro del Nido for their assistance with the animal experiments presented here and insights into the clinical applications of this technology. Funding for this work was provided by the US National Institutes of Health under grant NIH R01 HL073647.

References

[1] Baim, D.S.: Grossman's Cardiac Catheterization, Angiography, and Intervention, p. 992. Lippincott Williams & Wilkins (2005)

[2] Fukuda, T., et al.: Micro active catheter system with multi degrees of freedom. In: Proc. IEEE Int. Conf. Robotics and Automation, pp. 2290–2295 (1994)

[3] Jayender, J., Patel, R.V., Nikumb, S.: Robot-assisted catheter insertion using hybrid impedance control. In: Proc. IEEE Int. Conf. Robotics and Automation, pp. 607–612 (2006)

[4] Camarillo, D.B., Milne, C.F., Carlson, C.R., Zinn, M.R., Salisbury, J.K.: Mechanics Modeling of Tendon-Driven Continuum Manipulators. IEEE Trans. Robotics 24, 1262–1273 (2008)
[5] Yuen, S.G., Kesner, S.B., Vasilyev, N.V., del Nido, P.J., Howe, R.D.: 3D ultrasound-guided motion compensation system for beating heart mitral valve repair. In: Metaxas, D., Axel, L., Fichtinger, G., Székely, G. (eds.) MICCAI 2008, Part I. LNCS, vol. 5241, pp. 711–719. Springer, Heidelberg (2008)
[6] Bebek, O., Cavusoglu, M.: Intelligent control algorithms for robotic assisted beating heart surgery. IEEE Trans. Robotics 23, 468–480 (2007)
[7] Ginhoux, R., et al.: Active filtering of physiological motion in robotized surgery using predictive control. IEEE Trans. Robotics 21, 67–79 (2005)
[8] Nakamura, Y., Kishi, K., Kawakami, H.: Heartbeat synchronization for robotic cardiac surgery. In: Proc. IEEE Int. Conf. Robotics and Automation, pp. 2014–2019 (2001)
[9] Yuen, S.G., Novotny, P.M., Howe, R.D.: Quasiperiodic predictive filtering for robot-assisted beating heart surgery. In: Proc. IEEE Int. Conf. Robotics and Automation, pp. 3875–3880 (2008)
[10] Novotny, P.M., et al.: GPU based real-time instrument tracking with three-dimensional ultrasound. Medical Image Analysis, 458–464 (2007)
[11] Yuen, S.G., et al.: Robotic, Robotic Motion Compensation for Beating Heart Intracardiac Surgery. Int. J. Robotics Research 28(10), 1355–1372 (2009)
[12] Newman, M.F., et al.: Longitudinal Assessment of Neurocognitive Function after Coronary-Artery Bypass Surgery. New England J. Med. 344(6), 395–402 (2001)
[13] Kaneko, M., Yamashita, T., Tanie, K.: Basic considerations on transmission characteristics for tendon drive robots. In: Proc. Int. Conf. on Advanced Robotics, pp. 827–832 (1991)
[14] Nahvi, A., Hollerbach, J.M., Xu, Y., Hunter, I.W.: An investigation of the transmission system of a tendon driven robot hand. In: Proc. IEEE/RSJ Int. Conf. Intelligent Robots and Systems, pp. 202–208 (1994)
[15] Palli, G., Melchiorri, C.: Model and control of tendon-sheath transmission systems. In: Proc. IEEE Int. Conf. Robotics and Automation, pp. 988–993 (2006)
[16] Nordin, M., Gutman, P.: Controlling mechanical systems with backlash - a survey. Automatica 38, 1633–1649 (2002)
[17] Bassett, E.K., Slocum, A.H., Maslakos, P.T., Pryor, H.I., Farokhzad, O.C., Karp, J.M.: Design of a mechanical clutch-based needle-insertion device. PNAS 106, 5540–5545 (2009)
[18] Armstrong-Helouvry, B., Dupont, P.E., Canudas De Wit, C.: A survey of analysis tools and compensation methods for control of machines with friction. Automatica 30, 1083–1138 (1994)
[19] Recker, D.A., Kokotovic, P.V., Rhode, D., Winkelman, J.: Adaptive nonlinear control of systems containing a deadzone. In: Proc. IEEE Conf. on Decision and Control, pp. 2111–2115 (1991)
[20] Horowitz, R.: Learning Control of Robot Manipulators. Trans. of ASME 115, 402–411 (1993)

Towards a Verified Simulation Model for Radiofrequency Ablations

Andreas Weihusen[1], Lisa Hinrichsen[2], Thomas Carus[3], Rainer Dammer[2], Richard Rascher-Friesenhausen[1,2], Tim Kröger[1], Heinz-Otto Peitgen[1], and Tobias Preusser[1]

[1] Fraunhofer MEVIS, Bremen, Germany
[2] Bremerhaven University of Applied Sciences, Germany
[3] Cuxhaven Hospital, Germany

Abstract. The simulation of radiofrequency ablations (RFA) can predict the achievable coagulation area and thus provide useful information for treatment planning, especially in cases in which the heat distribution can be limited by vascular cooling effects. A strong reliability of the numerical simulation results is essential for clinical use.

In this paper, we present a novel experimental procedure for the verification of RFA simulation systems in a lifelike environment without requiring animal tests. RF ablations are performed within isolated, perfused porcine livers, the corresponding configurations are reconstructed and simulated on a computer, and the resulting pathoanatomical coagulations are compared to their simulated counterparts with consideration of vascular cooling effects. We have applied this procedure for an initial verification of an existing RFA simulation system. The results are presented and discussed in this paper.

Keywords: RF ablation, evaluation, simulation.

1 Introduction

Malignant diseases are a leading cause of death worldwide [1]. Over 50% of all patients develop liver metastases with significant morbidity and mortality [2]. Percutaneous image-guided thermal ablation therapies have been established as an important therapy alternative for the treatment of liver tumors if surgical resections are contraindicated [3]. Among these therapies, the radiofrequency (RF) ablation shows advantages in safety, effectiveness, and easy applicability [2] and thus has taken a significant role in the clinical routine.

Radiofrequency ablation (RFA) is a thermal procedure that destroys tumor cells by a local heating of the tissue. Blood vessels can limit the range of the ablation by heat dissipation and must be considered during the planning of the intervention [4]. A numerical simulation of the underlying biophysical and chemical processes considering these restrictions can provide an estimation and associated validation of the achievable coagulation area. Moreover, it can be used

N. Navab and P. Jannin (Eds.): IPCAI 2010, LNCS 6135, pp. 179–189, 2010.

to optimize the RF applicator placement [5]. For clinical use, a strong reliability of the simulation results is essential.

In this paper, we present a novel experimental verification procedure and its application to an existing numerical RFA simulation model described in [9] along with its implementation in a clinically usable research software system [14]. Our goal is the initial verification of the simulation's reliability in a lifelike setting without animal tests. For that, RF ablations are performed within perfused, isolated porcine livers obtained from a slaughterhouse. The corresponding experiment configurations are reconstructed and simulated with the software system, and the resulting coagulations are pathoanatomically analyzed and compared to their simulated counterparts.

A detailed description of the experimental environment and procedure is given in the next section, along with an introduction to the biophysical model and its implementation. The results of the initial experimental series are discussed in section 3. Conclusions are drawn in section 4.

Related Work: The simulation of thermal ablation therapies, and particularly RF ablation, has been considered by several authors [6] [7] [8] [9]. They primarily describe the modeling of the ablation process and the computational solutions of their models. A comprehensive review of RF ablation models is given in the overview article of Berjano [10]. Several groups have examined the vascular cooling effect during RF ablations in an experimental environment [4] [11]. Moreover, Lubienski et al. have developed a perfusion model in bovine livers for RF ablation bench testing [12]. Our work combines the experimental approach with the verification of a numerical simulation to achieve a reliability of the simulation for clinical use.

2 Methods

The reliability of a simulation system depends on both the incorporated biophysical model and the parameterization, including the reconstruction of the ambient vascular system relative to the electrode position. The biophysical modeling of the ablation process is introduced in 2.1, and the parameterization is described in 2.2. The lifelike environment is described in 2.3.

2.1 Biophysical Model

The biophysical model of our RFA simulation is an extension of the initial model of Stein [6]. It describes the process of tissue degradation by induction of a high-frequency alternating current with consideration of state-dependent material parameters, such as the electric and thermal tissue properties, and the biochemical properties of the proteins [9]. The basic model incorporates an iterative cyclic process of three basic parts which act simultaneously and interfere with each other (Fig. 1):

1. Electrodes are placed in the malignant tissue. The applied electric current heats the tissue due to the tissue's electrical resistance. The induced energy is computed using the electrostatic equation

$$\mathrm{div}(\sigma\nabla\phi) = 0 \tag{1}$$

where ϕ is the time- and space-dependent electric potential and σ is the state-dependent electric conductivity. The equation is equipped with specific boundary conditions at the electrodes and the boundary of the computational domain [9].

2. The evolving heat diffuses into the ambient tissue. The spatial heat distribution is calculated by the bioheat-transfer-equation. The dissipation of heat by blood circulation is modeled as a heat-sink term on the right hand side of this equation.

$$\rho\, c\, \partial_t T - \mathrm{div}(\lambda\nabla T) = Q \tag{2}$$

where ρ, c, and λ are the material dependent density, heat capacity, and thermal conductivity, respectively, and Q contains the heat sources and sinks. Again, we impose appropriate boundary and initial conditions to this equation [9]. For the temperature dependent evaporation of water from the tissue and the corresponding nonlinear behavior of the electric and thermal conductivity, we take special correction steps into account [9], which approximate the energy balance for the physical phase changes taking place.

3. The cell proteins are affected by the increasing heat and begin to denature. At a certain state, the cell denaturation is irreversible, and the (malignant) cells die. In our model, this temperature-dependent tissue degradation D is computed by the Arrhenius formalism[13]

$$D = A_A \int_0^t \exp\left(-\frac{E_A}{RT}\right) ds \tag{3}$$

where A_A and E_A are tissue-dependent Arrhenius constants and R is the universal gas constant. Due to computed changes in temperature, evaporation state, and cell degradation, the local biophysical parameters need to be adapted at each iteration step.

The simulation of the biophysical process is performed by the computation of the ablation state in time steps of 1 second. Each computation step requires the solution of the partial differential equations (1), (2) and (3), which are numerically solved using finite element methods on a uniform spatial grid. We use a grid size of 2^6+1 nodes in axial, sagittal and coronal direction, which is a good compromise between accuracy and performance.

2.2 Implementation

The initial parameterization is determined on the basis of contrasted CT images. The biophysical parameters of liver tissue and blood vessels are taken from

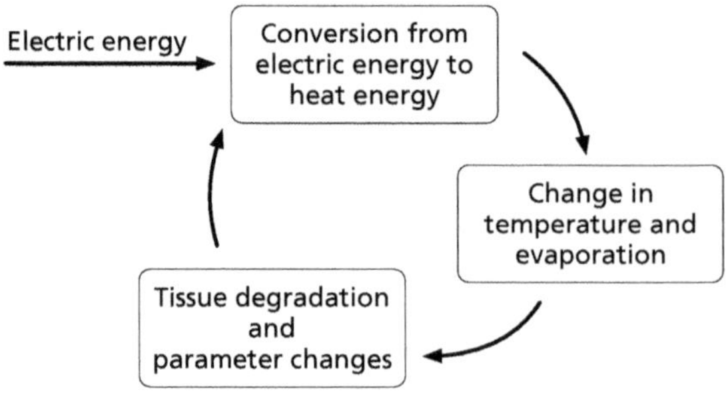

Fig. 1. Sketch of the iterative cycle of computation steps of the biophysical RFA model

Stein [6]. The reconstruction of the ablation settings from original CT data, including the RF applicator placement and the segmentation of the ambient vascular system, and the simulation are executed as follows:

First, the virtual RF applicators is placed at the target area within the CT image. The target position and the orientation of the RF applicator is defined by a pair of spatial coordinates, which are set interactively. The masks of the electrode and applicator shaft are incorporated into the simulation parameterization. The applicator placement additionally defines the position and range of the computational area, which is a subdomain of the original CT image.

Next, a segmentation of the vascular system is performed within the computational area. The segmentation method is based on a Bayesian background suppression of the liver tissue and a combination of thresholding and region growing [15]. The vessel segmentation can be interfered by radial image artifacts caused by the electrode material during the CT scan. These brighter artifacts can also be segmented using region growing with manually adapted thresholds and afterwards be suppressed from the vessel mask (Fig. 4). The resulting vessel mask is incorporated into the simulation parameterization.

Most RFA generator models provide an impedance feedback control for optimized energy induction. This feedback control is approximated by a simplified model in our simulation: The initial power is set by the user, after which the power is calculated by an impedance-dependent function at each computation step.

The computation is performed iteratively until the computed applied energy exceeds a given threshold. The simulation results in the spatial temperature distribution and the coagulation mask, which is a function of the spatial tissue degradation. The coagulation volume and the ablation time are also reported.

2.3 Experiment Setup

The applicability of the simulation model in a lifelike environment has been evaluated in an initial experimental study on isolated, perfused porcine livers obtained from a slaughterhouse. 21 ablations were executed in seven livers. The resulting coagulations were then analyzed pathoanatomically. The results were compared to the corresponding results of the simulation. The experimental workflow is organized as follows:

Preparation: The porcine liver must be first fixed to provide immobility of the organ during the experiment. For this purpose, we have constructed a cubic container with an embedded, perforated board on which the liver is fixated by plastic sticks (Fig. 2). Besides the fixation, the container serves as a drain box in the perfusion cycle and for the adjustment of the RF applicators. The size of the container is aligned to fit into a standard CT scanner. To avoid image artifacts during the CT scans, the container and the perforated board are built of acrylic glass.

Next, the perfusion is connected. The portal vein and hepatic artery are attached to elastic tubes of two different diameters, which realize the corresponding perfusion rates of 75% and 25%. Both tubes are connected to a perfusion device that provides a realistic pulsating organ perfusion [16] (Fig. 2, right side). For perfusion, we use saline solution at body temperature 37 °C, which heats the porcine liver to approximately 37 °C, too. The temperature is controlled by a heating unit placed within the perfusion device.

Finally three needle-shaped bipolar RF applicators [17] are placed at different positions in the liver and connected to the corresponding power generator. They are fixated by perforated acrylic glass strips, which are clamped at the top of the container. The applicator type is internally cooled. The overall length of both electrodes is 40 mm.

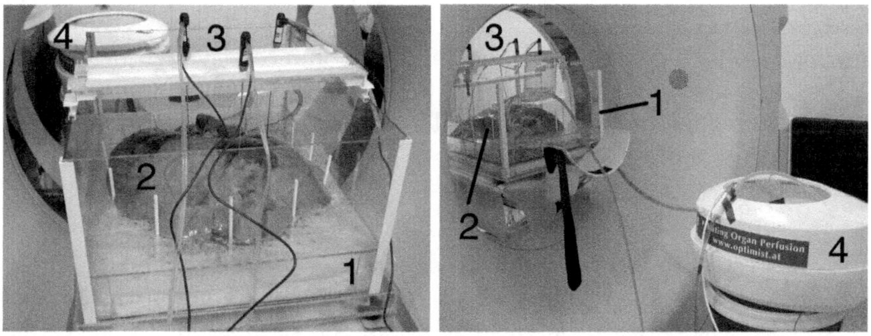

Fig. 2. Experimental setup with container (1), embedded liver (2), three RF applicators (3), and the pulsating organ perfusion (4) on the backside of the CT scanner

Execution: The experiment begins with an initial CT scan of the perfused liver with positioned RF applicators. The purpose of this scan is the image-based reconstruction of the applicator positions and the surrounding vascular system for the configuration for the numerical simulation, as described in section 2.2. Contrast agent is added to the saline solution to improve the visibility of the vessels in the acquired image.

The ablations are executed consecutively with one active applicator at a time using a standardized parameterization with an initial power of 40W and an applied energy of 15 kJ. During the ablation, no contrast agent is used to avoid accumulation within the coagulating tissue.

Afterwards, three liver tissue samples with enclosed coagulations are cut out and preserved for the subsequent pathoanatomical examination, using a formaldehyde solution as tissue fixative.

Analysis: The analysis of the individual experiments consists of two parts: the pathoanatomical examination of the real coagulations and the analysis of their simulated counterparts. The analysis aims at a comparison of the coagulation volumes and coagulation shapes with regard to the cooling effects caused by perfusion.

Each tissue sample is cut into slices. The first cut is along the RF applicators' direction, the next cuts are parallel with slice thicknesses between 5 and 10 mm. Pictures are taken from each slice for the comparison with the simulated shapes. The coagulation volume is approximated from the coagulation areas visible in each slice. First, the width and height are measured, and the area A is approximated by the ellipse calculated from these values. Next, a polynomial function $f(A)$ is interpolated using $(x, A(x))$ as nodes, where x denotes the distance to the center slice. The coagulation volume is finally computed as the integral of $f(A)$ between both roots.

The corresponding experimental settings are reconstructed on a PC for the parameterization of the numerical simulation, as described in section 2.2. The resulting simulated coagulation is visualized as a colored overlay within the image data to provide a visual examination of the shape adaptions due to cooling effects of nearby vessels. The computed coagulation volume is logged for comparison with the pathoanatomical results. Additionally, the quality of the local vessel segmentation is logged, considering under- or overestimations.

3 Results

As previously mentioned, the ablations were stopped at an applied energy of 15 kJ. The corresponding simulations terminated accordingly if the applied energy exceeded 15kJ. Based on this condition, the simulation can be verified in three ways: by a comparison of the coagulation volumes, by a comparison of the coagulation shapes, and also by a comparison of the ablation times, whereas volume and shape are more important verification criteria.

The results of each comparison step are discussed in the following sections. Particular attention will be given to accuracy of the vessel segmentation in section 3.2, because it affects the simulated coagulation volume significantly.

3.1 Examination of Ablation Times

The examination of the experimentally measured times of all 21 ablations shows a large dispersion of values (minimum 7:44 min., maximum 15:40 min., mean

10:10 min., standard deviation 1:55 min.) compared to the simulated times (10:33 min., 13:29 min., 11:51 min., 0:45 min.). On the one hand, the time differences can be caused by the simplified generator model in the simulation. On the other hand, we have observed a high variability of ablation times in the lifelike system, even when comparing the respective ablation times within each individual liver due to locally variant tissue characteristics. Because the measured time is less important than the size and shape of the achieved coagulation and due to the large dispersion, we discard the ablation time for the purpose of verification.

3.2 Comparison of Coagulation Volumes

Individual comparison: The volumes of all 21 coagulations are measured pathoanatomically as described in section 2.3 and compared to the volumes of their simulated counterpart (Fig. 3).

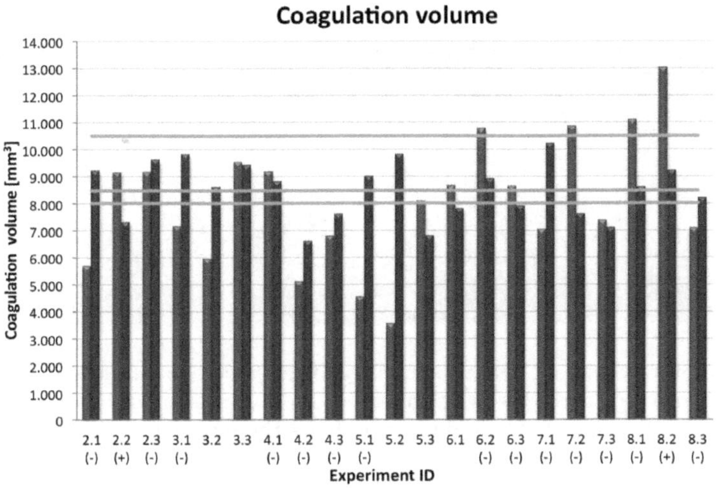

Fig. 3. Comparison of measured volumes (blue bars) and simulated volumes (red bars). The horizontal blue and the red lines show the corresponding mean values. The horizontal green line shows the volume of a simulated coagulation without vascular cooling as a reference. Cases are tagged with (+), if the vessel system is over-segmented, and with (-), if under-segmented.

Individual vascular cooling effects are clearly recognizable in both measured and simulated coagulation volumes (Fig. 3). Therefore, the volumes have to be compared with consideration of the segmentation accuracy, which may be limited due to the compensation of electrode artifacts (Fig. 4).

5 cases show accurate segmentation results. Considering the purpose of treatment planning, a reliable simulation should provide equal or smaller volumes than the measured coagulations. 3 cases fulfil this condition with at most 16% less volume, compared to the measured coagulation. In 1 case, the simulated necrosis expands partially across the liver rim (experiment 3.2), which is a shortcoming

of the simulation system. The measurement of the coagulation in experiment 5.2 was detracted by a decomposed tissue sample and thus is excluded from the examinations.

In 14 cases, vessels are partially ignored due to the compensation of electrode artifacts. This leads to a larger simulated volume in 8 cases compared to the measured volume. Especially in experiment 5.1, the real coagulation is strongly restricted by a large vessel in close vicinity to the electrode, which is covered by artifacts in the CT image and thus could not be segmented. 6 simulated volumes are unexpectedly smaller than the measured volume.

In 2 cases, not all artifacts could be suppressed. The corresponding simulated volumes are smaller than the measured ones in both cases.

In summary, we have 3 cases with an accurate vessel segmentation and promising results of the simulated ablation volumes. Two shortcomings of the implemention are the disregard of the liver rim and the sensitivity to artifacts of the vessel segmentation.

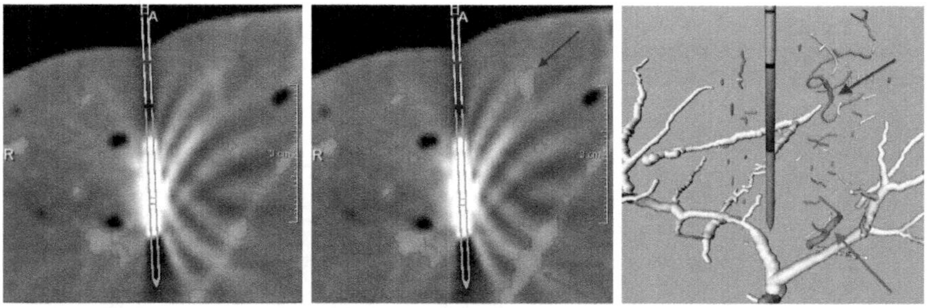

Fig. 4. Example of vessel segmentation quality: If the electrode artifacts are suppressed, one vessel branch (red arrow) is not segmented. If all vessels are segmented, additional artifacts occur (blue arrow). The right image shows the segmentation differences in 3D.

Overall comparison: Again a large dispersion of the coagulation volumes is observable (Table 1), according to the local variability of the tissue characteristics. The simulated coagulation volumes show a similar adaptivity of the model to the individual liver vascularization, but with less dispersion due to the limited parameterization options of the biophysical model.

Table 1. Dispersion of measured and simulated coagulation volumes

	Minimum	Maximum	Mean	Standard deviation
Measured volume	3556 mm^3	13013 mm^3	8018 mm^3	2361 mm^3
Simulated volume	6600 mm^3	10200 mm^3	8476 mm^3	1054 mm^3

3.3 Comparison of Shapes

To compare the experimental and simulated coagulation shapes, we first examined vessels in the pathological slices, which affected the coagulation shape in a recognizable way. Afterwards, we tried to identify the corresponding vessels in the segmentation masks (Fig. 5). Finally, we verified whether the simulated coagulation was affected by the vessel in a similar way as in the experiment.

We found 39 vessels which affected the experimental coagulation shape. The simulated coagulation shapes were affected by 27 of them (69 %). In 7 of these 27 cases, the simulated coagulation shape is similar to the experimental one (26 %). 8 cases show a stronger constriction of the simulated shape (30 %). 12 cases show a weaker constriction of the shape(44 %), but in most of these cases, the vessel segmentation is incomplete due to the compensation of electrode artifacts.

The shape comparison helps conclude that the simulation model is able to predict the vascular cooling effect with a slight tendency towards an underestimation of the coagulation size in the vicinity of vessels.

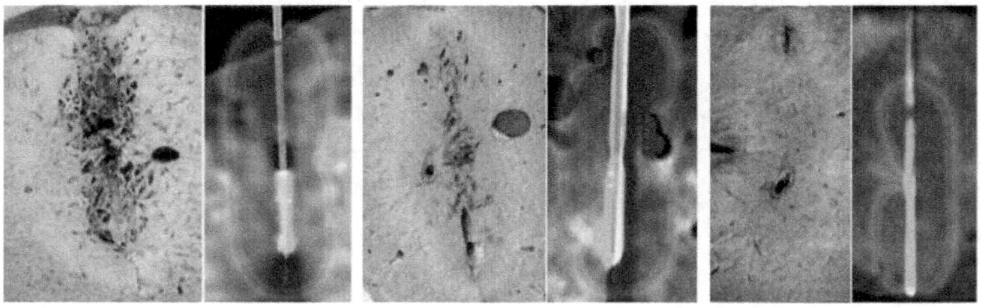

Fig. 5. Three examples for the comparison of experimental and simulated coagulation

4 Discussion

We have described an experimental procedure for the verification of RFA simulation systems in a lifelike system without requiring animal tests. The procedure has been applied for an initial verification of an existing RFA simulation system, which incorporates the simulation of the biophysical process as well as methods for the reconstruction of the ablation configuration from CT images.

We have evaluated the RFA simulation system on the basis of 21 RF ablations in isolated porcine livers with realistic perfusion and body temperature. The verification is performed by a comparison of the volumes and shapes of experimental and simulated coagulations. The most promising results are given by the shape comparison, which shows a similarity of measured and simulated coagulation shapes in the vicinity of vessels in 69%. In cases with appropriate segmented vessels, the comparison of the volumes shows approximately equal or slightly smaller coagulation sizes, which is promising, too. Two shortcomings of the implementation could be identified: The simulation disregards the liver rim, and the sensitivity of the vessel segmentation to electrode artifacts in CT. Because of that, a reliable accuracy of the simulation requires further improvements.

Improvements: The present segmentation method is prone to image artifacts caused by the electrodes in the CT scan. This problem can be solved by the use of more accurate segmentation methods or, alternatively, by the reduction of artifacts during the image acquisition: Coaxial needles can be used to mark the applicator positions during the CT scan, after which the inner needles can be replaced by the RF applicators.

The aforementioned measurement of the coagulation volumes from slices is only approximative. It can be refined using thinner slices and a precise measurement of the coagulated area within the slices instead of an ellipsoidal approximation. Each area of one coagulation can be manually segmented on the slice image. The corresponding 2D masks can later be matched to a 3D volume, which can be compared easily to the simulated counterpart.

The experimental results show the large variability of the tissue characteristics. Currently, the initial biophysical parameters could only be idealized values obtained from literature. The sensitivity of the model to these parameters is part of our current research. The proposed evaluation precedure is useful for the verification of each development step. An extension of the present environment, which provides the measurement of specific tissue parameters before the ablation, can optimize the initial conditions of the verification procedure.

5 Conclusion

The proposed environment is useful to verify simulation models for RF ablations as well as similar thermal procedures. It can also be used to verify improvements to the simulation model or for the comparison of optimized parameterizations. The main feature is the avoidance of animal tests, as long as a simulation model has proven to be accurate enough within this environment.

The initial experimental series provided valuable experience for optimization of both the simulation system and the verification procedure. A follow-up project is planned to continue the verification. Future work will focus on the optimization procedures discussed in section 4.

Acknowledgments. We would like to thank Dr. med. Oei and his team for the supply of the CT scanner and the image acquisition during all experiments. We also thank Prof. Dr. med. Heine and his team for the pathoanatomical analysis of the tissue samples. Finally we thank Klaas Rackebrandt and Christian Rieder for experimental and computational support.

References

1. World Health Organization: Fact sheet no. 297 "Cancer" (2009), `http://www.who.int/mediacentre/factsheets/fs297`
2. Pereira, P.L.: Actual role of radiofrequency ablation of liver metastases. European Radiology 17, 2062–2070 (2007)
3. Goldberg, S., Gazelle, G., Mueller, P.: Thermal ablation therapy for focal malignancy: A unified approach to underlying principles, techniques, and diagnostic imaging guidance. AJR 174, 323–331 (2000)

4. Lu, D.S.K., Raman, S.S., Vodopich, D.J., Wang, M., Sayre, J., Lassman, C.: Effect of vessel size on creation of hepatic radiofrequency lesions in pigs: assessment of the "heat sink" effect. AJR 178, 47–51 (2002)
5. Altrogge, I., Preusser, T., Kröger, T., Büskens, C., Pereira, P.-L., Schmidt, D., Peitgen, H.-O.: Multiscale optimization of the probe placement for radiofrequency ablation. Academic Radiology 14, 1310–1324 (2007)
6. Stein, T.: Untersuchungen zur Dosimetrie der hochfrequenzstrominduzierten interstitiellen Thermotherapie in bipolarer Technik. Fortschritte in der Lasermedizin, vol. 22, Müller and Berlien (2000)
7. Tungjitkusolum, S., Staelin, S.T., Haemmerich, D., et al.: Three-dimensional finite-element analyses for radio-frequency hepatic tumor ablation. IEEE Trans. Biomed. Eng. 49, 3–9 (2002)
8. Villard, C., Soler, L., Gangi, A.: Radiofrequency ablation of hepatic tumors: simulation, planning, and contribution of virtual reality and haptics. Computer Methods in Biomechanics and Biomedical Engineering 8, 215–227 (2005)
9. Kröger, T., Altrogge, I., Preusser, T., Pereira, P.-L., Schmidt, D., Weihusen, A., Peitgen, H.-O.: Numerical Simulation of Radio Frequency Ablation with State Dependent Material Parameters in Three Space Dimensions. In: Larsen, R., Nielsen, M., Sporring, J. (eds.) MICCAI 2006. LNCS, vol. 4191, pp. 380–388. Springer, Heidelberg (2006)
10. Berjano, E.J.: Theoretical modeling for radiofrequency ablation: state-of-the-art and challenges for the future. BioMedical Engineering OnLine 5 (2006)
11. Frericks, B.B., Ritz, J.P., Albrecht, T., Valdeig, S., Schenk, A., Wolf, K.J., Lehmann, K.: Influence of intrahepatic vessels on volume and shape of percutaneous thermal ablation zones: In vivo evaluation in a porcine model. Investigative Radiology 43 (2008)
12. Lubienski, A., Bitsch, R.G., Lubienski, K., Kauffmann, G., Duex, M.: Radiofrequency ablation (rfa): Development of a flow model for bovine livers for extensive bench testing. CardioVascular and Interventional Radiology 29, 1068–1072 (2006)
13. Arrhenius, S.: Über die Reaktionsgeschwindigkeit bei der Inversion von Rohrzucker durch Säuren. Z. Phys. Chem. 4, 226–248 (1887)
14. Weihusen, A., Ritter, F., Kröger, T., Preusser, T., Zidowitz, S., Peitgen, H.-O.: Workflow oriented software support for image guided radiofrequency ablation of focal liver malignancies. In: Proceedings of SPIE, vol. 6509, p. 650919 (2007)
15. Zidowitz, S., Drexl, J., Kröger, T., Preusser, T., Ritter, F., Weihusen, A., Peitgen, H.-O.: Bayesian Vessel Extraction for Planning of Radiofrequency-Ablation. In: Bildverarbeitung für die Medizin, pp. 187–191. Springer, Berlin (2007)
16. OPTIMIST Handelsges.m.b.H., Austria, `http://www.optimist.at`
17. RF-applicator CelonPro *Surge* 200-T40, Celon AG medical instruments, Germany, `http://www.celon.de`

Early Clinical Evaluation of a Computer Assisted Planning System for Deep Brain Surgeries: 1 Year of Clinical Assistance

Pierre-François D'Haese[1], Rui Li[1], Srivatsan Pallavaram[1], Todd Shanks[3], Peter Zahos[4], Joseph Neimat[2], Peter Konrad[2], and Benoit M. Dawant[1]

[1] Dept. of Electrical and Computer Engineering, Vanderbilt University, Nashville, TN, USA
[2] Dept. of Neurosurgery, Vanderbilt University Medical Center, Nashville, TN, USA
[3] Norton Neuroscience Institute, Louisville KY, USA
[4] New Jersey Neuroscience Institute, JFK Medical Center, NJ, USA
{pf.dhaese,benoit.dawant}@vanderbilt.edu

Abstract. Deep brain stimulation (DBS) is a surgical treatment involving the implantation of permanent electrodes connected to an implanted pulse generator, which sends electrical impulses to specific nuclei of the brain for treatment of movement and, more recently, of neurobehavioral disorders. A number of computer assisted surgery (CAS) systems are currently being developed to guide surgeons at various stages of DBS therapy. As these adjuncts become mature and ready for clinical application, their evaluation, in terms of clinical impact and ergonomic features, becomes a necessity. The goal of this paper is to provide an evaluation of the utility of the DBS planning system we have developed. We study how the automatically generated plans are used and modified by the end-users. The proposed criteria include the evaluation of the rigid registrations between the MR-T1 and T2 to the patient CT, the selection of the anterior and posterior commissures (AC-PC) and the target points. For each of these criteria, we check if the automatic plan was modified and, if so, by what degree. Our results show that the registrations were not modified in 95% of the cases; the AC and PC selections were modified in average by only 0.83mm and the sub-thalamic nucleus (STN) targets by 1.04mm.

Keywords: DBS, Deep Brain Stimulation, CAS, Computer Assisted Surgery.

1 Introduction

Since its approval in the United States in 2002, deep brain stimulation (DBS) has become an integral part of the treatment armamentarium for various movement disorders. Deep brain stimulation (DBS) surgery involves implanting electrodes which provide chronic electrical stimulation to deep brain nuclei. This stimulation is thought to regulate the neural signals sent between different nuclei and reduces the severity of the symptoms. DBS therapy involves three stages: pre-operative target localization, intra-operative electrode placement, and post-operative programming of the implant. Currently, the most common targets for movement disorder therapy are

N. Navab and P. Jannin (Eds.): IPCAI 2010, LNCS 6135, pp. 190–199, 2010.

the sub-thalamic nucleus (STN), the ventral intermediate thalamic nucleus (VIM) and the globus pallidus interna (GPi). These are selected by the surgeons either directly from MRI visualization, or indirectly by using internal landmarks such as the anterior and posterior commissures (AC-PC) or the red nucleus boundaries. During the surgery, the position of the target is refined to compensate for the patient's anatomical variability and brain shift. Target refinement is typically done using two types of intra-operative observations: micro-electrode recordings (MER) and stimulation response. The surgical team, variably including neurosurgeons, neurologists and neurophysiologists, analyzes the MERs and establishes functional borders of the structures of interest that will be stimulated to find an optimal location for the implant. During the stimulation phase, mild electrical currents are applied using stimulating electrodes to evaluate the clinical efficacy and side effect profile of stimulation in different regions of the mapped target. When a satisfactory position is found, the exploratory electrodes are removed and the permanent DBS implants are inserted. Subsequently, an implantable pulse generator (IPG) is placed under the patient's skin near the collarbone and connected to the final implants for stimulation. Finally, by programming the IPG, the neurologist adjusts the parameters of stimulation post-operatively. This involves selecting the stimulation contact(s) (each DBS implant has 4 independent contacts) and setting parameters including voltage, pulse width and frequency. These settings are optimized to produce the greatest therapeutic benefit.

The fundamental goal of computer assisted surgery (CAS) is to make the surgery patient-specific, more accurate, and reduce variations between surgeons. A number of methods and computer assisted systems for DBS therapy have been developed to assist surgeons at each of the stages of deep brain stimulation (DBS) therapy described above. Ideally, these components are integrated in a complete system such that sophisticated diagnostic technologies are used to create a patient-specific surgical plan. This plan is used to create or set the stereotactic frame and is available during surgery for predictive guidance. The plan, augmented with the electrophysiologic and stimulation data acquired during the surgery, is then passed to the post-operative system to guide the neurologist in tuning the implant stimulation parameters.

Computer assisted surgery systems for DBS planning can assist the surgeon in locating the optimal stimulation zone accurately via some form of guidance method. A wide range of guidance methods can be considered, including anatomical and histological representations as proposed by Chakravarty et al. [3], Yelnik et al. [7] or Bardinet et al. [8] or, probabilistic functional atlases (PFA) as introduced by Nowinski et al. [10], and atlases of intra-operatively acquired information as described by Finnis [4] or Guo [5]. Our group has described and retrospectively validated techniques by which a computer system can be used to predict anterior and posterior commissures (AC-PC) and optimal location for target [9, 11]. In 2006, Castro et al. [14] have also shown that atlas-based targeting was feasible with accuracy comparable to manual selection of targets.

Given the variety of these guidance methods, it becomes increasingly important to test and analyze them for CAS in a quantitative and context-dependent manner to determine which is most suitable for a given surgical task. The evaluation of such systems on a large number of patients can only be done when the system is being used routinely in the clinical setting. We have implemented a system that is integrated in the clinical workflow., This system has been used for several years at our institution and parts of which have recently been adopted by several other centers to assist the surgeons and neurologists in the planning, implantation, and programming phases of the DBS procedure. In this paper, we evaluate the clinical DBS planning system we have developed over the years and test its ability to assist the surgeons to create surgical plans.

2 Materials and Method

Computer-assisted surgery relies on the use of quantitative data rather than surgeon intuition to facilitate clinical decision-making. In order to gather the needed quantitative information, we have developed a database that contains image data for over 400 patients and we have a system in place in which two synchronized Oracle databases are running, thus guaranteeing availability of data 24/7. A suite of software has been developed to permit data entry and visualization during the pre-, intra- and post-operative phases of the process. We call this secure data repository along with the associated processing algorithms "CranialVault", and the software suite which permits access to this database as well as visualization tools CRAVE (CRAnialVaut Explorer). Communication with the database happens via the internet on secured and encrypted channels affording the users the flexibility to download and use the data from any computer anywhere. The system has been designed to follow HIPAA regulation (Health Insurance Portability and Accountability Act) to protect patients' data confidentiality.

CranialVault contains the following information for DBS patient treated at Vanderbilt University Medical Center or at external sites who have local IRB approval: (1) Pre-operative data includes CT images, MR images (typically T1-weighted without contrast agent, T1-weighted with contrast agent, and T2-weighted) as well as planned targets. (2) Intra-operative data acquired during the procedure includes somatotopic data (correspondence between the position of a receptor in part of the body and the corresponding region of the deep brain nuclei that is activated by it), response to stimulation, micro-electrode recordings and the location of electrode implantation. (3) Post-operative data includes CT images acquired immediately after the procedure, CT images acquired about a month after the procedure and programming data consisting of the clinically selected contact as well as stimulation parameters.

The database also contains what we refer to as atlases. These are MRI reference volumes (currently we use four), which are used to spatially normalize all the information we acquire in individual patients by mapping them from patient image space to the atlas space using registration techniques. We use multiple reference volumes as atlases because there is evidence in the medical imaging literature [2] that combining information from several atlases leads to more accurate results, when projecting information from atlases to patient volumes, than a single atlas. All data are stored in the native patient space and then projected onto the atlas space using registration. We also store manual segmentations of structures such as the thalamus, putamen, STN, SNr, GPi, ventricles, and red nucleus in the four MR image atlas volumes as well as the locations of landmarks like the AC and PC.

2.1 Computer Assisted Planning and Data Flow

Using the data contained in CranialVault and our registration algorithms, our system can be used to prepare all the information needed to plan a new DBS case. This includes (1) automatic localization of the AC and the PC, (2) prediction of the optimal position of the implant, (3) segmentation of anatomical structures, and (4) creation of electrophysiological maps.

Figure 1 illustrates the data and process flow used to create a CAS DBS plan for every patient undergoing this surgery at Vanderbilt. Once the images have been acquired, they are transferred and entered into CranialVault for processing. The images are all registered to the CT images. The MR-T1 are also registered to each of the atlases rigidly and non-rigidly.

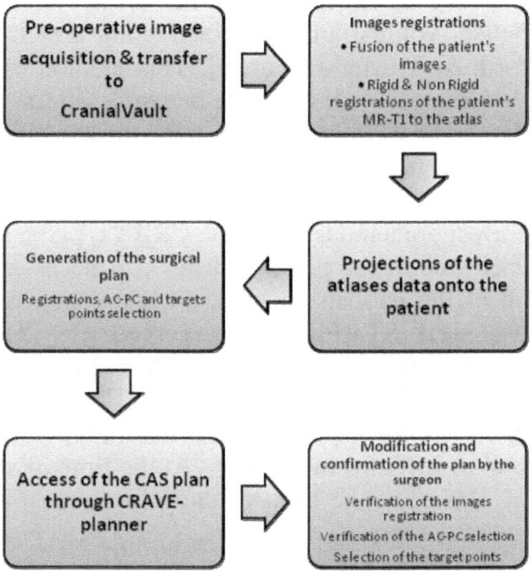

Fig. 1. Data and process for DBS surgery planning at Vanderbilt using CranialVault

Briefly, the non-rigid registration algorithms, which we call ABA (Adaptive basis algorithm) [1] is an intensity-based registration algorithm that uses the normalized mutual information as similarity measure [17]. It computes a deformation field that is modeled as a linear combination of radial basis functions with finite support. This results in a transformation with several thousands of degrees of freedom. Two transformations (one from the atlas to the subject and the other from the subject to the atlas) that are constrained to be inverses of each other are computed simultaneously. ABA reduces the computational complexity and improves the convergence properties of related B-splines-based approaches by identifying regions

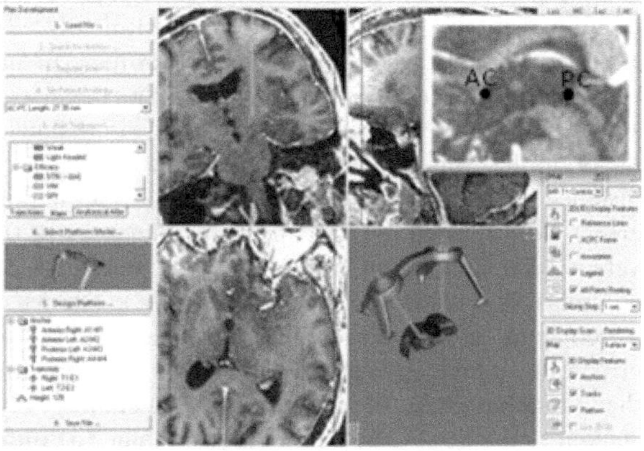

Fig. 2. Snapshot of an automatically created plan loaded in CRAVE-planner. The CAS plan contains the AC-PC, targets and entry points that define the trajectories. Anatomical and statistical maps are shown too. The overlapping pictures show a close up view of the automatically selected AC and PC on a sagittal view.

of mis-registration and adapting the compliance of the transformation locally. The algorithm arrives at the final deformation iteratively across scales and resolutions.

The data is then projected using the computed transformations from the atlases to a patient volume and combined using a method based on the STAPLE algorithm put forth by Warfield et al [6]. This method evaluates the performance of the mapping between each atlas and the patient's volume using segmented structures that surround the region of interest and weighs the contribution of each atlas to the results [12].

A surgical plan is finally created and stored in CranialVault. Once (s)he receives a notification that the plan is ready by email, the surgeon accesses the plan with the correct credentials using the CRAVE planner module (Figure 2). The surgeon verifies each step of the plan, modifies it if necessary and validates the plan for surgery. For all of the patients included in this study, a patient customized stereotactic platform was used (STarFix™ microTargeting™ Platform (FDA 510(K), Number: K003776, Feb 23, 2001, FHC, Inc.; Bowdoin, ME, USA); a recent study in the accuracy of this platform can be found in [15, 16]. Figure 2 shows an example of this device. Once the plan is confirmed, a virtual platform is created and its specifications are automatically sent to FHC for production. At the time of surgery, the customized platform will then be affixed to the head of the patient using pre-implanted anchors to guide the intra-operative probes.

2.1.1 Automatic Localization of the AC and PC

To predict the positions of the AC and the PC in a new patient, the positions of the AC and PC from each of the atlases are projected onto the patient and combined using the method described earlier. Early 2009 we published a retrospective validation of this method [11] and showed that we can predict the AC and PC points automatically more accurately than expert can do clinically. To establish this, we asked two experienced neurosurgeons to each select the AC and PC carefully in 20 patients. On each of those patients, we computed the mean of the selections to arrive at gold standards. We then measured the Euclidean distance between the gold standards and the point that was selected clinically (the clinical localization error) and the Euclidean distance between the gold standard and our automatic prediction (the atlas localization error). We reported in that paper a median error of 0.41 mm (Atlas vs. Gold Standard) versus 0.84 mm (Clinical vs. Gold Standard) for the prediction of the MC (middle commissure – centroid of AC and the PC). The MC is often used as the origin of the stereotactic reference system. Statistical analysis showed that the atlas localization error was statistically ($p<0.001$) smaller than the clinical error. The results also show that in about 80% of the cases the distance between atlas predictions and gold standard for the AC and PC was less than 1.0 mm which was true in only 25% of cases for the clinical selections. In 100% of the cases the distance between atlas predictions and the gold standard for MC was sub-millimetric while it is only true in about 70% of the cases for the clinical selections. More detailed results can be found in [11]. In this study, we test this method prospectively on new patients.

2.1.2 Automatic Prediction of the Target Points

Each target (STN, VIM, GPi …) in the atlas is defined as a cluster of final implant positions obtained by projecting these points from previous individual patients onto the atlases. Using the same method described earlier, we can project the centroid of a given cluster from each atlas onto the new patient and combine these projections to produce an optimal target prediction. In 2005, we tested this method on subjects that already underwent the surgery. We compared the automatic and manual selections of the target points by comparing them to the position of the implant chosen intra-operatively by the surgeon [9]. We reported an average Euclidian error of 1.7 mm for the automatic method compared to 2.4 mm when manual prediction was done without any assistance but this study was limited to 21 cases. In this paper we test our method prospectively on new patients.

2.2 Evaluation of the Planning Assistance

For each patient that underwent the procedure at Vanderbilt Medical Center and institutions part of the CranialVault project during the last year, the imaging data was transferred and processed, a surgical plan was created by our system prior to the surgery and provided for assistance to the surgeon at the time of planning. The surgeons were alone while reviewing and modifying the automatically generated plan.

We compare the three main aspects of the assistance system. 1) The automatic registrations: how many times the automatic registrations between the MRI sequences and the CT were used or modified; if modified, by how much and how it affected the position of the targets. 2) The automatic selection of the AC and the PC: we measure how many times the points were modified and the distance between their automatic and manual selections. 3) Finally, we compute the distance between the automatic and manual selection of the targets. The results are reported in the following section. Because both the stereotactic points and the targets stored in the plans are CT coordinates, if the final MRI to CT registrations are different from the planned registrations, i.e., if the user has modified the transformation computed by the system, the points cannot be compared. These cases were removed from the statistics presented in the results section.

2.3 Data

This study includes 80 patients who underwent a DBS procedure between January 1st 2009 and December 20th 2009 for a total of 144 implants (82 STN, 29 GPI and 33 VIM). With IRB approval each patient had pre-operative MRI (T1, T1+Contrast and T2) and CT. Typical CT images were acquired at kVp = 120 V, exposure = 350 mAs and 512x512 pixels. In-plane resolution and slice thickness were respectively 0.5 mm and 0.75 mm. MRI T1 (TR 7.9 ms, TE 3.65 ms, 256x256x170 voxels, with typical voxel resolution of 1x1x1 mm^3) using the SENSE parallel imaging technique (T1W/3D/TFE) and MRI T2 2D-TSE (TR 3000 ms, TE 80 ms, 512x512x45 with typical voxel resolution of 0.46x0.46x2 mm^3) were acquired on a Philips 3T scanner. All the images were processed and a surgical plan created for each patient. Because of another study, the automatic selections of the targets were kept hidden from the surgeon for 27 patients. For these patients, only the registrations and the automatic selections of the AC and PC were available. Ten patients were unilateral cases.

Four surgeons (PK, JN and TS at the Vanderbilt Medical Center and PZ at the New Jersey Neuroscience Institute) have used the computer assisted system planned for, 12, 35, 24 and 7 patients respectively.

3 Results

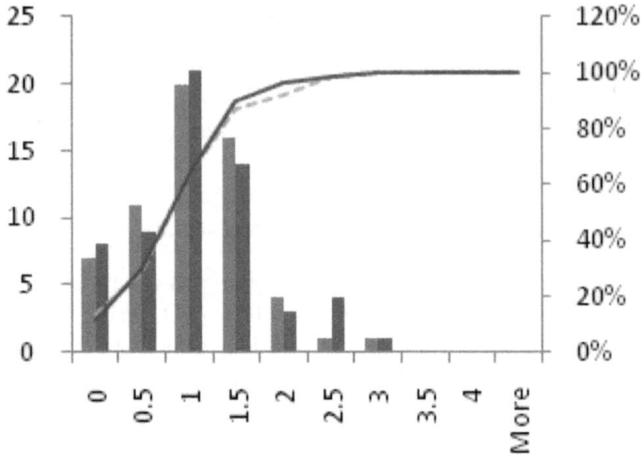

Fig. 3. Frequency and the cumulative frequency of the adjustment of the computer assisted selections of the AC (light gray/line) and the PC and PC (dark gray/dotted line)

On a total of 80 patients, 67 plans were made in time and used for computer assisted planning. For 13 patients, the plans were not used because the images were not transferred in time to our server, because the plans could not be created on time due to limited processing resources, or because the plan was done offline and the system could not then be accessed. These 13 cases were processed retrospectively and were not more complex than any other. On 134 registrations, counting both MR-T1 and MR-T2 to CT, 128 were used without any modifications; for the 6 remaining registrations, the surgeon decided to modify them manually or semi-automatically with the registration algorithm available in the planner. Table 1 reports the difference in translation Δ(tx, ty, tz) and rotation Δ(rx, ry, rz) between the pre-computed registrations and the registrations validated by the surgeons. The resulting error in mm on the AC, PC and target points due to the mis-registration is reported in Table 2.

Table 1. Average difference between translations (Tx, Ty, Tz in mm) and rotations (Rx, Ry, Rz in degrees) components of computer assisted registrations modified registrations by the surgeons

		Tx	Ty	Tz	Rx	Ry	Rz
T1->CT	Avg	0.03	0.13	0.36	0.24	0.06	0.02
T1->CT	Stdev	0.39	0.26	1.19	0.76	0.67	0.43
T2->CT	Avg	0.05	0.01	0.47	0.18	0.04	0.17
T2->CT	Stdev	0.03	0.24	0.69	0.69	0.22	0.23

Table 2. Median impacts of the mis-registration on the AC, PC, left and right targets

	Ace	PCe	LTe	RTe
T1->CT	1.02	0.61	0.30	0.77
T2->CT	0.77	0.52	4.51	4.38

Table 3 details the statistics of the modifications made to the computer selected stereotactic and target points. Figure 3 plots both the frequency and the cumulative frequency of the differences between the computer assisted and the final selections of the AC and the PC.

Table 3. Modifications made to the pre-selected stereotactic and targets points

	Stereotactic points			Targets		
	AC	PC	ALL	STN	GPI	VIM
Avg.	0.83	0.83	1.94	1.04	2.56	3.47
StdDev.	0.57	0.60	1.79	0.96	1.07	2.38

4 Discussion

As discussed earlier, the goal of this paper is to evaluate the usefulness of our computer assisted planning system in real clinical use. Over the past few years we validated different parts of our guidance system and presented encouraging results on being able to provide accurate selection of AC-PC and targets to the surgeon. However, putting all the pieces together to create a complete computer assistance system and getting the surgeons to trust and use the system clinically was a difficult step. In this study we present the results we have obtained after one year of clinical use of our computer assistance system for planning DBS procedures by four different surgeons. We have shown that pre-computed registrations of the patient's MRIs to the pre-operative CT were used without modification in 95% of the cases. 5% of the registrations did not satisfy the surgeon and were manually modified.

For the cases successfully aligned, our results show that the AC and PC automatic selections were modified in average respectively by 0.83±0.57mm and 0.83±0.60mm. 15% of the computer selections of the AC and PC were used without modifications, 63% where modified by less than 1mm and 90% by less than 1.5mm. For comparison, the inter-surgeons variability for the selection of the AC and PC was estimated at respectively 1.53±1.44mm and 1.45±1.24mm by Pallavaram et al. in [11].

Finally, our results show that the automatic selections of the targets have been modified in average by 1.04±0.96mm, 2.56±1.07mm and 3.47±2.38mm, respectively, for the STN, GPI and VIM cases. The adjustment for the STN is thus on the order of one voxel, which we consider to be good. The lager modifications we have observed for the other targets could have several explanations. Automatic targeting is based on statistics computed from the final intra-operative position of implants from prior surgeries but the pre-operative target chosen by the surgeon may be different. For instance, surgeons may select a target that has a clear electrophysiological signature and then move the electrode by a fixed offset intra-operatively. One example is targeting for the ventralis caudalis (VC) borders for VIM cases because sensory effects can be observed intra-operatively in this structure. The final DBS lead is then placed anteriorally.

Even though the accuracy of our VIM and GPI targets need to be improved, these are encouraging results that suggest the feasibility of producing automatically generated plans customized to each patient. As the whole system is based on the information contained in CranialVault fed by the experience of top neurosurgeons, this could make the DBS surgery patient-specific, more accurate, and reduce variations between surgeons.

In our study, we have compared automatic and manual pre-operative target positions. We could also have compared these to the final implant position. But we have documented the fact that brain shift during the procedure may be substantial [18]. The final implant position thus reflects adjustments made by the surgical team to compensate for this shift. Comparison of pre-operative and intra-operative positions is thus not a good measure of planning accuracy.

The system is also designed to be easily extended and modified. The database is currently running on a single server but it can be distributed on several. More importantly, the various algorithms that operate on the data (e.g., registration, segmentation, etc) can be modified or replaced and new algorithms added. Because we keep all the raw data we can also reprocess them if a better algorithm is proposed. The system architecture we have developed is thus extremely well suited for the rapid clinical evaluation of new algorithms and techniques. For instance, we are currently investigating new methods to improve the prediction of VIM and GPI by combining statistical information from the atlas with anatomical structures such as the optic tracts. We are also expanding CranialVault to gather and process data from other sites. Our long term vision is to develop a central repository for DBS surgery.

The system as a whole is a research system that has not reached the stage of a commercial product but a standalone version of the planning system has been licensed to FHC, Inc., which manufactures the StarFix platform in use at Vanderbilt. This module is not connected to the database and it does permit automatic planning. BMD and RL receive royalties from this licensing agreement.

Acknowledgments. This research has been supported, in parts, by NIH R01EB006136.

References

1. Rohde, G.K., Aldroubi, A., Dawant, B.M.: The adaptive bases algorithm for intensity-based non rigid image registration. IEEE Trans. on Medical Imag. 22(11), 1470–1479 (2003)
2. Rohlfing, T., Maurer, C.J.: Multi-Classifier framework for atlas-based image segmentation. Paper read at IEEE Computer Society Conference on Computer Vision and Pattern Recognition, Washington D.C., USA (2004)
3. Chakravarty, M.M., Bertrand, G., Hodge, C.P., Sadikot, A.F., Collins, D.L.: The Creation of a Brain Atlas for Image guided Neurosurgery Using Serial Histological Data. Neuroimage 30(2), 359–376 (2006)
4. Finnis, K.W., Starreveld, Y.P., Parrent, A.G., Sadikot, A.F., Peters, T.M.: Three dimensional database of subcortical electrophysiology for image-guided stereotactic functional neurosurgery. IEEE Trans. on Medical Imaging 22(11), 93–104 (2003)
5. Guo, T., Finnis, K.W., Parrent, A.G., Peters, T.M.: Development and application of functional databases for planning deep-brain neurosurgical procedures. In: Duncan, J.S., Gerig, G. (eds.) MICCAI 2005. LNCS, vol. 3749, pp. 835–842. Springer, Heidelberg (2005)

6. Warfield, S.K., Zou, K.H., Wells, W.M.: Simultaneous Truth and Performance Level Estimation (STAPLE): An algorithm for the validation of image segmentation. IEEE Trans. on Medical Imaging, 903–921 (2004)
7. Yelnik, J., Bardinet, E., Dormont, D., Malandain, G., Ourselin, S., Tandé, D., Karachi, C., Ayache, N., Cornu, P., Agid, Y.: A three-dimensional, histological and deformable atlas of the human basal ganglia. I. Atlas construction based on immunohistochemical and MRI data. Neuroimage 34, 618–638 (2007)
8. Bardinet, E., Bhattacharjee, M., Dormont, D., Pidoux, B., Malandain, G., Schüpbach, M., Ayache, N., Cornu, P., Agid, Y., Yelnik, J.: A three-dimensional histological atlas of the human basal ganglia. II. Atlas deformation strategy and evaluation in deep brain stimulation for Parkinson disease. J. Neurosurg. 110, 208–219 (2009)
9. D'Haese, P.-F., Cetinkaya, E., Konrad, P.E., Kao, C., Dawant, B.M.: Computer-Aided Placement of Deep Brain Stimulators: From Planning to Intraoperative Guidance. IEEE Trans. on Medical Imaging, 1469–1478 (2005)
10. Nowinski, W.L., Belov, D., Benabid, A.L.: An Algorithm for Rapid Calculation of a Probabilistic Functional Atlas of Subcortical Structures from Electrophysiological Data Collected during Functional Neurosurgery Procedures. Neuroimage 18, 143–155 (2003)
11. Pallavaram, S., Dawant, B.M., Koyama, T., Yu, H., Neimat, J.S., Konrad, P.E., D'Haese, P.-F.: Validation of a fully automatic method for the routine selection of the anterior and posterior commissures in MR images. Journal of Stereotact. Funct. Neurosurg. 87, 148–154 (2009)
12. D'Haese, P.-F., Pallavaram, S., Niermann, K., Spooner, J., Kao, C., Konrad, P.E., Dawant, B.M.: Electrophysiological atlas based fully automatic selection of DBS target points: a multiple atlases approach. In: MICCAI (Medical Image Computing and Computer Assisted Intervention), Palm Springs, California, USA (2005)
13. Pallavaram, S., Yu, H., Spooner, J., D'Haese, P.-F., Bodenheimer, B., Konrad, P.E., Dawant, B.M.: Inter-surgeon variability in the selection of anterior and posterior commissures and its potential effects on target localization. Journal of Stereotact. Funct. Neurosurg. 86, 113–119 (2008), doi:10.1159/000116215
14. Castro, F.J., Pollo, C., Cuisenaire, O., Villemure, J.-G., Thiran, J.-P.: Validation of experts versus atlas-based and automatic registration methods for subthalamic nucleus targeting on MRI. International Journal of Computer Assisted Radiology and Surgery 1(1), 5–12 (2006)
15. Balachandran, R., Mitchell, J.E., Dawant, B.M., Fitzpatrick, J.M.: Accuracy Evaluation of microTargeting Platforms for Deep-Brain Stimulation Using Virtual Targets. IEEE Transactions on Biomedical Engineering 56, 37–44 (2009) [PMID: 19224717]
16. D'Haese, P.-F., Pallavaram, S., Konrad, P.E., Neimat, J.S., Fitzpatrick, J.M., Dawant, B.M.: Clinical accuracy of a customized stereotactic platform for deep-brain stimulation after accounting for brain shift. Journal of Stereotac. Funct. Neurosurg. 88, 81–87 (2010) [PMC Journal - In Process]
17. Studholme, C., Hill, D.L.G., Hawkes, D.J.: Automated 3-D Registration of MR and CT Images of the Head. Medical Image Analysis 1(2), 163–175 (1996)
18. Pallavaram, S., Dawant, B.M., Remple, M.S., Neimat, J.S., Kao, C., Konrad, P.E., D'Haese, P.-F.: Effect of brain shift on the creation of functional atlases for deep brain stimulation surgery. Int. J. CARS (2009), doi:10.1007/s11548-009-0391-1

Author Index

GPSR Compliance

The European Union's (EU) General Product Safety Regulation (GPSR) is a set of rules that requires consumer products to be safe and our obligations to ensure this.

If you have any concerns about our products, you can contact us on ProductSafety@springernature.com

In case Publisher is established outside the EU, the EU authorized representative is:

Springer Nature Customer Service Center GmbH
Europaplatz 3
69115 Heidelberg, Germany

Batch number: 09474016

Printed by Printforce, the Netherlands